Communicatic in the Cla:

An Introduction for Professionals in School Settings

Fourth Edition

William O. Haynes, PhD, CCC-SLP
Professor
Department of Communication Disorders
Auburn University

Michael J. Moran, PhD, CCC-SLP
Professor
Department of Communication Disorders
Auburn University

Rebekah H. Pindzola, PhD, CCC-SLP
Professor
Department of Communication Disorders
Auburn University

JONES AND BARTLETT PUBLISHERS
Sudbury, Massachusetts
BOSTON   TORONTO   LONDON   SINGAPORE

World Headquarters

Jones and Bartlett Publishers
40 Tall Pine Drive
Sudbury, MA 01776
978-443-5000
info@jbpub.com
www.jbpub.com

Jones and Bartlett Publishers
Canada
6339 Ormindale Way
Mississauga, Ontario L5V 1J2
CANADA

Jones and Bartlett Publishers
International
Barb House, Barb Mews
London W6 7PA
UK

Jones and Bartlett's books and products are available through most bookstores and online booksellers. To contact Jones and Bartlett Publishers directly, call 800-832-0034, fax 978-443-8000, or visit our website, www.jbpub.com.

Substantial discounts on bulk quantities of Jones and Bartlett's publications are available to corporations, professional associations, and other qualified organizations. For details and specific discount information, contact the special sales department at Jones and Bartlett via the above contact information or send an email to specialsales@jbpub.com.

Copyright © 2006 by Jones and Bartlett Publishers, Inc.

All rights reserved. No part of the material protected by this copyright may be reproduced or utilized in any form, electronic or mechanical, including photocopying, recording, or by any information storage and retrieval system, without written permission from the copyright owner.

Library of Congress Cataloging-in-Publication Data

Haynes, William O.
  Communication disorders in the classroom : an introduction for professionals in school settings / William O. Haynes, Michael J. Moran, Rebekah Pindzola. — 4th ed.
    p. cm.
  Includes bibliographical references and index.
  ISBN 0-7637-2743-1 (pbk.)
  1. Children with disabilities—Education—United States. 2. Language arts—Remedial teaching—United States. 3. Speech disorders in children—United States. 4. Communicative disorders in children—United States.   I. Moran, Michael J., Ph. D. II. Pindzola, Rebekah H. (Rebekah Hand) III. Title.
  LC4028.H39 2006
  371.9'0446—dc22
                                                                                    2005011485

Production Credits
Executive Editor: Jack Bruggeman
Editorial Assistant: Katilyn Crowley
Production Director: Amy Rose
Associate Production Editor: Kate Hennessy
Marketing Manager: Emily Ekle
Associate Marketing Manager: Laura Kavigian
Manufacturing Buyer: Therese Connell
Cover Design: Kristin E. Ohlin
Composition: Auburn Associates, Inc.
Printing and Binding: Malloy, Inc.
Cover Printing: Malloy, Inc.

Printed in the United States of America
09 08 07 06 05   10 9 8 7 6 5 4 3 2 1

Contents

Preface

Most of us take the ability to communicate for granted. We communicate every day for a wide variety of purposes. Yet most people are not aware of the vast complexity of the communication process. For instance, it takes the action of about 100 muscles to say even a simple word such as *pop*. These muscle actions must be coordinated in simultaneous and serial movements at a speed of about 13 speech sounds per second! In addition to the actual production of speech, a person must think of something to say (cognitive activity), select words and sentence structures (language ability), and adapt the utterance to the appropriate communication context (noisy versus quiet room, child versus adult listener, and so on). The steps in this process are accomplished in fractions of seconds. Unfortunately, many conditions, both physical and behavioral, can interfere with this complicated process and create a communication impairment. These speech, language, or hearing disorders have the potential to affect a student communicatively, socially, psychologically, and academically.

This fourth edition of *Communication Disorders in the Classroom: An Introduction for Professionals in School Settings* provides an updated portrait of the far-reaching impact that a communication impairment has on the lives and academic success of students in preschool all the way through adolescence. For the past 15 years, this text has been used by training programs in the disciplines of education, special education, and communication disorders as an example of how professionals from these diverse areas can cooperate in helping students with speech, hearing, and language problems in an academic setting. Federal legislation and current educational trends have changed school systems significantly during the past decade. Today, a typical classroom may have children with a variety of disabilities included with normally developing students. This current trend toward inclusion of students with disabilities in the normal classroom is predicted to increase even more with continued changes in legislation and educational philosophy. Thus, it is not unusual to enter a classroom and find a child with a mobility impairment, a child with hearing loss, a student with a serious medical condition, a child with brain injury, students with attentional and learning problems, and many with communication disorders. As a result of inclusion, both regular and special education teachers have more demands placed upon them than ever before. Not only are they required to teach academic content, but they also must make numerous adjustments in their teaching styles and interaction patterns to accommodate students with various disabilities. In this technological age, the amount of information to be taught to students doubles in less than a decade. This information explosion, coupled with increased demands associated with inclusion, makes the job of a teacher challenging, sometimes frustrating, and occasionally impossible. This textbook provides background information and suggests a variety of strategies that can make educational professionals more effective as they deal with students with communication impairments.

We take great pride in the fact that instructors from a variety of backgrounds have used this textbook. For example, in some universities, the Department of Communication Disorders offers a service course designed for teachers that acquaints them with speech, hearing, and language problems likely to be encountered in the public school environment. Specialists in speech-language pathology typically teach these courses. In other universities, the Department of Special Education may offer a course focusing on a variety of disabilities with communication disorders as a major topic. Sometimes, these departments offer a specific course on communication disorders taught by a special educator who may or may not have a background in speech-language pathology or audiology. Finally, speech-language pathologists working in schools may find this text a valuable resource manual for providing information to classroom teachers in nontechnical language. We have tried to incorporate certain components into the text that will make the book useful to regular educators, special educators, and speech-language pathologists. Our primary aims in this regard are the following:

- Provide state-of-the-art information—A specialist in the particular subject area wrote each chapter in this book. The authors have had many years of clinical experience in their areas and have studied application of speech-language pathology in public school settings.
- Minimize jargon—The fields of communication disorders and education have many technical and professional terminologies. Unfortunately, such technical jargon often does more to separate professionals than it does to facilitate cooperation and understanding. We have attempted in this book to use only terms that teachers need to know to understand a particular disorder, or terms that they may encounter on reports, individual educational programs (IEPs), and in meetings.
- Keep the goals in mind—This book has six major goals:
  - Acquaint teachers with general background information on the types of communication disorders likely to be encountered in their classrooms.
  - Familiarize teachers with the roles of the speech-language pathologist in the public school setting.
  - Give teachers an understanding of how speech-language pathologists assess and treat students in the school setting.
  - Illustrate how teachers and speech-language pathologists can work together in assessing and treating students both in and out of the classroom.
  - Give teachers concrete suggestions on how to interact with children experiencing communication disorders in a classroom context.
  - Show the importance of communication, linguistic, and metalinguistic skills to academic success.

To accomplish these goals, each chapter contains a section on the nature of the communication disorder, assessment issues, direct and indirect treatment options, and suggestions for teachers.

We hope that teachers and speech-language pathologists will continue to find this text informative, clear, and relevant to their work.

chapter one

Communication Disorders in the Schools: Background, Legal Issues, and Service Delivery Models

BACKGROUND INFORMATION: THE COMMUNICATION DISORDERS PROFESSIONAL

Communication takes many forms, some verbal and some nonverbal. **Language** is a major part of the human communication system as it includes words and the rules for organizing them. **Speech** is the process by which sound is shaped into meaningful units, such as words, and audition is the process of hearing what is said. A multitude of factors can interfere with the normal development of speech, language, and audition. Acquired damage, as from traumatic injuries and diseases, also can affect a person's ability to use speech and language or to hear it. These constitute **communication disorders**. Disordered communication can affect a person's lifestyle in a negative way.

Audiology and speech-language pathology are professions that play primary habilitative and rehabilitative roles for children and adults with communication disorders. These communicative specialists often work closely with many professionals such as physicians, neurologists, dentists, classroom teachers, psychologists, occupational therapists, physical therapists, nurses, and special educators. From this brief discussion, it may be obvious that specialists in speech-language pathology and in audiology can work in a variety

1

of settings, such as hospitals, community clinics, rehabilitation centers, private practices, and school systems. According to recent surveys (American Speech-Language-Hearing Association, 2003) about 56% of speech-language pathologists work in school settings, and 35% are employed in health care facilities such as hospitals and other residential facilities. The remaining 10% are either in private practice or university settings. Credentials for employment in these job settings may differ. The **American Speech-Language-Hearing Association** (ASHA) is the national certifying body for professionals in the fields of audiology and speech-language pathology.

Audiologists focus on problems of hearing, and perform diagnostic, habilitative, and rehabilitative services. A subspecialty in the field of audiology trains educational audiologists to best perform these services in the public school environment. In states that do not yet hire educational audiologists, the speech-language pathologist (SLP) or the school nursing staff may be responsible for screening hearing and making appropriate referrals to audiologists. The SLP would then be involved in providing appropriate rehabilitative services for students identified as hearing impaired. Chapter 10 will discuss common audiological problems and the management of the hearing-impaired child in the classroom.

Speech-language pathologists diagnose and treat both the problems of speech and the problems of language. Disorders of speech include voice disorders, stuttering, and articulation or phonology disorders. Some of these are illustrated below.

Heather, an 11th grader, has a vivacious personality that makes her popular with classmates and a natural choice for the cheerleading squad. By midseason she was experiencing frequent bouts of laryngitis. Her voice has become consistently husky. The speech-language pathologist assessed Heather's voice and determined that it was indeed lower pitched than most girls of this age and that her voice was consistently hoarse. Subsequent examination by a physician specializing in disorders of the throat revealed the presence of vocal nodules. The doctor recommended voice treatment by the speech-language pathologist at Heather's school to determine if the nodules could be reduced through therapy instead of surgical intervention.

Juan's hesitant speech has been evident since the first grade; however, now that Juan is in the sixth grade, the problem has become socially and academically crippling. The teacher has stopped calling on him to answer questions in class. The long pauses Juan takes to get the first word started are embarrassing for the teacher, the student, and the entire class. When Juan speaks, it is with great effort. His eyes usually squint shut and his mouth becomes contorted or frozen in unusual postures; sounds eventually emerge only to become halted again. Juan's circle of friends has dwindled to one or two. He is the loner of the sixth grade class, and the teacher believes him to be shy. The school's new speech-language pathologist is excited to work with Juan and feels that much can be done to ease his stuttering.

Billy has just started first grade. When shown a picture of a robot and asked to talk about it he says, "Da a bi ma. He fai i pa. He kuh ti. Oo, he mi." Billy clearly has trouble putting speech sounds together; this may be termed an articulation disorder or a phonological disorder (a distinction will be made in Chapter 3). The child attempted to say, "That's a big monster. He flies in space. He crushes things. Oo, he's mean." The speech-language pathologist, after studying the nature of Billy's speech errors, explains to the parents and classroom teacher a proposed intervention regime to help Billy learn to not omit the ends of words and substitute sounds. The agreed upon plan sets a goal of intelligible speech for Billy.

Speech-language pathologists also diagnose and treat language disorders in children, adolescents, and adults. Language disorders may be developmental or acquired. Consider the following illustrative cases:

Maria is a child of four who was born with Down syndrome. Prior to her enrollment in special education services, she verbalized little. Communication often involved pointing, grunting, or an occasional attempt at a 1-syllable word. Maria still does not communicate at a level appropriate for her chronological age, yet she is making progress. The collaboration within the classroom between the teacher and the speech-language pathologist has proved fruitful. Maria now produces multiword utterances such as: "More milk," and "Joe outside."

Butch not only got his driver's license when he turned 16, he also got a motorcycle. Unfortunately, three months later he was involved in a traffic accident. He survived, and his broken bones, cuts, and bruises healed well enough. The traumatic injury to his brain, however, left consequences. After acute hospitalization and some rehabilitation, Butch reentered school. Never before had he had difficulty understanding a teacher's instructions, but now he seemed confused and at a loss as to what to do. Additionally, there was poor comprehension when Butch read his textbooks. When he spoke, Butch seemed to drift from the topic at hand and often had trouble thinking of the words he wished to say.

Subsequent chapters in this book will address in more detail disorders of speech and language teachers are likely to encounter in the school-age population. While **speech-language pathologist** is the preferred title for these communication disorders specialists, other titles are also in use. In the environment of young children, the title *speech teacher* or *speech therapist* often proves popular. In clinical settings, *speech clinician* may be more typical. Still, it should be remembered that the professionally accepted name is *speech-language pathologist*. To be less cumbersome, we have used the abbreviation SLP in the present text.

COMMUNICATION DISORDERS IN THE SCHOOLS: CASELOAD ISSUES

The intent of this book is to provide classroom teachers and special education personnel with information on communication disorders so that they can better serve students with specific speech, language, or hearing problems. You may well wonder how many students have disorders of communication. In the 50 states and the District of Columbia for the 2000–2001 school year, a total of 5,775,772 students (aged 6 to 21 years) received special education services (U.S. Department of Education, 2000). Over 50% of students being served by special educators in the public schools had learning disabilities as their primary handicap. Students who were primarily speech or language impaired accounted for 18.9% of the total served, and students with hearing impairments accounted for 1.2%. Clearly then, students with learning disabilities and communication disorders constitute the bulk of handicapped students served in the schools with other categories of handicapping conditions being less prevalent (e.g., mentally retarded, emotionally disturbed, multihandicapped, orthopedically impaired, visually handicapped, and so on). The astute reader will no doubt have noticed that all the incidence figures reported above are for children above the age of 5 years. According to the law, schools must provide services for preschool children between the ages of 3 and 5 years. Many school systems have expanded this mandate to also include the birth-to-3-years population.

Because speech and language disorders are more prevalent in preschool age children, this population expands the potential caseload of the school-based SLP considerably. It is important to note that of the students who are classified as learning disabled, mentally retarded, multihandicapped, and orthopedically impaired, a large proportion of these youngsters have an accompanying communication disorder in speech, hearing, or language. These students are classified according to their primary disability (e.g., mental retardation) and are not included in the 18.9% of speech/language-impaired students previously mentioned because this figure represents only those students whose primary classification is a speech or language disorder. Thus, the SLP has a large number of cases who have speech, language, or hearing impairment as their primary disability, and also a very large population of other children whose primary classification represents another category, but who are likely to be receiving speech or language treatment as part of their special education program. As a result of the large caseloads, the number of SLP positions in public school systems can be expected to increase nationwide over the next few years. According to the U.S. Bureau of Labor Statistics, the employment rate for the profession of speech-language pathology is expected to grow significantly for the next decade. A 27% increase in job openings is predicted to compensate for the shortfall in available SLPs to serve ever growing caseloads of children and adults. All teachers, but especially elementary and special education personnel, can fully expect to have students with significant communication disorders in their classrooms at some time.

Results from the 2003 ASHA Omnibus Survey indicate that the average caseload size for speech-language pathologists working in the schools full time is 53 with a range from 15 cases to 110 cases. Average caseload size varies significantly by state. For example, on the ASHA Omnibus Survey of 2003, the lowest average caseload was North Dakota with 32, and the highest was Indiana with 75. As will be seen later in this book, SLPs may utilize any of several available service delivery models. Some students are seen individually, others in groups, and some goals are accomplished by integrating treatment into classroom activities. The 1992 ASHA Omnibus Survey indicates that speech-language pathologists have a mean of 49 individual sessions and 83 group sessions per month. Nearly 71% of their caseload consists of students above the age of 6 years, 26% represents 3- to 5-year-olds, and almost 3.5% are in the birth-to-age-2 years group. Additionally, a wide range of severity of communication disorders was represented in the studied SLPs' caseload: 23% of students exhibit severe impairments, 51% moderate impairments, and 26% mild impairments.

Subsequent chapters of this book will describe the various prevalence figures associated with each type of communication disorder. The frequency of occurrence, say, of language impairments is vastly different from that of voice disorders. The ASHA Omnibus Survey (2003) summarized data representing each disorder type on the typical SLP's caseload. Table 1-1 shows this information. The percentages exceed 100 because of co-occurring disorders. For example, a student may exhibit both a language and articulation disorder. It is easy to see from Table 1-1 that the SLP must have expertise across many disparate areas. The implication for teachers is that this diverse group of students will also be present in their classes.

LEGAL ISSUES: PUBLIC LAWS AFFECTING STUDENTS WITH COMMUNICATION DISORDERS

State and local education agencies must now follow federal mandates to provide children and youth who have disabilities with appropriate and free edu-

Table 1-1 Percent of School-Based SLPs Providing Regular Services to Each Disorder Group and the Average Number of Clients Representing the Category on the Caseload

Diagnostic Category	% of SLPs Who Report Regularly Providing Services	Mean # of Clients in Category on Caseload
Aphasia	6.0	4.5
Articulation/phonology	91.8	23.9
Attention deficit disorder	65.4	7.5
Autism/pervasive developmental disorder	77.4	5.0
Cognitive disorder	43.6	10.6
Swallowing disorder	13.8	4.0
Fluency disorder	67.5	2.5
Hearing disorder	45.8	3.2
Learning disability	72.4	16.5
Mental retardation	70.9	10.8
Motor speech disorder	4.7	4.1
Augmentative communication	50.8	4.8
Reading/writing	37.7	14.0
Language impairment	61.1	17.2
Verbal apraxia	59.4	3.1
Voice disorder	33.8	1.9

Source: Adapted from ASHA Omnibus Survey 2003

cation. Several public laws are responsible for these sweeping reforms in public education:

- PL 94-142—Education for All Handicapped Children Act, which includes the Individuals with Disabilities Act (IDEA)
- PL 99-457—Education for All Handicapped Children Act Early Interventions Amendments of 1986
- Section 504 of the Rehabilitation Act (1973)
- Americans with Disabilities Act of 1990—This act and its amendments mandated that reasonable accommodations be provided by any institution including schools to students with disabling or handicapping conditions.

We will briefly discuss each of these mandates because they provide a legal basis for provision of services to students with communication disorders. Understanding the law helps to explain many of the procedures SLPs and teachers engage in during a school year. The majority of processes in place for helping children with disabilities are not simply arbitrary; they are established by law.

Individuals with Disabilities Education Act (IDEA) of 1997

The Education for All Handicapped Children Act (PL 94-142) mandated in 1977 that all handicapped children between the ages of 3 and 21 years receive a free, public education that is appropriate to their need. PL 94-142 has been amended five times over the years and the guidelines were embodied in the Individuals with Disabilities Education Act (IDEA) of 1997. Needless to say, disorders of communication may adversely affect educational achievement. Therefore, students with speech, language, or hearing disorders are covered under IDEA and entitled to free and appropriate individualized services. All handicapped children and their parents are guaranteed, under this law, **due process** with regard to **identification, evaluation,** and placement. This includes the identification, evaluation, and placement for disorders of communication as well as other handicapping conditions. These procedures are performed by a team of school professionals in cooperation with the student's parents. Neidecker (1987) explains the rights and responsibilities of the parents at any team meeting:

> Due process gives the parents the right to have full status at the meeting. They have a right to question why any procedure is necessary,

why one may be selected over another, how a procedure is carried out, and whether or not there are alternative procedures. If parents disagree with the recommended procedures they have the right of review with an impartial judge (pp. 39–40).

Although this is a federal law, individual states were allowed latitude in developing rules and regulations to comply with IDEA. Educational procedures, therefore, vary from state to state. Although this law has far-reaching consequences for the delivery of school services, only some of the key points of the law that affect the work of the speech-language pathologist will be mentioned here. The National Dissemination Center for Children and Youth with Disabilities (NICHCY) has a great site on the Internet that includes a detailed training package on the law (www.nichcy.org). Part of the law specifies that a team of educational personnel and the parents must develop an **individualized education plan**, or **IEP**. In the case of a student with a communication disorder, the speech-language pathologist would be a member of the team. The team also includes the parents, teachers and, when appropriate, the student. The 1997 IDEA has emphasized that the regular classroom teacher participates in the IEP process. Although IEP forms differ among school districts, certain information must be contained in each. Table 1-2 lists the IEP components adapted from the National Dissemination Center for Children and Youth with Disabilities. After being developed, the IEP is signed by the team members, and is reviewed and typically updated annually. The new IDEA 2004 is piloting multiyear IEPs that include goals for three years and must be reviewed annually and at transition points. Of course, IEPs can be reviewed and revised more often at the request of a parent or teacher.

IDEA also stipulated that the student with a disability be provided educational services in the **least restrictive environment**. This means the student should be educated to the maximum extent possible in the regular class with normal peers, if the classroom has the least barriers to successful learning. We shall return to this concept of least restrictive environment later in the chapter when we discuss service delivery models that the speech-language pathologist may adopt. Suffice it to say that the local education agency is responsible for providing the appropriate educational programs, in the least restrictive environment, for all handicapped students. When the school cannot provide the appropriate evaluation or educational placement based on what the student needs, the local school system must pay to secure those services, possibly by contractual arrangement. Payment may include services,

Table 1-2 Components of the Individualized Education Plan

1. A statement of the present level of performance
2. A statement of annual goals
3. Short-term instructional objectives
4. Specific special education and related services to be provided
5. Extent of participation in the regular educational program
6. Projected date for initiation of services
7. Anticipated duration of services
8. Appropriate criteria to determine if objectives are achieved
9. Evaluation procedures to determine if objectives are achieved
10. Schedules for review
11. Assessment information
12. Placement justification statement
13. Some statement of how special education services are tied to the regular education program

transportation, tuition, and room and board if the student is placed in a residential or tuition-based program as the least restrictive environment (Neidecker, 1987).

More amendments to the law have included children with autism and traumatic brain injury, and state that these students may qualify for special education services, rehabilitation counseling, and social work. In addition, assistive technology devices and services have been added with a requirement that schools should make these available, if required, as a related service, or that a supplementary aid or service be provided in the regular classroom environment. An assistive technology device is any item or piece of equipment, whether acquired commercially, off the shelf, modified or customized, that is used to increase, maintain, or improve the functional capabilities of students with disabilities. Common types of assistive technology devices in school settings include: augmentative communication boards, FM systems or auditory trainers for the hearing-impaired, Braille materials, and access to large print or computers for students who are mobility impaired. Some of these devices are explained more fully in Chapter 12.

Every student receiving special education services must have a statement of transition service needs on their IEP by age 14 years (or younger, if appropriate). Transition service plans should include information regarding the responsibilities of participating agencies, and must include activities for the student that are designed to promote movement from school to postschool environments. These environments may include postsecondary education, vocational training, employment, adult education, independent living, adult services, and/or community participation.

A comprehensive evaluation must be conducted, and an IEP must be developed prior to the initiation of appropriate services. The speech and language services may be classified as either a primary **special education service** or a **related service**. If a student already qualifies for another type of special educational program, then the speech and language services are regarded as a related service for federal funding purposes. No matter how many special education services or related services a student receives, only one IEP should be developed that includes all services. Related services can be provided only for a student who has qualified for a special education service. The purpose of related services is to enable the student to benefit from special education. Parents and teachers should understand, then, why a student with even a mild problem is classified as requiring special education.

Education of the Handicapped Act Early Intervention Amendments of 1986

Some of the first amendments to the Education of the Handicapped Act were the Early Intervention Amendments of 1986 (PL 99-457). This served to broaden and strengthen the mandate for providing services to preschool children between the ages of 3 and 5 years. Additionally, federal incentive grant monies were made available to stimulate phasing-in services for the birth-through-age-2 years populations. Speech-language pathologists traditionally have treated these very young children in private practices, community and university clinics, and hospital settings. The school SLP, as provided under PL 99-457, is now responsible for providing early intervention programs.

This is an exciting and challenging aspect of the public school SLP's job for several reasons. First, considering the population of preschool handicapped children as a whole, the vast majority have a communication delay even if their primary handicap is a hearing impairment, cognitive deficit, motor problem, or the like. Second, school systems do not have a captive audience in terms of identifying these children; they are not attending the public schools. Thus, locating, identifying and screening preschool children with communication disorders will necessarily entail much community and agency interaction. The school SLP should be a member of an early intervention team from the school system who is responsible for working with parents, day care centers, pediatricians, health departments, private practices and other children's services. Through cooperative community efforts, preschool children with communication delays will be identified. IEPs for these children may reflect several agencies' roles and responsibilities in the provision of services. Service delivery for this population: (1) could be home-based, day care-based, center-based, or a combination of these; (2) vary in intensity; and (3) may require more coordination with agencies and parents.

Infants and toddlers (from birth to 3 years) must be screened and evaluated utilizing parents or caregivers. The early intervention team then must develop an **individualized family service plan** (**IFSP**) for the children who qualify. The family of the infant or toddler is the primary focus of the intervention plan, and the plan must be reviewed and revised as needed (at least every six months). PL 99-457 is a noncategorical law, meaning that children can qualify for services under the general term "developmental delay" and would not necessarily be labeled or categorized as they are under IDEA (i.e., hearing impaired, mentally handicapped, and so forth).

The law encourages the parent training necessary in the total treatment of these young children. Consequently, teachers and speech-language pathologists are becoming more involved in the development and supervision of innovative parent-training programs.

No Child Left Behind Act of 2001

In 2002 President George W. Bush signed the No Child Left Behind (NCLB) Act (PL 107-110) into law. The NCLB requires states to assess students in grades 3–8 and once again in grades 10–12 in the areas of math and reading using measures selected by individual states. The purpose of the testing is to measure the annual yearly progress (AYP) of individual children and school systems on reading and math goals. Test scores from individual school systems must improve for *all* students including minorities, low-income students, and students with disabilities. If a student is not making sufficient AYP for two consecutive years, the law provides for giving parents a choice of schools and supplemental educational services (e.g., tutoring). The law also mandates that teachers of core academic subjects are "highly qualified" in terms of their educational qualifications, certification, or licensure. With regard to students with disabilities, the NCLB as well as the IDEA require that these students participate in the state accountability and assessment system. As previously stated, IDEA requires that the IEP developed by a team of professionals and the parent include some description of how a child will be assessed to determine if goals are being achieved. In most cases, students with disabilities will be able to participate in the typical means of assessment (e.g., standardized tests) with appropriate accommodations. In the case of severely involved students, typically those with the most significant cognitive impairments, there is a provision for use of an alternate assessment aligned to an alternative achievement standard. The NCLB assumes that alternate assessments should not be necessary for more than 1% of students in the school system. The ultimate goal of NCLB is 100% student proficiency by 2014.

Individuals with Disabilities Education Improvement Act of 2004

In 2004 the original IDEA was reauthorized as the Individuals with Disabilities Education Improvement Act (PL 108-446). With the addition of the word *Improvement* to the title, one would think that the new acronym would be IDEIA, however, the vast majority of governmental agencies and national/state education agencies still refer to the new law as IDEA 2004. IDEA 2004 does not go into effect until July 2005, so IEPs written before that time will comply with IDEA 1997 standards. One of the goals of IDEA 2004 was to align the new law more closely with NCLB. Some important areas that have changed, or been added to IDEA 2004, that mainly affect IEPs are as follows:

- Alignment with NCLB
  - The IDEA 2004 includes a definition of a "highly qualified provider" for special education teachers.
  - The new law mandates that all students must be taught using the same academic standards.
  - In accord with NCLB, all students must participate in grade-level assessments or alternate assessments.
- Initial evaluation and consent for services
  - School systems may pursue an initial evaluation of a child identified by **child find** through a mediation process in cases where parents refuse consent or fail to respond.
  - If parents refuse to consent to the provision of special education services, the school shall not pursue mediation procedures to override them.
  - Initial eligibility determination must occur within 60 days from the parents' consent to evaluate their child (there are some exceptions for students who move frequently, such as migrant workers).
  - Parents and professionals may decide that a 3-year reevaluation is not necessary, but the IEP team must still have a meeting. Reevaluations do not need to take place more than once a year unless the IEP team requests it.

- IEPs
  - A new provision was added for an addendum to the IEP for when the goals are amended instead of writing a whole new IEP.
  - All annual goals must be measurable.
  - Although a description of transition services in the IEP were mandated at age 14 years in the original IDEA, this has been changed to age 16 years.
  - The IEP can be amended without calling a new IEP meeting if the parents and school system agree.
  - School systems may not require a student to take medications as a condition for attending classes or determining eligibility for special education.
  - The IEP must be developed within 30 days of eligibility determination.
  - There are new regulations regarding transferring from one school to another.
  - School systems are not required to pay for assistive technology devices that require surgical implantation (e.g., cochlear implants).
- Safeguards
  - A summary of procedural safeguards must be given to parents once a year, upon initial referral, during due process or upon request
  - New regulations on student discipline are included in IDEA 2004.

Section 504 of the Rehabilitation Act of 1973

"No otherwise qualified person with a disability in the United States . . . shall, solely on the basis of disability, be denied access to, or the benefits of, or be subjected to discrimination under any program or activity provided by any institution receiving federal financial assistance." Since public schools receive federal financial assistance, they are prohibited from denying a person with a disability the opportunity to participate or benefit from programs or services or otherwise limiting a qualified person with a disability in the enjoyment of any right, privilege, or advantage. Under Section 504, a person with a disability is defined as someone with a physical or mental impairment that substantially limits one or more major life activities. The term "substantially limits" means the person is unable to perform a major life activity, or is severely restricted as to the condition, manner, or duration under which a major life activity can be performed in comparison to the average person. Some students who do not meet the categorical criteria for special education services will be entitled to reasonable accommodations under Section 504.

For example, students who are identified as having attention deficit disorder (ADD) or attention deficit-hyperactivity disorder (AD-HD) qualify for services under Section 504 and should have a 504 Plan which delineates any accommodations needed by the student.

Americans with Disabilities Act

The Americans with Disabilities Act (ADA) was enacted July 26, 1990, providing "comprehensive civil rights protection for *qualified individuals with disabilities*." An individual with a disability is a person who has a physical or mental impairment that substantially limits a major life activity, or has a record of such impairment, or is regarded as having such impairment. The ADA applies to public entities and includes any state or local government, and any of its departments, agencies or other instrumentalities; thus, it applies to public schools. Specifically, all programs, services, and activities of schools are covered (e.g., fieldtrips, parent meetings, standardized exams, lab classes, etc.). Participation in programs, services, and activities may not be denied simply because the person has a disability. Students with disabilities must be in integrated settings, unless separate or different measures are needed to ensure equal opportunity (e.g., a specially designed recreational program for students with mobility impairments may be permitted, but students with disabilities cannot be refused participation in other recreational programs). Unnecessary eligibility standards or rules which deny students with disabilities an equal opportunity to enjoy programs, services, and activities must be eliminated and reasonable modifications must be made to policies, practices, and procedures, unless a fundamental alteration of the program would result. Auxiliary aids and services must be furnished when necessary to ensure effective communication, unless an undue financial burden or fundamental program alteration would result. Additionally, special charges cannot be placed on students with disabilities to cover the cost of barrier removal or auxiliary aids, and a student with a disability may choose not to accept a reasonable accommodation.

Communication has a special role in implementation of the ADA. Schools must ensure that communications with students who have hearing, vision, or speech impairments are as effective as for other students, and when necessary, auxiliary aids must be provided. Auxiliary aids include services or devices such as: qualified interpreters, assistive listening devices, telecaptioning, telecommunication devices (TDDs), videotext, taped textbooks, brailled materials, and large print materials. Auxiliary aids must be provided at no cost to the student. Students with hearing or speech impairments must be able to directly access emergency phone services, including 911.

THE ROLE OF THE SPEECH-LANGUAGE PATHOLOGIST IN THE SCHOOL SYSTEM

Public school SLPs hold unique and interesting positions within the school system hierarchy. Superintendents are responsible to the school board and, in turn, may have a number of assistant superintendents, depending upon the size of the system. The special education director is responsible to the upper level of superintendents and oversees the provision of special education services in the entire school system. Under the special education director in large school systems that employ 10 or more SLPs, usually one SLP will be designated as the speech pathology coordinator and would have the responsibility of managing speech pathology staff and services throughout the school system. In smaller systems, a senior SLP may be designated for leadership purposes, but usually all of the SLPs report directly to the special education coordinator who would then be responsible for the speech pathology program as well as other special education services. The SLP often works with more than one building principal, since many SLPs serve multiple schools. It is most helpful to keep the principals informed of the services being provided in the building, schedules, and any problems which arise. A well-informed principal can provide support in situations where it is needed. In addition to daily interactions with teachers, the SLP frequently works with support personnel (psychologists, social workers, nurses, physical or occupational therapists, and so forth) and agency and community professionals.

The actual work settings and job responsibilities of speech-language pathologists within the school system can vary greatly. The following three vignettes illustrate this broad range.

Mr. James works at Glen High School and Marymont Junior High. His caseload consists of 8 hearing-impaired students working on curriculum language and social interaction skills, 6 stutterers ranging in severity from mild to severe, 14 students with specific learning disabilities (SLD) who attend a communication skills class, 10 students who are in the program for the mentally handicapped and are working on functional communication skills necessary for vocational placement, and 2 students who are working for improved voice quality (one has nodules and the other is hyper-nasal). In addition to the case management of each of these individual students, Mr. James has a variety of other responsibilities. He heads the high school committee on the coordination of special services and is a member of the school-based intervention team at the junior high. Because he is skilled in sign language, he assists throughout the system in interviews, evaluations, or IEP meetings involving students or parents who use sign language for communication. The director of special education has recently asked Mr. James to develop a series of videotapes in which the system's special education procedures, parent's rights, and due process are explained fully in sign language.

Mrs. Sarnoff is an SLP for the Piedmont School District. She serves an elementary school in the mornings and a middle school in the afternoons. This allows her to see the severe cases every day. At the elementary school, she works in the early childhood class and the multihandicapped class using a collaborative consultation approach with the teachers. She integrates classroom curriculum content into all of the therapy sessions. This means that she must be in touch with the teachers, know what is being taught, and what subject areas and skills are most in need of support. Ten of Mrs. Sarnoff's cases are preschoolers who come into the schools for speech and language services. She works closely with the parents, training them to facilitate their child's communication skills. Mrs. Sarnoff also serves on the school-based support team at both schools. These teams process the prereferral concerns of teachers, providing appropriate intervention strategies. They also process all referrals for evaluation. Mrs. Sarnoff works closely with the teachers in her buildings, and is always willing to discuss their concerns. Several of the children in the multihandicapped class use augmentative communication devices. Mrs. Sarnoff evaluated the children and was instrumental in obtaining the appropriate device for each child. She is training the children, parents, and teachers to use these devices interactively. Mrs. Sarnoff has had advanced training in this area and serves as a consultant to the region regarding augmentative communication.

The East Regional Early Intervention Team consists of a physical therapist, social worker, early childhood special educator, and speech-language pathologist. Katherine Smith, the SLP, works with the team in the infant and toddler program. The infants are brought to the Hope Center where the team works with the parents by evaluating, demonstrating, and coaching to increase responsiveness of parent and infant. Infant referrals come from parents, neonatal high-risk nurseries, pediatricians, and agencies. Often a member of the team is asked to come to the hospital neonatal intensive care unit to meet parents and begin a supportive relationship. Katherine has found this to be an interesting aspect of her job. She also has organized a parent support group and attends these meetings as a facilitator. Katherine works in the toddler class where an early childhood special educator works with the 2- to 3-year-olds on a daily basis. Katherine has specific goals for each child and reviews these frequently with the teacher. They work together integrating communication and curriculum goals. All of the infants and toddlers have an individualized family service plan (IFSP) developed by the team and the parents after an assessment of family and child strengths and needs. Katherine is also a member of the transition team which facilitates the movement of parents and children from one program to another (e.g., from infant to toddler program, from toddler to preschool program, and from preschool to school-age services). She maintains records on all of the children, and attends weekly early intervention team meetings which often include persons from other agencies who are serving the parents and child (e.g., health department, children's services, human resources, and such). If the parents of a developmentally delayed infant cannot come to the Hope Center, or the toddler cannot be transported, Katherine or another team member makes regular home intervention visits.

As you can see, there is great diversity within the public school setting. This is one of the exciting aspects of the profession of speech-language pathology. Yet all three SLPs share some common responsibilities. First, SLPs must manage each individual case from the initial screening or referral to a final determination that a maximum level of progress has been attained. Second, SLPs must manage their caseload as a whole by summarizing individual case data for compliance, planning, and reporting purposes. These summarized data, by school and total caseload, are given to the special education director (or speech pathology coordinator) who is responsible for program management. All SLPs are thus involved in three levels of management (individual student, caseload, and program levels) regardless of the size of their school system. Some of the specific responsibilities involved in planning, directing, and providing services to students with communication disorders will now be discussed.

Case Finding

Case finding, most commonly called **child find**, refers to the preliminary identification of students with potential communication disorders. Case finding usually involves two procedures: screenings and/or referrals. **Screenings** are quick assessments of a student's communicative abilities, and if a problem is suspected, then a second screening may be scheduled or plans for a diagnostic assessment may be set into place. Some cases are identified by a referral from another professional. Sometimes parents refer their own children for screening. In most states an active effort has been made to provide materials (e.g., flyers, posters) for the public that outline normal development in critical areas (e.g., language, social, self-help, hearing, cognitive) and symptoms that would indicate the need for a screening by a professional.

Procedures for locating preschoolers with potential communication disorders will range from "preschool roundups" in small towns to media blitzes in larger metropolitan areas. Mass screenings in the schools take an inordinate amount of time and really are not cost effective. It is much more prudent to put time and effort into quality teacher in-services, screenings upon teacher request throughout the year, and effective communication with teachers (e.g., good rapport, working relationships, and the like). In addition, the laws require that there be no lapse in services. Thus, speech and language services for children who are already identified must be initiated the first week of the school year, making mass screenings more difficult to conduct.

Referral is a widely used method of case finding. Referrals can be made by anyone who has the student's welfare in mind and suspects a problem. This would include the parents, family doctor, school nurse, school counselor, principal, the individual student, and, of course, the teachers. Referrals should be encouraged by the speech-language pathologist. The procedures and opportunities for requesting a screening or making a referral should be presented to teachers, parents, and other professionals periodically. The success of a referral system is dependent on the ability of teachers to identify potential disorders of communication. There is evidence that without training, many communication problems can be effectively identified by teachers. On the other hand, some disorders such as voice problems and subtle language problems may not be as readily identified by teachers (Sommers & Hatten, 1985). The information provided in this textbook should go far in helping you recognize and understand a myriad of communication disorders so that you can be a more effective referral source.

Evaluation

The process of initial evaluation involves formal and informal testing of the student who has failed the screening or has been referred. Results of the assessment process usually yield a diagnosis (e.g., language disorder, fluency disorder, or categorizing a student as performing within normal limits). If the student is diagnosed with a communication disorder, the evaluation will include an estimate of severity.

According to IDEA all students with disabilities must receive a comprehensive multidisciplinary evaluation to determine if the child is eligible for special education. Eligibility must be determined prior to placement in a special education program, and written parental permission is required for this testing. The speech-language pathologist must comply with the law and be sure that test instruments are valid, not racially or culturally discriminatory, and administered in the student's native language. Tests can be standardized (norm referenced, criterion referenced), nonstandardized (e.g., language sample) or, most appropriately, a combination of both.

The evaluation may be conducted over several days and should focus on the suspected area of deficit in detail. The SLP should do a global communication assessment as well, including articulation skills, language competencies, and the normalcy of fluency, voice, and hearing. There also should be an examination of the speech mechanism to look at anatomical structure and function. Case history information from the parents, educational and behavioral observations from the teacher, and classroom observation of the student can be important. Additional information (such as level of cognitive functioning) obtained from school personnel may be helpful in interpreting the assessment data.

It should also be pointed out that assessment is ongoing. Once a student is found eligible and subsequently placed in a treatment program, progress must be constantly monitored by the speech-language pathologist and the classroom teachers. These periodic reevaluations let the SLP know the success or failure of therapeutic techniques and the need to change or modify the program. The need for dismissal from services also is determined by this ongoing evaluation process.

Participation in Meetings for Case Staffing and Eligibility Determination

It should be remembered that the purpose of the initial evaluation is to obtain information regarding a student's communication skills that can be presented to the eligibility committee who will determine if placement would be appropriate in a speech, language, and/or hearing program in the school. After the testing, the SLP must be prepared to describe to the eligibility committee how a student's communication disorder interferes with educational performance and the ability of the student to profit from classroom instruction. We often hear tales of students who clearly have difficulties in school or with communication, the parents are convinced that their child has a problem, and sometimes even the professionals who do the evaluation suspect an impairment, yet the child does not "qualify" for special education services. How can such a thing occur? One reason is that each school system operates under federal, state, and local guidelines. Eligibility determination ultimately is accomplished by combining these three levels of administrative regulations. It is not unusual for a child to qualify for services in one state, only to be ineligible when the family moves to another state. It is a shame when administrative guidelines override the concerns of parents and professionals. If a student is diagnosed with a particular problem, it is unfortunate if he or she cannot receive appropriate services just because of administrative regulations. Yet it happens often enough that parents have formed support groups, and the legal profession has offered consultative services for parents who feel that the school system has not provided appropriate services to their children. Sometimes we just do not spend enough time and effort in evaluation of students. Ehren (1993, p. 20) states:

> Eligibility often shapes caseloads in ways that seem inconsistent with the state of the art. . . . In lieu of making a diagnosis, we ascertain whether the student meets eligibility criteria. Evaluation, then, becomes an eligibility determination process, rather than a process to describe a student's communication status. . . . First we need to make a diagnosis, next, recommend the need for service; then, discuss eligibility. Diagnosis should drive eligibility; eligibility should not dictate the diagnosis. Eligibility criteria should be viewed as the last hoop to jump through in identifying a student.

Participation in staffing and placement decisions regarding the student is another responsibility of the speech-language pathologist. As a member of the placement team, the SLP reviews the data on individual students and participates in the development of the individualized educational plan (IEP) or individualized family service plan (IFSP) for each student. Parents must give written permission for placement prior to the initiation of services.

Delivery of Treatment

Although called by different names (e.g., therapy, intervention, remediation, habilitation/rehabilitation services) treatment refers to the actual delivery of services. **Treatment** may be **direct**, with the speech-language pathologist working directly with the student, or **indirect**, with the speech-language pathologist working with others (such as the classroom teacher or parent) to develop, improve, or maintain communication abilities of the student.

Treatment principles for each of the disorders of communication frequently encountered in the schools will be discussed in subsequent chapters of this book. In essence, however, treatment involves the instructional activities for the improvement of the communication deficit. The SLP must be accountable and able to show that the program of treatment is progress directed by maintaining accurate student data. In some school systems, the SLP may be fortunate to have the assistance of paraprofessionals. **Paraprofessionals**, also known as communication aides, speech-language pathology assistants, or support personnel, can carry out some of the more routine treatment procedures established by the SLP. These aides are, however, limited by their educational qualifications and school system guidelines as to how much assistance they can render.

As a teacher, you should support the speech-language treatment programs of your students. Participate whenever possible by working closely with the SLP (such as through sharing curricular topics, monitoring the use of techniques, assisting in carryover, and numerous other ways which will be discussed throughout this book). In general, allow your classroom to be a real-life situation where the student can practice newly learned communication behaviors or strategies.

SERVICE DELIVERY MODELS

Whenever a child in the public schools receives treatment for a communication disorder it is almost always a team effort. A general guideline is that the more severe the case, the more team members will be involved. For example, a child who has cerebral palsy and a hearing impairment may require many different types of services from a broad range of professions (e.g., audiology, physical therapy, occupational therapy, SLP, classroom teacher, social worker, etc.). On the other hand, a child with a learning disability may be seen by the LD teacher, regular classroom teacher, and the SLP. Finally, a child whose only problem is misarticulation of the s̲ sound may only be seen by the SLP and classroom teacher. Teams can operate in a variety of ways as they work with children, and there are several common models almost always cited in this regard which will be discussed below.

Multidisciplinary, Interdisciplinary, and Transdisciplinary Team Models

Indirect as well as direct approaches to providing services typically involve parents, teachers, and other professionals acting as a team that participates in assessing, treating, and evaluating a treatment program. Three models of team approaches can be viewed as a spectrum with the **multidisciplinary model** on one end, the **transdisciplinary model** on the other end, and the **interdisciplinary model** in the center (Figure 1-1). On the multidisciplinary end of the spectrum, there tends to be less cooperation among team members in terms of planning and implementation of a remedial program. There is also less communication among team members on this end of the continuum and more "fractionalizing" of the child, meaning he or she is taken out of class for speech, then for work on a learning problem, then for counseling about academic adjustment, and so forth. As we approach the transdisciplinary end of the continuum, more group cooperation in planning and implementation and much greater communication exists. Many goals have been incorporated into the child's daily classroom routine, and perhaps other team members have worked with the classroom teacher regarding how to use specific strategies in the child's daily activities. This accomplishes the educational objectives without constantly removing the child from his classroom.

We can see that one thing common to all three approaches is that they use a variety of professionals. For instance, a regular classroom teacher, audiologist, SLP, psychometrist, and special educator may be involved with a case in all three approaches. A second similarity is that all three approaches deal with both assessment and treatment of the child's problem. The differences among the approaches, however, are the focus of the present section. Initially, we will discuss the multidisciplinary and interdisciplinary models.

The multi- and interdisciplinary approaches maintain the independence of each discipline in terms of doing separate evaluations and holding separate treatment sessions with the child. For planning purposes, both multi- and interdisciplinary approaches involve each professional making separate sets of annual goals and short-term objectives, although they make up one individualized educational program. When implementing the IEP, the multi- and interdisciplinary approaches either carry out the goals independently, or in the latter approach, incorporate some goals of other team members when

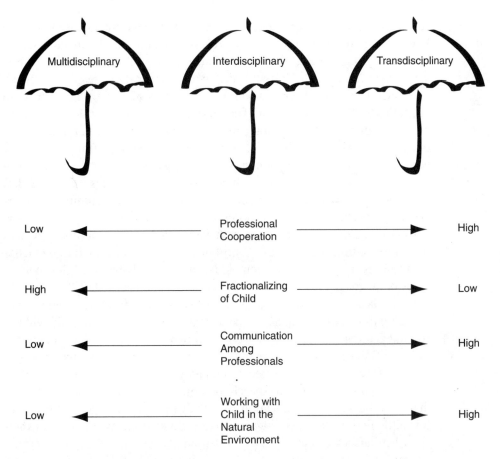

Figure 1-1 Three Models of Service Delivery

possible. This tends to fractionalize the child and his program of treatment. It has often been said that it takes more than a staple punched through a pile of separate reports to make an integrated program. Yet, this is what often happens in a multidisciplinary approach. Even though the IEP may contain goals in many areas, often team members focus only on the goals that apply to their own disciplines. It is not uncommon for one professional to be unaware of the specific goals that another team member has targeted at a given point in time or of the child's progress in that area. Another criticism of these models is that it may not be clear exactly which member of the team is accountable for working on certain goals and evaluating programs.

In the transdisciplinary model, the assessment and treatment options are developed by the professionals and family together. It is important to remember, however, that regardless of the assessment–treatment model, the IEP must be developed jointly by professionals and family members. The transdisciplinary model emphasizes such interactions more than others. There is much consultation and discussion during the assessment period; team members may observe the child in a variety of settings in addition to collecting individual test data. The guiding philosophy is that team members are committed to working together *across discipline boundaries* to make the intervention effective. A prominent concern in transdisciplinary models is the notion of a primary service provider. In most cases, one professional sees a child more often than do other professionals during the day. The classroom teacher, for instance, has many more opportunities to interact with a particular child and observe behavior than the SLP. As such, the teacher and classroom environment have much to offer in terms of evaluation information for the SLP. Who knows more than the child's teacher about his typical communication skills, problem-solving strategies, consistency of language errors, intelligibility, fluency, and social skills?

The classroom environment and teacher are also primary considerations in the treatment of speech and language problems because the child will use communication skills in the classroom throughout the day. In most cases, the SLP sees children with communication disorders for individual sessions. This is especially true in the beginning phases of treatment. When the child leaves the classroom to go to speech therapy, the SLP must *contrive* activities that resemble real communication, especially in the later stages of treatment. It is difficult to justify spending time creating a natural environment for therapy when one already exists in the classroom. Often, children can effectively learn to use correct sentence structure, speech sounds, fluent speech, and good vocal habits in the confines of the speech room. However, as soon as the child returns to the classroom environment, these skills are often forgotten. An enduring complaint of SLPs for decades has been that it is relatively easy to *establish* a new communication skill, but it is most difficult to *generalize* these skills to the child's natural environment. The classroom teacher, as a team member, can be of crucial assistance here.

If close communication between the SLP and the teacher occurs, the teacher can assist in facilitating **generalization** of newly established behaviors. For example, a child with a language problem who omits *is* from sentences such as "He is my friend," can easily be trained by the SLP to remember the *is* in therapy sessions. Yet, the child goes back to the classroom and continues to say sentences without the *is* included in them. If the teacher could remind the child to include *is* in classroom conversation, the child would rapidly learn that this piece of language is important and finally generalize it into daily communication. Cooperation of team members is not a one-way street. For example, imagine that a particular child scores low on vocabulary tests administered by the SLP indicating the child should have some vocabulary enrichment. The SLP could consult with the classroom teacher and begin to train vocabulary words related to the child's academic work. For example:

> An SLP that we know was working with a student on building vocabulary and the production of a correct s sound. The SLP asked the teacher which areas of the child's academic performance were weak, and the teacher indicated that the child was particularly struggling in the understanding of city government. The SLP borrowed a textbook from the teacher and centered part of the child's therapy sessions around the topic of government, introducing related new vocabulary words and monitoring the child's s sound during discussions they had about how the city was run.

This example underscores the symbiotic relationship between professionals. One final note about cooperation among professionals is necessary. Historically, professionals of various types have felt that certain training was their exclusive province. This type of "turfism" tends to be counterproductive. The most important goal is that the child develops skills, eradicates maladaptive behaviors, and learns specific information and strategies for problem solving. It makes no difference whatsoever if a child's grammar is corrected by the SLP, a teacher, or a parent. The critical point is that the problem is remediated. If a child learns certain concepts about classroom work from the SLP, he is further ahead, and the teacher should not feel that his or her territory has been encroached upon.

Types of Service Delivery Offered by the Speech-Language Pathologist

The SLP working in the school environment can offer a continuum of services to help students with communication disorders. There are a number of terms that are commonly used to refer to different types of services.

Direct and Indirect Services

When the SLP is working with children individually or in small groups, it is called direct service. These direct services can be performed in the classroom, or they can be provided in a treatment room located elsewhere in the school building. When the SLP works with the student outside the classroom, either individually or in a group, this is sometimes called a *pullout* model of service delivery. Most SLPs have offices or treatment rooms in which they can work with an individual child or small group for several treatment sessions per week. If the children are grouped, they are often chosen because they are all working on the same types of problems (e.g., groups of children with stuttering problems or language disorders). While some SLPs are assigned exclusively to a single school building, others are itinerant in that they travel among several schools, providing services to each. Whether the SLP is itinerant or not, he or she should maintain close communication with all teachers regarding the students seen in treatment. Direct services in which the SLP removes the students from the classroom environment have advantages and disadvantages. One positive aspect is that the SLP can work with the student in an environment free from distractions, and this is helpful in establishing many communication behaviors (e.g., teaching a new sound to the child). Another advantage is that certain therapy approaches involving drills or specialized equipment can be more easily implemented outside of the classroom. On the other hand, if the student is removed from the classroom, several times a week, he or she can miss valuable academic lessons while in speech-language treatment sessions. Direct services provided in the classroom can be of help to both the communication disordered child as well as the teacher. The SLP can help the teacher by assisting with classroom activities, giving them a communication slant that is beneficial to all members of the class. Direct services provided in the classroom assist in the generalization of goals gained in a therapy room into the natural environment.

In most school systems, there is a mixture of direct and indirect services provided by the SLP. Some children are seen exclusively with direct services, others receive a combination of direct and indirect, and still others receive all of their treatment in the indirect mode. The configuration of services received depends on the caseload, teacher cooperation, the particular philosophy of the SLP, and guidelines set by the school system and state department of education.

Interestingly, the ASHA Schools Surveys conducted in 1992 and 2003 indicated, "Except for the birth-to-2-years age group, the most frequently used service delivery model was the traditional pullout, followed by the classroom-based model. For the birth-to-2-years age group, the most used model was the collaborative consultation model." Although it is true that many states are currently emphasizing use of indirect and collaborative models of service delivery, the ASHA data suggest that the majority of public school speech-language pathologists surveyed indicate that direct services are still prevalent.

Indirect Services: A Consultative or Collaborative Approach

Speech-language pathologists use a variety of assessment–treatment models to deal with both children and adults who have communication disorders (Damico, 1987; Frassinelli, Superior, & Meyers, 1983; Fujiki & Brinton, 1984; Marvin, 1987). As previously mentioned, in the traditional direct service model, the child is removed from the classroom and seen individually or in a group by the SLP. Parents, teachers, and administrators have become so accustomed to this direct service model that they may find it unusual to deal with other modes of treatment, such as a consultative or a collaborative mode. Basically, collaboration is a three (or more) person chain of service. For instance, the consultant (SLP) provides professional service to the child indirectly through the teacher. Collaboration as a practice, is not new. Speech-language pathologists have made suggestions to teachers and parents for decades regarding how they can assist in treatment progress. We have now begun to realize that different children may require different levels of direct or indirect involvement by the SLP, and that there is a continuum of services that can be offered. Consultation models have been shown to be effective and workable in school systems (Ferguson, 1991; Magnotta, 1991; Montgomery, 1992; Moore-Brown, 1991).

A teacher might ask "For what kind of case would I be the primary interventionist?" One example might involve a child who is nonverbal in a preschool class. A primary goal for this child is to increase communication attempts through pointing and physically regulating the teacher (e.g., putting the teacher's hand on a toy to wind it up) in natural daily activities. This would be a difficult goal for the SLP to work on outside of the classroom. Yet, the teacher would not have to do anything extra for the child in terms of preparation, beyond simply attending to the child's pointing during certain activities and allowing the child to physically regulate him or her to make needs known. The SLP then would evaluate the occurrence of communication attempts at different points in therapy and prescribe changes in the teacher–child interaction.

In another example, the consultant (SLP) might make an in-service presentation on a topic in dialectal variation, such as the occurrence of African-American English features in the language of minority children. A teacher attends the in-service and later has a student who indicates that he or she wants to learn to write some short stories in a standard English form and eliminate elements of African-American English from the story. He or she also indicates a desire to learn to shift styles, speaking standard English on certain occasions and then shifting back to African-American English when desired. The teacher might agree to monitor the writing and speaking in certain situations, and let the student know when dialectal features occur. In this case, the teacher really does all the assessment, intervention, and evaluation of the program with only some advice and information from the SLP consultant. Since this student is a dialect speaker, he or she did not have a clinically significant communication disorder, so no IEP would be necessary in this case.

This collaborative model highlights enhanced communication and problem solving among professionals, and the plan for assessment and intervention actually springs from these discussions. It is probably a basic fact that people tend to participate more fully in an intervention program if they have had some role in determining its course. A teacher who has a good idea about how to approach a problem of a communication-disordered child in the context of the classroom is more likely to carry it out than if he or she is asked to do a particular task by the SLP. When this child is served exclusively by the classroom teacher with the SLP acting as a consultant, the IEP must reflect the provision of indirect services only.

One can see that the continuum of services that the SLP can offer varies considerably in terms of teacher and SLP involvement. Almost any variation on the above models is possible, and the particular configuration of treatment responsibilities decided upon for a particular child depends on some of the following variables:

1. Types of goals for a particular case, and the child's point in the therapy program (whether he or she is just beginning treatment or nearing dismissal)
2. Willingness of the SLP to be flexible in service provision
3. Willingness of the teacher to consider alternative models of service
4. Time available for consultation meetings for both parties

Although most children can benefit from direct service by the SLP, we have tried to make the point that in many instances the SLP can best deal with cases by working collaboratively with the teacher or parents. Some other specific examples of cases that might be treated effectively with collaboration are illustrated below:

Case 1: One common example of a case suited to collaborative models is a child who habitually abuses his or her vocal cords by frequently yelling, screaming, and using the voice improperly. It is difficult to see how the SLP could monitor this behavior if the child is seen only individually in an isolated therapy room. The teacher sees the child more than the SLP and can monitor instances of vocal abuse and discourage them. The major input of the SLP would be to introduce proper vocal hygiene practices to the child, inform the teacher and parents of those practices, and monitor changes in the child's vocal quality over time.

Case 2: Any child who is speaking in utterances less than three to four words in length is a natural candidate for indirect or collaborative treatment. These children require continuous stimulation of certain language forms and need to be naturally reinforced for use of correct language in real communicative situations (e.g., give the child objects he asks for; look at things he labels). The SLP could isolate this child and contrive activities similar to those already occurring in the classroom; however, this appears to be nothing more than reinventing the wheel. The teacher is with the child during his daily activities and can not only model appropriate language, but also reinforce the use of utterance types as suggested by the SLP. A very powerful technique known as *recasting* involves restating a child's incorrect utterance in a correct manner. For instance, if a child says "Him my friend," a teacher or parent could say "Yes, he is your friend." Many research projects have demonstrated that recasting can effectively promote the use of correct language forms in children with language disorders (Paul, 2001). This is a technique that does not take much extra time, and can be naturally incorporated into any interaction with a child.

Case 3: A final example of appropriate use of indirect or collaborative therapy involves a child with any type of communication disorder who is in the generalization portion of speech-language therapy. The SLP can train the child's speech and language behavior to only a certain level, and then it is time for the child to use these new skills in natural situations. We often see children who produce impeccable s sounds in conversation with the SLP in the therapy room, only to misarticulate in the classroom or at home. Similarly, children who stutter are frequently fluent with the SLP, but fail to use their fluency-enhancing techniques in real situations.

In summary, these are just a few of the almost endless examples of how the classroom environment is critical to the generalization of nearly everything the SLP trains in children with communication disorders.

Myths Surrounding the Collaborative and Consultative Models

Although a collaborative approach to dealing with communication disorders has logical and practical advantages, many administrators, teachers, and even SLPs are resistant to change. It is always easier to remain with the inertia of past practices. Also, people believe in several myths that are difficult to debunk.

The first myth is that individual therapy services are always better than services delivered in the context of a classroom or home environment. It is true, that for many cases, individual therapy time is clearly important. This is especially true in the beginning stages of therapy, but becomes less true as the program progresses.

Jeff had been in individual therapy sessions for almost a year working on his r sound. His enthusiasm was waning, and the SLP had difficulty keeping him motivated. One day, she decided to put Jeff in a group of two other children working on articulation problems. They played some competitive games in therapy as they worked on speech sounds, and Jeff responded well to the challenge. He was determined to make more correct r sounds than anyone else in the group.

We need to integrate the child into classrooms and groups so that skills learned in therapy will generalize. Also, most children with language disorders are best dealt with in the classroom where real situations and peer-modeling can occur. Isolation might actually be a detriment to such cases.

The teacher was surprised when the SLP said that she would rather work with Carrie in the classroom than take her to the speech therapy room. Carrie had been diagnosed as mentally retarded and spoke in 1- to 2-word utterances. The SLP wanted to expand Carrie's sentence length to three to four words. Every day, the SLP came into the classroom and stayed close to Carrie as she performed her class projects in art, music, and story time. Whenever Carrie said something in a 1- to 2-word utterance the SLP would expand it to three to four words. So, if Carrie said "Want ball," the

SLP would say "I want ball." This type of stimulation was carried on throughout all the activities, and every time Carrie would say a 3-word sentence on her own, the SLP would repeat what the child had said in an excited tone.

The second myth has to do with the notion that certain problems are best dealt with by the particular professional that has expertise in a given area. In essence, the SLP should be the only one to deal with communication disorders, the psychologist should be the only one to deal with behavior problems, and so on. This issue is complex because the problems that children have are very complex. Most of the time, these problems affect the child in many areas. For instance, if the child has an emotional problem, it will be manifested in the classroom, in speech therapy, in music class, in physical education, at home, and on the playground. The behavior disturbance or emotional conflict teacher obviously cannot be present in all of these situations. However, if all of the educational team members are familiar with the child's problem, the intervention program, and the goals to be accomplished by the youngster, everyone can facilitate the child's progress. If a child has a communication disorder, it is not just the province of the SLP because the difficulty in communicating will be present in the classroom, at lunch, at home, and at recess. Thus, the more people familiar with the problem and the methods of correcting it, the better. The practice of only one team member dealing with a problem is unrealistic and not very economical as a treatment approach.

A third myth, that professionals have a territory which must be protected from others, is very much related to the second myth just discussed. Clearly, we are all members of a team that has the best interests of the child at heart. It is naïve to think that communication is the province only of the SLP or that reading is to be dealt with only by the teacher. Many children are helped with reading by parents, other professionals, and even other children. Almost any area from communication and motor skill to emotional development overlaps so much with all professional areas that it is counterproductive to think of encroaching on someone's territory.

The fourth myth is that people who advocate the collaborative model are just trying to get out of doing the work themselves. It is important to note that in a consultative model, the person doing the intervention should not take on tasks that would interfere with his or her primary mission. For instance, a teacher (whose main job is teaching) should not be expected to carry on speech or language therapy sessions or make treatment materials for such procedures. The collaborative model suggests that the teacher can incorporate communication goals into his or her already existing activities, but not design special tasks dealing with speech or language. For example, a teacher might have a reading group in which children read aloud. If a member of the group has been working on a problem pronouncing the r sound (e.g., _wabbit_ for _rabbit_), then the teacher might consult with the SLP about it. The teacher would then know if the child is capable of making the sound correctly during conversation, but simply forgets most of the time. The teacher might volunteer, as a collaborator, to monitor the r sound during reading group and ask the child to say it correctly when it is produced in error. Another example might be a preschool teacher who has planned an art activity. In class he or she has a child who is working with the SLP on combining two words in sentences (e.g., red crayon, want paper). The teacher might volunteer to stimulate or model certain word combinations during the art activity or try to get the child to answer questions using 2-word utterances. At the very least, the teacher could naturally reinforce the child for using any spontaneous word combinations by responding to his comments during the art activity and at other points during the school day. One can readily see that these applications of the collaborative model involve little extra planning and additional work on the part of the teacher and has great benefits for the student. Remember also that collaboration is a two-way street. The speech-language pathologist will participate in collaborative activities involving classroom work when incorporating reading, phonemic awareness, writing, spelling, and academic content into treatment sessions for children with a variety of communication disorders. These activities can be included in a therapy session by the SLP without extensive preparation and within the context of established goals for communication.

Conducting Collaboration: Some Practical Advice

One might get the impression that collaboration is less complicated and takes less time than providing direct services. Usually, this could not be farther from the truth. In fact, collaboration when well done, can actually take more time than direct services. Collaboration is not something that should be "dabbled" with by teachers and SLPs. The process involves thorough assessment of the child, establishing goals, determining who will be responsible for different aspects of the treatment program, and evaluating the effectiveness of the program. As you can see, collaborating correctly involves spending some time in meetings and documenting the process. Following are some guidelines that have been gleaned from a variety of sources in the collaboration literature (Damico, 1987; Ferguson, 1991; Frassinelli, Superior, & Meyers, 1983; Fujiki & Brinton, 1984; Magnotta, 1991; Marvin, 1987; Montgomery, 1992; Moore-Brown, 1991).

- Administrative matters
  - Decide on a set time and place for a meeting. The time and place should be agreeable to all team members. This formalizes the process so that members are not simply dabbling in the case. If you are going to approach a problem with a concerted effort, it should not be done in an informal manner, leaving many important issues and responsibilities to chance.
  - Formalizing the process with a written collaboration plan also makes team members accountable to school administrators who may ask questions about indirect services in terms of numbers of cases, types of cases, and faculty time spent on such enterprises.
- Attitudinal variables
  - Be a good listener and show respect and consideration for the other team members' expertise, questions, opinions, decisions, concerns, or goals involving the child.
  - Be positive. Look at consultation as a way to bring about positive change for the child.
  - Let the other team members know when you think they have a good idea (reinforce other team members).
- Conducting the meetings
  - In discussing the child, see that every member of the team has a chance for input.
  - When different areas of concern are discussed, let the expert in each area lead the discussion. This has been called "situational leadership." For instance, if the issue is language, perhaps the SLP should lead the discussion. If the discussion turns to performance in reading or how to get certain language behaviors to occur in the classroom, the teacher should take the lead.
  - Team members should withhold solutions until all areas of concern and possible approaches have been discussed. When a team member proposes a solution to the child's problems before the team has fully discussed it and all members have had input, it is no longer a team approach. This is a major problem to guard against, because it is a human tendency to want to be the first with the resolution to a prob-

lem and not make the solution a true group effort. The contributions of team members should be viewed as suggestions and parts of a puzzle to be combined for a total program.

o When discussing the needs of the child, each team member should not use words or phrases that would confuse other team members. We refer here to the use of professional jargon that may not be understandable to other team members. Use of jargon not only interferes with good communication, but also subtly places other team members in lesser positions because then the specialist has to explain or lecture the team on the terms. Every profession has its jargon and biases, so it is good to avoid specialized terms when possible.

o Talk about specific goals for the child. The team should discuss ways that these goals can be reached in all environments.

o When the goals and evaluation procedures have been discussed, the team should make all parties accountable for the ultimate success of the program. The team should define roles and expectations of each team member so that confusion will not arise. Each team member should clearly understand what his or her role in the program will be and what is to be done by each person.

o The plan should be recorded on a form or on a written protocol outlining the goals, procedures, and roles of each team member. This protocol should be filed in the child record for future reference.

o The team should reconvene after the plan has been in effect for a period of time to evaluate progress and make alterations to goals and procedures.

In preparing for the current revision of this text, we interviewed speech-language pathologists and asked them for their views on barriers they have faced in implementing a collaborative model. One major barrier was lack of time for meetings. Often it is difficult to find the time for team members to get together. Some SLPs said they use e-mail to communicate about some aspects of collaboration among team members. Others said that they make time by meeting after school, or scheduling meetings at available times during the day. The other major barrier reported by the SLPs we interviewed was that some (a minority) teachers are simply not oriented to collaboration. Some perceive themselves as being too busy or feel that working on communication disorders is not their job. They may be used to the direct service model, and may not be interested in collaboration. Trying to force someone into a service delivery model they do not believe in can often lead to sabotage, lack of cooperation, and ineffective services for the child we are trying to help. The lessons are to use collaborative models with those professionals who are amenable to participating and make a concerted effort to make these collaborations successful. Also, success tends to breed further success. Once a collaborative model has been successful with a teacher, he or she is more likely to participate in future cases and the whole process will be easier because it is familiar to all team members.

We have tried in this chapter to provide an overall view of the possible ways that classroom teachers and speech-language pathologists might interact in providing services to students with communication disorders. Teachers should expect to come in contact with the SLP in referrals, evaluation, and treatment. We hope that when the SLP comes to meet with you concerning children in your class that you will develop a productive and enjoyable professional as well as personal relationship.

THE ROLE OF THE CLASSROOM TEACHER IN IDENTIFICATION, ASSESSMENT, AND TREATMENT

Consider the following vignettes of three teachers:

Mrs. Thomas has taught kindergarten for 12 years. She has been concerned for some time about little Rachel, who appears to have a great deal of difficulty following directions. Carefully sequenced instructions were given for making a pinwheel out of a stick, construction paper, and a metal pin. Rachel ended up with a "ball" of construction paper that was poised on the end of the stick like a perverted magic wand. Mrs. Thomas requested a hearing test for Rachel from the speech-language pathologist, and it was found that she has a significant hearing loss caused by recurring ear infections. Since she received an evaluation by an audiologist and wore her new hearing aid, she has had little trouble with comprehending instructions.

Mrs. Carson has dealt with Reginald for two years—once during his first time through third grade and again when he had to repeat it. She has put in literally hundreds of hours observing whom he likes and who likes him. She knows to whom he talks and the topics of conversation. She not only knows what he's learned, but *how* he's learned, what motivates him, what he can do, what he cannot do, what makes him cry, and who his favorite baseball player is.

For instance, she knows that Reggie has difficulty in meeting a strange adult for the first time and that whenever he is asked to perform a task, it is always wise to present the instructions twice. After obtaining permission to evaluate, the new SLP asked if he could take Reggie for an hour to do some tests of the child's language ability. Unfortunately, he never asked Mrs. Carson any questions before removing Reggie for his tests. When the SLP brought Reggie back, he announced that Reggie had failed all of the language tests and did not talk to the SLP when he tried to obtain a conversational sample from Reggie. Mrs. Carson was not surprised. Her input about how to deal with Reggie would have made the evaluation much more effective.

Bob Brooks is a teacher who becomes uncomfortable whenever he thinks of watching and listening to Emilio Chavez. Emilio has a severe stuttering problem and produces long, torturous blocks accompanied by facial grimaces and inspiratory gasps. Bob has discussed this with the SLP and knows it was not a good policy to avoid calling on a child who had a stuttering problem. So, now it was time to ask Emilio a question and see the look of a trapped animal quickly eclipse the child's face. Bob knows Emilio is in speech therapy and the technique he is supposed to use is a slowed-down, stretched type of speech that prolongs vowel sounds to increase fluency. As Emilio began to answer, he pressed his lips tightly together, and his head began to jerk in a series of rapid arrhythmic movements that lasted almost half a minute. Mr. Brooks finally said, "Remember to start out slowly and prolong the vowels like you do in speech class." Emilio stopped, tried to relax, and was able to answer the question appropriately with much less abnormality in his speech as he slowly glided from one vowel to the next.

These three vignettes illustrate the participation of teachers in three important aspects of dealing with communication disorders: identification of cases, evaluation of children's communication skills, and treatment of communication problems. In the examples involving case detection and treatment, the teacher succeeded in helping the communication-disordered child. In the case involving evaluation, the SLP failed to profit from the expertise of the teacher before evaluating a child. If he had only asked the teacher some questions, the evaluation would have been more efficient and would have provided more information. It is, of course, up to the individual classroom teacher, the school administration, and the SLP to determine specific roles and duties in the real world. If teachers could incorporate even some of the information included in this text into their daily interactions with children and SLPs, gains could be seen in several areas. First, the children with communication disorders would be detected, evaluated, and treated more quickly and effectively. Second, SLPs would be able to perform their jobs more efficiently and be able to focus maximum effort on the cases that require the most attention. Third, teachers would be able to have an even greater impact on their students. Finally, as a member of the educational team, teachers would develop strong professional relationships with other disciplines.

Children in the public school system who are enrolled in special education make up a highly heterogeneous group. There are children who represent almost every exceptionality, and public school professionals are expected to be able to diagnose and treat these problems and prescribe appropriate educational programs. In addition to representing a disparate variety of handicapping conditions, these children also manifest a full range in severity of their disorders. No single professional can hope to have expertise in assessment and remediation for every kind of physical, cognitive, language, speech, emotional, or educational problem. It is because of this diverse population and the monumental literature available about each type of disorder that public school professionals generally incorporate a team approach when dealing with special education cases. In subsequent chapters, we will outline many specific ways that teachers and SLPs can cooperate in helping students with communication disorders.

REFERENCES

ASHA [American Speech-Language-Hearing Association]. (1984). Guidelines for caseload size for speech-language services in the schools. *ASHA, 26*(4), 53–58.

ASHA [American Speech-Language-Hearing Association]. (1992). *1992 omnibus survey caseload report: SLP.* Rockville, MD: Author.

ASHA [American Speech-Language-Hearing Association]. (2003). *2003 omnibus survey caseload report: SLP.* Rockville, MD: Author.

Damico, J. (1987). Addressing language concerns in the schools: The SLP as consultant. *Journal of Childhood Communication Disorders, 11,* 17–40.

Ehren, B. (1993). Eligibility, evaluation and the realities of role definition in the schools. *American Journal of Speech-Language Pathology, 2*(1), 20–23.

Ferguson, M. (1991). Collaborative/consultative service delivery: An introduction. *Language, Speech & Hearing Services in Schools, 22,* 147.

Frassinelli, L., Superior, K., & Meyers, J. (1983). A consultation model for speech and language intervention. *Journal of the American Speech-Language-Hearing Association, 25*(11), 25–30.

Fujiki, M., & Brinton, B. (1984). Supplementing language therapy: Working with the classroom teachers. *Language, Speech & Hearing Services in Schools, 15*, 98–109.

Kurpius, D. (1978). Consultation theory and process: An integrated model. *Personnel and Guidance Journal, 6*, 335–338.

Magnotta, O. (1991). Looking beyond tradition. *Language, Speech & Hearing Services in Schools, 22*, 150–151.

Marvin, C. (1987). Consultation services: Changing roles for SLPs. *Journal of Childhood Communication Disorders, 11*(1), 1–16.

McCormick, L. (1984). Extracurricular roles and relationships. In L. McCormick & R. Schiefelbusch (Eds.), *Early Language Intervention*. Columbus, OH: Charles E. Merrill.

Montgomery, J. (1992). Implementing collaborative consultation: Perspectives from the field. *Language, Speech & Hearing Services in Schools, 23*, 363–364.

Moore-Brown, B. (1991). Moving in the direction of change: Thoughts for administrators and speech-language pathologists. *Language, Speech & Hearing Services in Schools, 22*, 148–149.

Neidecker, E. A. (1987). *School programs in speech-language: Organization and management*. Englewood Cliffs, NJ: Prentice-Hall.

Paul, R. (2001). Language Disorders from Infancy Through Adolescence: Assessment and Intervention. St. Louis, MO: Mosby.

Peters-Johnson, C. (1992). Professional practices perspective on caseloads in schools. *ASHA, 34*, 12.

Schetz, K. F., & Sheese, R. J. (1989). Software that works in school settings. *ASHA, 31*(1), 65–68.

Schien, E. (1978). The role of the consultant: Content expert or process facilitator. *Personnel and Guidance Journal, 6*, 339–343.

Sommers, R. K., & Hatten, M. E. (1985). Establishing the therapy program: Case finding, case selection, and case load. In R. J. Van Hattum (Ed.), *Organization of speech-language services in schools*. San Diego, CA: College-Hill.

U.S. Department of Education. (2000). To assure the free appropriate public education of all children with disabilities: Fourteenth annual report to Congress on the implementation of the Individuals with Disabilities Education Act.

Woodruff, G., & Hanson, C. (1987). *Project KAI*. Funded by U.S. Department of Education, Special Education Programs.

TERMS TO KNOW

American Speech-Language-Hearing Association (ASHA)

audiologists

child find

communication disorders

due process

evaluation

generalization

identification

individualized education plan (IEP)

individualized family service plan (IFSP)

interdisciplinary

language

least restrictive environment

multidisciplinary

paraprofessionals

referrals

related services

screenings

special education services

speech

speech-language pathologists

transdisciplinary

treatment (direct and indirect)

STUDY QUESTIONS

1. Discuss the importance of federal special education laws from PL 94-142 to IDEA 2004. What are some of the main points of each public law?

2. What is the individualized education plan? What are some of its components? How is the IEP developed?

3. Why is it important that teachers make referrals to speech-language pathologists? What are the requisite skills needed to be able to make these referrals?

4. Differentiate between direct and indirect treatment services.

chapter *two*

Normal Aspects of Communication

INTRODUCTION

To better understand the communication disorders reviewed in the following chapters, it is helpful to first understand some basic aspects of normal communication. Human communication is a very complex process, many aspects of which are not yet fully understood. It is not even possible to talk about "normal" communication without specifying for whom it is normal. The ability to communicate is a developmental skill. We do not expect an infant to be able to communicate as well as a first grader, and we do not expect a first grader to communicate as well as a college student. Children exhibit different levels of communication skills at various stages of their development. Teachers should be aware of these different levels of communication skills because expecting too much can lead to frustration on the part of the student and the teacher, and expecting too little can result in a failure to identify early signs of a communication disorder.

There are several terms which will be used throughout this book that are important to understand. These terms are **communication**, **language**, and **speech**. Many people use these terms as if they were interchangeable and say *communication* when they mean *language* or *language* when they mean *speech*. It is essential that you understand what is meant by each of these terms and the differences among their meanings.

COMMUNICATION

Communication is the broadest of the three terms and refers to an exchange of ideas or feelings. Speech and language are means of communicating, but human beings communicate in many ways. Artists communicate through their art. A painting or a sculpture can communicate feelings or ideas in a very effective manner. Those of us with less artistic skill can communicate through gestures, body positions, or facial expressions. A tight jaw and a clenched fist communicate one meaning, while a smile and a wink communicate quite another. The most common way for human beings to communicate, however, is the way we are communicating now, through language.

LANGUAGE

Language can be defined in many ways. Perhaps the best definition of language for the purposes of this chapter comes from Bloom (1988). She defines language as: "A code whereby ideas . . . . are represented through a conventional system of arbitrary signals for communication" (p. 2). According to this definition, to communicate through language, a person must first have an idea, arrange some symbol system in such a way that another person can process those symbols and draw from them the intended meaning.

Several conditions must be met to communicate using language. First, the person sending the message must have an idea to communicate. If you were asked to discuss agricultural practices in Estonia prior to World War I, you probably would have some difficulty because you may not have much of an idea to communicate. As children grow, their knowledge and understanding of the world also grow. As a result, they have more ideas to express and more things to communicate. A second condition is that the communicator must be familiar with the symbol system used to express ideas. If you have studied a foreign language, you know that it is easier to say what you want to say in your native language than in the new language, even though your idea is the same. It takes time and practice to master a new symbol system. As you will see in Chapter 3, children master their language symbol systems in developmental stages. It is important to remember that language is not only expressed, but for communication to occur, language must also be received. When we send a message, we are using **expressive language**; when we receive a message, we are using **receptive language**. We are communicating with you (we hope) through language. We are using expressive language, putting our ideas into symbols. You are using receptive language, processing those symbols so you can understand what our ideas are. If you understand what our ideas are, then we have communicated. The process involved in expressive language is **encoding**, putting ideas into code, and the process involved in receptive language is **decoding**, taking ideas out of code. To communicate through language, both the encoder and the decoder must know the same code. If you speak only English and you try to explain something to someone who speaks only Mandarin Chinese, any communication would probably result from gestures and facial expression rather than from language because you do not share a common linguistic code with your listener. It does not matter how slowly or how loudly you say the words. The other person will not be able to understand you because he or she does not have knowledge of the code. Even if a student in your class speaks English, if that student does not have knowledge of the words you are using, slower, louder speech will simply serve to frustrate both teacher and student.

Because language is such a broad topic, it is sometimes helpful to specify certain aspects or subcomponents of language. Five subcomponents are typically identified. **Semantics** is the component of language having to do with meaning. From the teacher's perspective, this component is roughly equivalent to vocabulary. Our vocabularies expand throughout our lives. It is hoped you are adding to your vocabulary as you read this chapter. During childhood however, vocabulary grows rapidly. Between the ages of 2 and 4 years, it seems as if the child learns a new word every day. As with all components of language, the semantic component has both an expressive and receptive aspect. Like adults, children usually understand more words than they use. It is not correct to assume that a student does not understand a word simply because he or she never uses it. On the other hand, because a student uses a word in one context, it does not mean that he or she understands all of the possible meanings associated with that word, or even is aware that the word has other meanings. A *loud* jacket, a *sharp* student, or a *school* of fish might not convey the same meaning to a child that they do to an adult. In the same way, idiomatic expressions such as, "You're pulling my leg," or "She went to pieces," may suggest some unusual images to a student who knows all the words but on a less abstract level.

Syntax is the component of language which has to do with the way we put words together to make sentences. This includes rules regarding the acceptable order of words in sentences. Syntax is related to those skills that teachers refer to as grammar. As children develop, syntax develops. Children begin with single words and move to 2- and 3-word utterances. Gradually they are able to use questions, tenses, different forms of the verb *to be*, compound and complex sentences, and other advanced syntactic structures. Consider the complexity of the following sentence: "By this time next year you will have been in first grade for three months." A student who is not yet able to deal with such complex sentence structure will not be able to adequately decode the message.

Phonology is the component of language which deals with putting sounds together to make words. The sounds of a language are called **phonemes**, and there are certain ways in which phonemes can and cannot be combined to make words. For example, in English certain consonants can be combined in a cluster at the beginning of words, such as <u>fr</u> in *from*, <u>bl</u> in *blue*, and <u>scr</u> in *scream*, but we never begin a word with a <u>pb</u> or a <u>dg</u> combination. In the early stages of phonological development, it is quite common for children to avoid the use of any consonant clusters, so a word such as *green* may be produced as *geen*, and *stop* may be produced *top*. In very young children this is part of the normal development of phonology.

Morphology deals with the use of morphemes. A morpheme is the smallest unit of language that conveys meaning. A word such as *boy* is a morpheme. When the phoneme <u>s</u> is added to the word *boy*, the <u>s</u> means more than one. In this case, because the <u>s</u> conveys meaning, it is also a morpheme. In addition to signifying a plural form, an <u>s</u> can also indicate a possessive form when it follows an apostrophe, but in either case, the <u>s</u> has to be attached to another morpheme to have meaning. Morphemes which have to be attached to other morphemes are called **bound morphemes** and include plural- and tense-markers, as well as prefixes and suffixes such as <u>un</u> in *undress,* or the <u>ly</u> in *quickly*. Morphemes such as *boy*, which are meaningful when standing alone, are called **unbound** or **free morphemes**. A child's language development is often reflected in the number of morphemes used in each utterance.

Pragmatics has to do with the effective use of language in various contexts. Skills such as appropriately initiating a conversation, taking turns during conversation, and assessing how much information your listener needs to be able to understand your message are all part of pragmatics. It is very common for children to think that everyone shares their knowledge of people, places, and things. So when asked, "Where did you go on vacation," a child might say something like, "Billy's house." It is then left to the listener to ask, "Who is Billy?" and, "Where does he live?" As pragmatic skills increase, the child will be able to answer such a question by saying, "I went to visit my cousin Billy in Ohio."

There are two features of language which are important to point out. Language is **rule based**, and it is **generative**. By rule based, we mean that there are certain rules which all speakers of a language know and obey. We are not talking here of the rules you learn in junior high English class regarding split infinitives and dangling participles, but rules of which you may not even be aware. You simply know them as a speaker of your language. Some examples will help illustrate this point. You know that the prefix in means *not*. So if something is not accurate, it is inaccurate, and if it is not tolerable, it is intolerable. But what if something is not possible? You do not say inpossible; you say impossible. Why does the n become an m in this word? While you make the change somewhat automatically, you may not understand why you make the change. (It is simply more efficient to move from an m to a p than from an n to a p because the lips are together for m and p but apart for n). Here is another example of a phonological rule. Each of the following are words in English, with one exception. Which one is not a word in English?

1. monogenesis 2. palpus 3. rowel 4. fugacious 5. ssssseeeellpn

It shouldn't take very long for you to select number five. *Ssssseeeellpn* is clearly not a word in English. It is likely that some who read this chapter might have difficulty defining words one through four. Even if you did not know the meaning of the words (i.e., there was no semantic component to guide you), you were still able to identify the nonword. What was the phonological rule which was obeyed by the first four choices but violated by the fifth? After some thought, you might be able to say something about the syllable structure or too many consonants together without a vowel, but you probably cannot state a rule that you memorized somewhere in your educational history. As a speaker of English, you knew immediately that choice five was not a word. If we change the order of the letters so that "ssssseeeellpn" becomes "sleeplessness," you now recognize it as a word all too familiar to most college students.

Here is an example of a syntactic rule. Which of the following is an acceptable sentence?

1. The old miles were lived clearly on a clean plate.
2. Plate on old the clearly lived miles a clean were.

As in the previous example, it should not be hard for you to choose. Number one is a sentence, while number two is simply a jumbled string of words. What makes number one a sentence and number two a nonsentence? Once again, while it would be very difficult to rattle off a rule, you know that the sequence of words in number two do not qualify as a sentence. The words in number one, on the other hand, do form a sentence, even though the sentence is without meaning. As children develop their language skills, they must learn the rules of the language. During early stages of development, they do not have all of the adult rules, or they may operate under a different set of rules which allows them to communicate, but in a simpler fashion than adults. Consider the child who refers to his feet as *foots*. Here is a child who has learned the rule: "If more than one, add s." Assuming normal language development, the child will learn the exceptions to that rule later.

The other characteristic we mentioned was that language is generative. Once we learn the rules of the language, we can make and understand sentences which we have never heard before. You probably never heard the preceding sentence before, but you were able to understand it. The last time you took an essay test, you probably created sentences which you never used before (and in some cases may never use again). Children display this generative aspect of language very early in their development when they make sentences such as "All gone milk." Parents may repeat this utterance, but in most cases the sentence was first created by the child. An example of how children use their knowledge of linguistic rules to generate novel sentences was proved by the son of one of the authors. After a request that he behave, the boy responded, "But Dad, I am being have." It is this generative aspect of language, the ability to create new sentences, which makes language such a powerful tool for communication.

Language is most frequently expressed through two avenues: writing and speaking. The more common avenue for most people is speech.

SPEECH

Speech is the process of producing sound patterns in order to communicate. For most people, speech is a relatively effortless process. However, speech is a complicated action requiring the coordination of several processes. Five basic processes associated with speech are respiration, phonation, resonance, articulation, and cerebration. While these processes work together to produce speech, it is helpful to describe each separately.

Respiration

Respiration refers to the inhalation and exhalation of air from the lungs. Quiet breathing, as you are probably doing now, is an automatic function. When your body senses the need for oxygen, your chest cavity expands by the contraction of chest muscles and the **diaphragm** (the muscle that separates the chest cavity from the abdominal cavity). Expanding the chest cavity causes the lungs to expand. The increased size of the lungs results in lower pressure inside the lungs than outside, and air rushes in to balance the pressure. When you exhale, you relax the diaphragm and chest muscles, allowing the lungs to return to their resting position. As the size of the lungs decreases, the pressure inside becomes greater than outside, and air is forced out until the pressure inside the lungs once again equals the pressure outside. Beyond this function of exchanging carbon dioxide and oxygen, respiration also serves as the driving force for speech. Breathing for speech is a much more complicated process than quiet breathing. When using connected speech we allow only brief pauses to take a breath. Inhalation for connected speech then must be faster than inhalation for quiet breathing. Exhalation for speech is even more complex. Connected speech requires frequent changes in loudness and stress patterns. All of these changes require adjustments in the amount of air pressure provided by the respiratory system. Too much pressure results in speech that is too loud or in stress being placed on the wrong syllable. Too little pressure results in speech that is hard to hear or difficult to understand. Sometimes, we are almost out of air, but we don't want to pause to take a breath. So we force air out beyond the point where we would ordinarily stop to inhale. All of these adjustments must be done quickly enough to support rapid connected speech, and all must be coordinated with the activity of the other speech structures. Several abdominal, chest, and back muscles are used during exhalation for speech to provide just the right amount of air at just the right time to support a smooth flow of speech.

As air leaves the lungs, it travels through the trachea. Directly atop the trachea is a structure composed of cartilage and muscle, which some people call the voice box, but which we shall call the **larynx**. The larynx has several functions. One function is to prevent food or liquids from entering the trachea and eventually the lungs. The explosive coughing that one experiences after swallowing something "the wrong way" is a result of the larynx fulfilling its role as protector of the lower airway. Another function of the larynx is the production of voice. The process of producing voice is called phonation and is the next basic process of speech to be discussed.

Phonation

Phonation is the production of voice (be careful not to confuse phonation with phonology). Voice is produced in the larynx. The position of the larynx in relation to the lungs and trachea can be seen in Figure 2-1. The larynx forms what many people refer to as the *Adam's apple*. If you place your fingers on each side of your Adam's apple and produce a prolonged "eeeeeee," you should feel some vibration. What you feel is the rapid vibration of the vocal cords or, more accurately, the vocal folds. The vocal folds are two bands of muscle which run horizontally from the front to the rear of the larynx (see

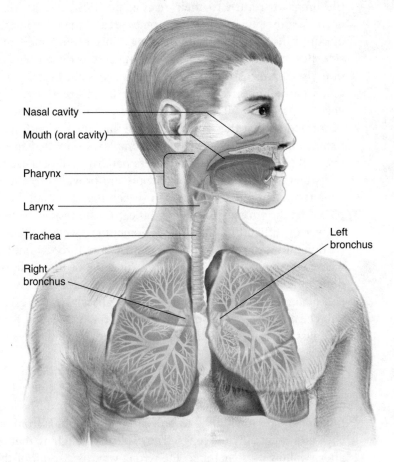

Nasal cavity

Mouth (oral cavity)

Pharynx

Larynx

Trachea

Right bronchus

Left bronchus

Figure 2-1 Relative Position of the Lungs, Larynx, and Pharynx
Source: Chiras, D. (2002). *Human biology: Health, homeostasis and the environment* (4th ed., p. 203). Jones and Bartlett. Reprinted by permission.

Figure 2-2). It is this vibration of the vocal folds which produces voice. The position and action of the vocal folds is sometimes difficult to visualize. It may be helpful to use the following hand analogy. With your index and middle fingers, make a V for victory (or the peace sign for old hippies). Now hold your fingers in a horizontal plane so that you are looking at the fingernail side. You now have an analogy of the vocal folds. They are attached in a V shape in the front but are free to move together and apart at the rear. During quiet breathing, the vocal folds are apart, or **abducted**, allowing air to pass into and out of the trachea and lungs. To produce voice, the vocal folds must be brought together, or **adducted,** following inhalation. In this position, the vocal folds lie in the path of the exhaled air. The airflow from the lungs sets the adducted vocal folds into vibration, causing a buzzing sound which serves as the basis for what will eventually be heard as voice. The rate of vibration, or cycles per second, determines the **frequency** of the voice.

We perceive frequency as **pitch**. A high-pitched voice is associated with faster vibratory rate (more cycles per second), and a low-pitched voice is associated with a slower rate of vibration (fewer cycles per second). While a rubber band is not a perfect analogy for a vocal fold, it should help to clarify the pitch-changing mechanism of the larynx. As a child, or in an idle moment as an adult, you've probably plucked a rubber band producing a sound. As you stretch the rubber band, it becomes longer, thinner, and tighter (or more

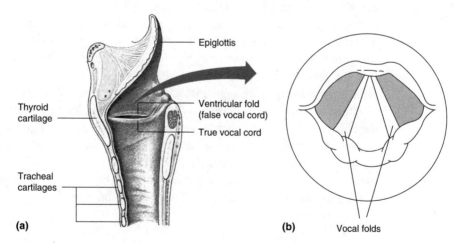

Figure 2-2 The Larynx and Vocal Folds
Source: **(a)** Chiras, D. (2002). *Human biology: Health, homeostasis and the environment* (4th ed., p. 209). Jones and Bartlett. Reprinted by permission. **(b)** Illustration by Mark J. Moran.

tense), and the sound produced by plucking it increases in pitch. That is roughly what happens to the vocal folds when a speaker increases vocal pitch. When you raise your pitch, you stretch the length of the vocal folds, which makes them thinner and increases the tension. A low pitch is associated with shorter, thicker, more lax vocal folds. While there is no significant pitch difference in the voices of young boys and girls, adult males have a lower pitch than adult females. The pitch difference between the sexes in adults is a result of the growth of the larynx during puberty.

In addition to pitch, another aspect of voice which we frequently alter is **loudness**. Just as pitch is the perceptual aspect of frequency, loudness is the perceptual aspect of **intensity**. Intensity is controlled primarily by the amount of air pressure with which the vocal folds are blown apart. Imagine that you are going to yell to a friend across a parking lot. Your friend is far away and the parking lot is noisy, so you will have to yell loudly. What is the first thing you do as you prepare to yell? For most people, the answer would be to take a deep breath. The large volume of air in the lungs resulting from the deep inhalation, along with forceful contraction of abdominal, chest, and possibly back muscles, provides the powerful exhalatory air stream needed for a loud voice.

Pitch and loudness by themselves do not completely describe a person's voice. Two people producing a sound at the same pitch with the same loudness would still sound different. The factor which gives each of our voices a certain uniqueness is the factor of **voice quality**. Quality is not as easy to define as pitch and loudness. While pitch and loudness are each perceptual aspects of single physical characteristics (frequency and intensity), quality is the perceptual aspect of several physical characteristics. To further complicate matters, we are not certain of all the physical characteristics that contribute to quality. Although pitch can be described as high or low, and loudness can be described as loud or soft, there is a plethora of terms used to describe quality. Terms such as *hoarse, harsh, breathy, rough, raspy, rich, mellow, flat,* and *throaty* are all attempts to describe voice quality. While we do not understand all of the factors which affect voice quality, most authorities agree that voice quality is related not only to the process of phonation, but also to the next process to be discussed, resonance.

Resonance

The sound we hear as a person's voice is not the same sound that was produced at the larynx. The sound has to pass through the **vocal tract**, which is the area from the larynx to the end of the lips or, sometimes, the end of the nostrils (see Figure 2-3). The size and shape of the vocal tract has an effect on

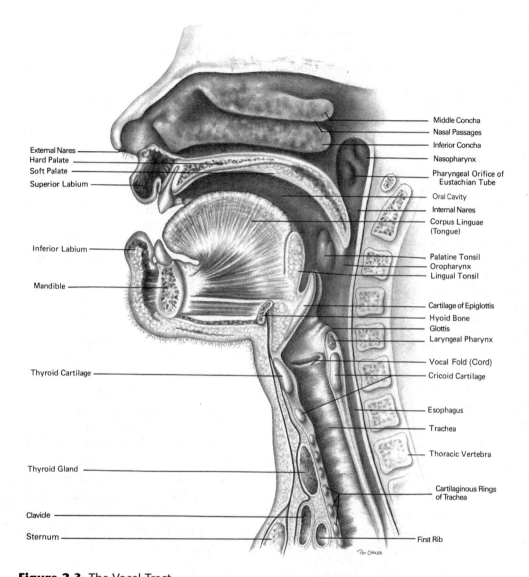

Figure 2-3 The Vocal Tract
Source: Donnersberger, A., & Lesak, A. (2000). *A laboratory textbook of anatomy and physiology* (7th ed., p. 332). Jones and Bartlett. Reprinted by permission.

the sound which we finally hear. The effect of the size and shape of the vocal tract on the sound which passes through it is **resonance**. An example of resonance is provided by a common childhood activity. Children often amuse themselves and others by talking into the cardboard tube from which paper towels or plastic wrap is dispensed. Holding the tube in front of the mouth results in a different sound. By holding the tube in front of the mouth, the child has effectively lengthened his vocal tract, and the sound that is finally released into the air is quite different than if it had been released at the lips. Perhaps the most important aspect of resonance to understand at this point is oral versus nasal resonance. For most speech sounds in English, the nasal cavity is closed off from the oral cavity by the upward and backward movement of the soft palate or **velum**. Only the m, n, and ng sounds are produced with the velum down (open). If other sounds, especially vowels, are produced with the velum down, the voice has a nasal quality and the person sounds as if he or she is "talking through the nose." If there is an obstruction in the nasal cavity which prevents the sound from passing through the nose on m, n, and ng, the person has a denasal quality and sounds as if he or she has a head cold. Problems of nasal resonance will be discussed further in later chapters. It is also in the vocal tract that speech sounds or phonemes are produced by means of the next process to be discussed, articulation.

Articulation

As mentioned in the previous discussion of language, phonology deals with the rules for putting speech sounds together to make words. **Articulation** is the physical production of the speech sounds. Speech sounds are produced by altering the flow of air from the lungs. The way in which the airflow is altered and the place in which it is altered determine which sound is produced. The body structures used to alter the flow of air through the vocal tract are called the **articulators**. Some articulators are movable and some are immovable. The articulators are listed in Table 2-1, and some may be seen in Figures 2-1 and 2-3. These structures produce all of the sounds of speech.

Before discussing individual speech sounds, there is a problem which must be solved. We wish to talk about speech sounds, but because we are communicating through written language, we must use a written symbol to represent each speech sound. Unfortunately, English is not a phonetic lan-

Table 2-1 The Articulators

Movable Articulators	Immovable Articulators
Lips	Teeth
Mandible	Alveolar ridge
Tongue	Hard palate
Soft palate (velum)	
Larynx	
Pharynx	

guage. By that, we mean that the letters of the alphabet do not always represent the same sound. For example, the c in *Cindy* is produced as an s, but the c in *candy* is produced as a k, and the two c's together in *Gucci* are produced as a ch. In other cases, the same sound may be represented by several different letters. The f sound can be represented by the letter f, but it is also represented by the ph in *Philadelphia* and the gh in *enough*. In these examples, we have been able to identify the sound we meant by referring to another letter, but that is not always the case. What sound does the s represent in *vision*? How can we differentiate the th in *the* from the th in *think*?

It is difficult to describe the sound without producing it. That is one of the limitations of written language: we cannot make the sounds we wish to describe. In the field of communication disorders, we solve this problem by using the International Phonetic Alphabet. In this alphabet, there is a symbol for each speech sound, and each symbol represents one and only one speech sound. It is beyond the scope of this text to teach the International Phonetic Alphabet, so when the written letter does not represent clearly the sound we intend, a key word will be used as an illustration (e.g., j as in joy). That way, we can use your speech to communicate our message.

There are two major categories of speech sounds or phonemes: vowels and consonants. Consonants are produced with a greater degree of obstruction in the vocal tract than are vowels. To produce a consonant sound, we must use two articulators to obstruct the flow of air in just the right way to produce the sound that we recognize as a consonant. Consonant sounds are distinguished from each other on the basis of three production features (see Table 2-2). The **manner of articulation** describes *how* the airflow is altered. The air can be completely blocked and then suddenly released, as is the case for p, b, t, d, k, and g. Because these sounds often have an explosive quality to their production, they are sometimes called **plosive** consonants, but they are not always exploded. For example, in the word *hat*, the final t is rarely exploded, especially in connected speech such as "My hat blew off." The aspect that all of these consonants do have in common is the complete stoppage of air at the beginning of production. Therefore, we will refer to these sounds as **stop consonants**. Another way to alter the airflow is to force it through a narrow opening. Forcing air through a narrow opening results in a friction noise, and consonant sounds made this way are called **fricatives**. Examples of fricatives are f, v, th (voiced as in *the* and unvoiced as in *thin*), s, z, sh and h, and the sound made by s in the word *vision*. Some sounds combine features of stops and fricatives and are called **affricates**. In English, there are two affricates: the ch sound as in *church*, and the j sound at the beginning and end of *judge*. Most speech sounds are made with the nasal

Table 2-2 Manner, Place, and Voice Characteristics of Consonants

| Place | Manner | | | | |
	Stop	Fricative	Affricate	Nasal	Semivowel
Bilabial	p, b*			m*	w*
Labio-dental		f, v*			
Lingua-dental		th (thin), th (the)*			
Lingua-alveolar	t, d*	s, z*		n*	l*
Lingua-palatal		sh s (vision)*	ch, j (joy)*		r*, y*
Lingua-velar	k, g*			ing*	
Glottal		h			

*Indicates voice

cavity closed off from the oral cavity by the velum. There are three sounds in English made with the velum open, allowing sound into the nasal cavity. The consonants m, n, and ng are called **nasals**. There are a group of consonants that are made with the vocal tract too constricted to be vowels but not as constricted as the other consonants. These sounds are called **semivowels**, because they are vowel-like but are still considered consonants. Semivowels are l, r, w, and y.

The second production feature used to distinguish among consonants is the **place of articulation**. The place of articulation indicates *where* in the vocal tract the alteration of the air stream occurs. Place of articulation is determined by the articulators used to produce the sound. For example, p, b, and m are made with both lips together. Because Latin names make every- thing sound a bit more scholarly, we call these sounds **bilabial** (two-lip) sounds. So p and b are bilabial stops, while m is a bilabial nasal. The sounds f and v are made with the lower lip between the teeth, so these sounds are **labio-dental**. The th sounds are made with the tongue between the teeth and are called **lingua-dental**. The ridge immediately behind the upper front teeth is the **alveolar ridge**. Several sounds are made with the tongue touching the alveolar ridge. These sounds, t, d, s, z, and l, are called **lingua-alveolar**. Mov- ing back, the next place of articulation is between the tongue and the hard palate. Sounds made in this place: sh, ch, the s sound in *vision*, and the j sound in *joy*, are called **lingua-palatal** sounds. The k and g are made with the tongue against the soft palate. We have already used palatal to mean hard palate, so we must use the term velar (referring to the velum). The k and g are **lingua-velar** sounds. (Note the spelling difference between alveolar and velar). Finally, at least one sound, h̲, is made at the glottis, so it is known as a **glottal** sound.

The third production feature used to distinguish among consonants is **voicing**. Some consonant sounds are voiced, while others are voiceless. Voiceless consonants are p̲, t̲, k̲, s̲, th̲ (as in *think*), sh̲, ch̲, and h̲. Voiced consonants are b̲, d̲, g̲, m̲, n̲, ng̲, v̲, z̲, th̲ (as in *the*), j̲ (as in *joy*), l̲, r̲, w̲, and y̲. Sounds that have the same manner and place of articulation but differ in voicing are called **cognates**. For example, s̲ and z̲ are both lingua-alveolar fricatives, but s̲ is voiceless and z̲ is voiced. Therefore, z̲ is the voiced cognate of s̲. The phonemes are organized by manner, place, and voice characteristics in Table 2-2.

Vowels are not as easy as consonants to classify. Vowels tend to be more continuous with each other, while consonants are more discrete. We cannot use the manner or voice features to distinguish among vowels because all vowels are made in the same manner (the manner of vowel production is called vocalic) and all vowels are voiced. That leaves only place. While we have said that vowels are produced with a relatively unobstructed vocal tract, the articulators do assume certain positions to produce each vowel. Vowels are classified according to tongue position. Say the vowel ee̲ as in *feet*, then quickly change to oo̲ as in *too*. Do this several times and note the direction in which your tongue moves. When you say ee̲ your tongue should be toward the front of the mouth and when you say oo̲ it should move to the back. The ee̲ is a **front vowel**; the oo̲ is a **back vowel**. Now do the same thing with ee̲ and a̲ as in *at*. Which way does the tongue move? It should move from high in the mouth for ee̲ to low in the mouth for a̲, so ee̲ is a **high vowel** and a̲ is a **low vowel**. It is on the basis of high and low and front and back that we distinguish among vowels. Vowel classifications are presented in Table 2-3.

Table 2-3 Vowel Classifications

	Front	Central	Back
High	m<u>ee</u>t		t<u>oo</u>
	h<u>i</u>t	b<u>u</u>t	f<u>oo</u>t
to	m<u>a</u>de	h<u>er</u>	n<u>o</u>
Low	r<u>e</u>d		l<u>aw</u>
	h<u>a</u>t		f<u>a</u>ther

A **diphthong** is a sound produced by the joining of two adjacent vowel sounds in the same syllable. The sounds represented by the <u>ow</u> in *cow*, the <u>oy</u> in *boy*, and the <u>i</u> in *mine* are the three primary diphthongs in English.

The muscle movements required to make the speech sounds and the rules used to put the sounds together to make words are governed by the nervous system. The critical role of the nervous system will be discussed as the process of cerebration.

Cerebration

Cerebration refers to the role of the nervous system in speech. The nervous system plays two distinct roles in speech. First, there is the cognitive-linguistic role. That role is supplying the ideas to be communicated, and managing the rules which are to be used to communicate those ideas. The other role involves the motor aspect of speech. The impulses which move and control the muscles of respiration, phonation, and articulation originate in and are carried by the nervous system. The nervous system can be divided into two portions: the central nervous system (or **CNS**) and the peripheral nervous system (or **PNS**). The CNS consists of those parts of the nervous system encased in a bony covering: the brain and spinal cord (see Figure 2-4). What we typically call the brain is actually several structures. The uppermost sec-

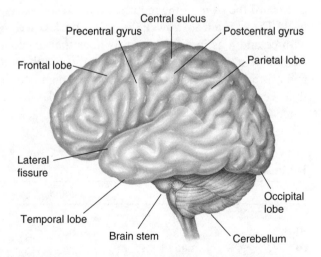

Figure 2-4 The Brain
Source: Chiras, D. (2002). *Human biology: Health, homeostasis and the environment* (4th ed., p. 255). Jones and Bartlett. Reprinted by permission.

tion is the cerebrum. The outer covering of the cerebrum, the **cerebral cortex**, is where most of the activity takes place. The cerebrum is divided into two halves or hemispheres. It appears that these hemispheres have different functions. In most people, the left hemisphere is associated with intellectual functions including language and speech. The right hemisphere is associated more with spatial relations, musical patterns, and nonlanguage functions. Each hemisphere is further divided into four lobes: the frontal, parietal, occipital, and temporal lobes (see Figure 2-4). The frontal lobe is associated with speech, and the temporal lobe is associated with hearing. The cerebral cortex sends signals to, and receives signals from, the rest of the body via nerve fibers.

The PNS consists of the parts of the nervous system that exit the bony covering and carry signals to and from the muscles and organs. Signals are carried to and from the muscles and organs of speech and hearing by fibers known as **cranial nerves**. The cranial nerves originate in the brain stem and innervate (i.e., carry signals to and from) most of the muscles above the shoulders. There are 12 pairs of cranial nerves (one member of each pair on each side of the body). The cranial nerves are quite complex and innervate nonspeech structures as well. All we hope to do here is to point out that these nerves serve as the connection between the nervous system and the speech structures.

The five processes of respiration, phonation, resonance, articulation, and cerebration allow human beings to put language into coded sound patterns. But communication cannot take place unless there is a way for others to decode those sound patterns. The way in which we usually decode the speech signal is through our sense of hearing.

HEARING

You will recall from our earlier discussion that speech is a sound pattern. The process used to receive sound is *hearing*. For us to hear a sound, three elements must be present. Small (1973) describes these elements in the following manner: First, there must be a sound source. This could be a car horn, a falling tree, or the speech-production mechanism. Second, there must be a conducting medium to carry the sound away from the source. This medium is usually air, but if you've ever put your ear to a railroad track or lived in an apartment with thin walls, you know that sound can travel through materials other than air. Finally, there must be a mechanism to receive the sound. The mechanism humans use to receive sound is the **audi-**

tory system. The part of the auditory system with which you are most familiar is the ear. It is the ear that changes the sound waves created by the speaker and carried through the air into nerve impulses that can be sent to the brain to be interpreted or decoded.

There are two aspects of sound that we need to mention briefly at this point: frequency and intensity. You should recall from our discussion of voice that frequency is the aspect of sound that we perceive as pitch. Frequency is measured in units called **Hertz (Hz)**. Intensity is the aspect of sound we perceive as loudness. Intensity is measured in **decibels (dB)**.

The ear consists of three parts: the **outer ear**, the **middle ear**, and the **inner ear**. These parts of the ear are shown in Figure 2-5.

The Outer Ear

The outer ear is made up of the part of the ear you see on the side of the head. This structure, made mostly of cartilage covered by flesh, is the **pinna**. Inside each pinna, leading into the head is a canal known as the **external auditory meatus**. Within the external auditory meatus are two structures

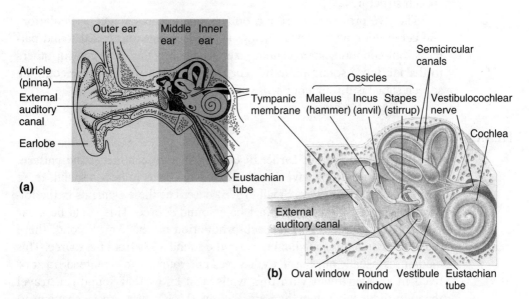

Figure 2-5 The Outer, Middle, and Inner Ear
Source: Chiras, D. (2002). *Human biology: Health, homeostasis and the environment* (4th ed., p. 290). Jones and Bartlett. Reprinted by permission.

which aid in protecting the ear from dust and other tiny particles. These structures are tiny hairs, which are visible upon close inspection of the ear, and tiny glands which secrete **cerumen**, a substance better known to most people as *ear wax*. Cerumen serves an important function in protecting the ear from foreign particles. Some people do produce too much cerumen, and it should be removed by a physician. Attempts to remove cerumen by cotton swabs or fingers often result in pushing the cerumen further into the canal, where it hardens and forms a barrier affecting hearing. The outer ear does not play as important a role in hearing as the other parts of the ear. The pinna apparently serves to gather the sound waves from the air and funnel them down the canal to the middle ear.

The Middle Ear

At the end of the external auditory meatus is a thin membrane known as the ear drum or, more properly, the **tympanic membrane**. The tympanic membrane separates the outer ear from the middle ear but will be considered here as part of the middle ear. Behind the tympanic membrane is a cavity known as the middle ear space. There are several structures within the middle ear space, the two most important of which are the **eustachian tube** and the **ossicles**. The middle ear space would be airtight except for the fact that it is ventilated by the eustachian tube. The eustachian tube leads from the middle ear to the **pharynx** and allows air into and out of the middle ear space. This serves to balance pressure on each side of the tympanic membrane. You have probably experienced your ears "popping" in an airplane or as you drive up or down a mountain road. As altitude increases, the air pressure decreases. The result is more air pressure in the middle ear than on the outside. This can be painful and cause reduced hearing sensitivity. As you yawn, talk, or chew gum, the eustachian tube opens, allowing air to escape from the middle ear until the pressure is balanced. With a decrease in altitude, the pressure outside becomes greater, and the eustachian tube opens to allow more air into the middle ear. As will be discussed in the chapter on hearing problems, eustachian tube malfunction and resulting middle ear disorders are quite common among children.

The other major structure of the middle ear is a chain of tiny bones. As you no doubt learned in elementary school, there are three bones in the middle ear. These bones are sometimes called the hammer, anvil, and stirrup because of their appearance, but the true names of these bones are the **malleus, incus**, and **stapes**. Together, these bones are known as the ossicles or the **ossicular chain**. The ossicles are attached to the tympanic membrane on one end and to a portion of the inner ear known as the **oval window** on the other end. As sound waves travel down the external auditory meatus they hit against the tympanic membrane, causing it to vibrate. The vibration of the tympanic membrane, in turn, sets the ossicular chain into motion, causing it to push in and out on the oval window transmitting the pressure wave to the inner ear.

The Inner Ear

The inner ear consists of two portions: the **vestibular** portion, which is related to balance, and the **cochlea,** which is associated with hearing. It is in the cochlea that the pressure wave is changed to a nerve impulse by the action of a specialized structure called the **organ of Corti** (see Figure 2-6). The organ of Corti extends almost the entire length of the snail-shaped cochlea. The cochlea is filled with fluid in which the organ of Corti rides.

When the ossicles of the middle ear move in response to sound, they create waves in the cochlear fluid. The waves cause **hair cells** in the organ of Corti to move in a shearing action. The shearing of the hair cells produces the nerve impulses which are carried along the auditory nerve and eventually to the brain. The organ of Corti is structured in such a way that different parts of the organ respond to different frequencies. The outer portion responds to high frequencies, and the inner portion responds to low frequencies. This is a very fortunate arrangement for receiving speech sounds. The frequency range of human hearing is approximately 20 to 20,000 Hz. Most speech sounds have the bulk of their energy between 500 and 2000 Hz. Because the speech frequencies are closer to the low end of the range than to the high end, the portion of the organ of Corti which responds to these frequencies is near the inner, most well-protected portion. This arrangement provides maximum protection for the portion of the cochlea most important to speech.

After the organ of Corti converts the sound wave to a nerve impulse, that impulse is carried over nerve fibers up to the temporal lobe of the cerebral cortex. The right ear sends signals to the left temporal lobe, and the left ear sends signals to the right temporal lobe. Once the nerve impulse reaches the cortex, it can be processed so that meaning can be attached. What was once a pressure wave in the air, then a series of nerve impulses, is now perceived as poetry, humor, anger, obscenity, or any other message which can be conveyed through speech. What was once an idea in one person's mind is now an idea in another's mind. Communication has occurred.

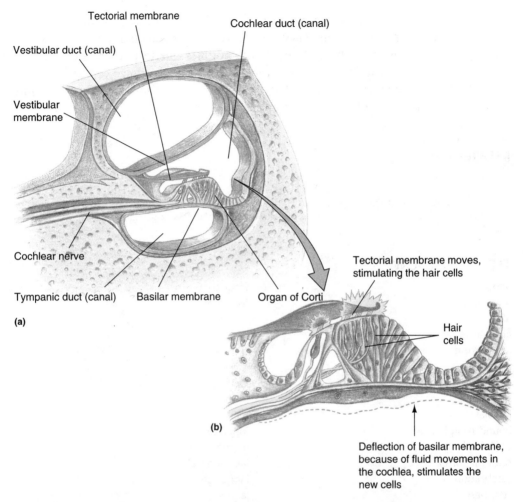

Figure 2-6 A Cross-Section Through the Cochlea Showing the Position of the Organ of Corti
Source: Chiras, D. (2002). *Human biology: Health, homeostasis and the environment* (4th ed., p. 291). Jones and Bartlett. Reprinted by permission.

CONCLUSION

Even from this rather brief discussion, you can see that the ability to communicate effectively through language and speech is a complex skill, requiring the coordination of several physical and intellectual functions. As with any complex process, there are many opportunities for things to go wrong. We all occasionally stumble over a sound or have difficulty finding the right word. Our voice sometimes deserts us, and we sometimes hear noises that exist only in our head. Normal does not mean perfect. There are, however, problems with communication that are outside the range of normal, problems which must be considered communication disorders. The rest of this book deals with these communication disorders.

REFERENCES

Bloom, L. (1988). What is language? In M. Lahey (Ed.), *Language disorders and language development*. New York: Macmillan.

Small, A. (1973). Acoustics. In F. Minifie, T. Hixon, & F. Williams (Eds.), *Normal aspects of speech, hearing, and language*. Englewood Cliffs, NJ: Prentice-Hall.

TERMS TO KNOW

abducted
adducted
affricate
alveolar ridge
articulation
articulator
auditory
back vowel
bilabial
bound morpheme
CNS
cerebral cortex
cerebration
cerumen
cochlea
cognate
communication
cranial nerves
decibels (dB)
decoding
diaphragm
diphthong
encoding
eustachian tube
expressive language
external auditory meatus

frequency
front vowel
fricative
generative
glottal
hair cells
Hertz (Hz)
high vowel
incus
inner ear
intensity
labio-dental
language
larynx
lingua-alveolar
lingua-dental
lingua-palatal
lingua-velar
loudness
low vowel
malleus
manner of articulation
middle ear
morphology
nasals
organ of Corti

ossicles

ossicular chain

outer ear

oval window

PNS

pharynx

phonation

phoneme

phonology

pinna

pitch

place of articulation

plosive

pragmatics

receptive language

resonance

respiration

rule based

semantics

semivowel

speech

stapes

stop consonant

syntax

tympanic membrane

unbound morpheme (free)

velum

vestibular

vocal tract

voice

voice quality

voicing

STUDY QUESTIONS

1. Identify and describe the five basic processes of speech.

2. Compare and contrast quiet breathing and breathing for speech.

3. Describe the mechanisms by which a speaker increases vocal pitch and loudness.

4. How do vowels differ from consonants? How are consonants classified? How are vowels classified?

5. Provide several examples of words in which the same letter represents different sounds. Provide examples of words in which different letters represent the same sound.

6. Describe the cognitive and the motor function of the brain in spoken communication.

7. Identify the major structures of the ear and describe their role in normal hearing.

chapter three

The Development of Language and Phonology

We often take for granted the process of a child learning how to talk. A newborn child cannot speak, yet in the space of only one year says his/her first words. Four short years later he/she has learned most of the basic language structures of the culture. Although the language acquisition process continues well beyond this age (Nippold, 1988), the child has moved from being nonverbal to producing complex and compound sentences involving embedding and conjoining in a relatively short time. This takes place with little direct help and often a great deal of distraction. When children reach school age, they can produce almost all of the basic sentence structures and speech sounds that are used by adults. Some, as discussed in this text, do not acquire language and speech sounds normally and this affects their ability to perform socially, communicatively, and academically. The present chapter is designed to provide a basic understanding of the order in which language and speech sounds are acquired by normally developing children. We present this information for two main reasons. First, in assessment of a child's language and sound system we must determine where he or she is in the developmental process. So, when we talk about various language and articulation assessment measurements in later chapters a basic knowledge of development is helpful. Second, the speech-language pathologist (SLP) will probably use the normal developmental order as a major consideration in selecting therapy targets to work on with children who have language or articulation disorders. The first part of the chapter deals with language development and the final portion considers the acquisition of the sound system.

EARLY COMMUNICATIVE DEVELOPMENT: GESTURES AND LANGUAGE

This section is dedicated to giving the classroom teacher a basic appreciation of the process and order of early communication development. We include this portion because, without an understanding of the aspects involved in communicative development, one cannot understand the types of children with limited language, how they are assessed, and how they are helped in intervention. We must say at the outset that the acquisition of communication is an extremely complex unfolding of highly interrelated abilities that is not fully understood. We do know, however, that certain components must be in place for the developmental process to occur, and we also know the basic order in which some of these aspects mature. Thus, the process of early communicative development may be grossly divided into two parts: 1) the basic building blocks of communicative development, and 2) the development of verbal communication. We will briefly discuss each of these two important areas.

Basic Building Blocks of Communicative Development

A contractor knows that the integrity of the house being built depends on a firm foundation. If the structure is built on a footing that is not level, or is cracked in places, problems will become apparent as the building progresses. Similarly, in the development of communication, there are a number of basic building blocks upon which the language acquisition process rests. We use the acronym **BACIS** (pronounced like *basis*) to reflect the basic building blocks or the basis of communicative development. Figure 3-1 shows the bases of communicative development and mentions some specific acquisitions in each area. Read the figure from the bottom to the top. The five areas, biological, access to a language model, cognitive ability, intent to communicate, and social ability, need to be in place prior to communication development. Upon these bases, actual communication develops from early gestures to the later use of complex sentences. It is important to mention

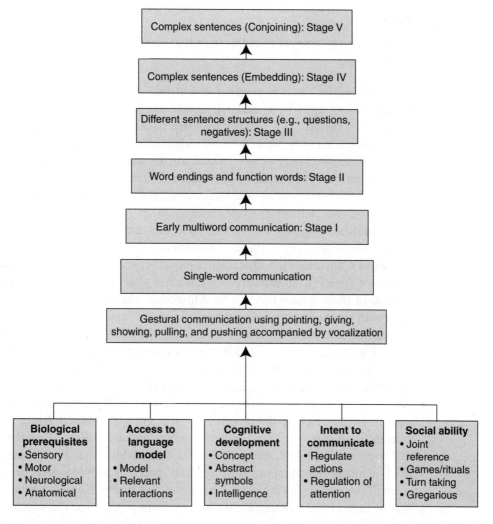

Figure 3-1 The BACIS of Language Development and Steps in the Language Acquisition Process

here that the building blocks for communication are developing simultaneously and influence each other in development. For instance, motor development allows a child to explore the environment, and this exploration facilitates cognitive and social development. We will briefly discuss each building block area.

Biological Bases

There are many prerequisites of language that could be considered biological in nature:

- *Sensory abilities*—It is imperative that a child possess adequate abilities to sense information from the environment in order to develop communication. This is important because we listen to others producing language, and we see what they are communicating within the environment. Thus, normal vision and hearing are critical for the development of language. There is much literature that shows those children with hearing or even visual impairments are at risk to develop communicative abilities at a slower rate (Kretschmer & Kretschmer, 1978).
- *Motor abilities*—When we use our speech mechanism to produce language, there are very complex adjustments that must take place. As shown in Chapter 2, the articulators move very rapidly to produce the variety of speech sounds in English. Children who do not have voluntary control of their speech mechanism will not develop oral language. Children with cerebral palsy, for instance, often have fine motor coordination difficulties, and some may never be able to produce oral language intelligibly. They may, however, be able to use a communication board or some electronic device to transmit their ideas to others. If a child is going to learn the oral production of language, motor ability must be intact.
- *Neurological status*—Language appears to be a skill that is developed only in species having the largest and most complex brains. When the human brain is damaged, typically the most complex skills are lost first. For instance, if an adult has a stroke, the first abilities that are impaired are fine motor coordination, language, and speech. If a child suffers brain damage prior to or during the birth process and begins life with a neurological impairment, we can almost always count on problems in developing communication.
- *Anatomical structure*—To produce normal oral language, the speech mechanism needs to be complete and intact. Children who are born with abnormalities of the mouth, face, or vocal tract experience difficulty in orally producing language, as will be seen when we discuss cleft palate in Chapter 11.

Access to a Language Model

For children to learn the language of their culture, they must have access to caregivers who model simplified language in relevant, appropriate situations.

It only makes sense that a child must have a pattern to follow in communication development. In extreme cases of children who were raised by psychotic parents or even by wolves in the wild, the result is the absence of linguistic verbal communication (Brown, 1958; Curtiss, Fromkin, Krashen, Rigler, & Rigler, 1974). If there is no one to act as a model in using language, no language will be learned. There is a great deal of research that shows that parents tend to simplify the length and complexity of their language when talking to children (Owens, 2005; Shulman & Haynes, in press). The normal language-learning child listens attentively to parents or other caregivers during play and soaks up the new words and sentences like a sponge. Without these interactions, the child does not develop language.

Cognitive Ability

Cognition is a very complex area, and the specific relations between language acquisition and cognitive development are only just being discovered. While we are not certain about the exact nature of the cognition-language relationship, we do know that certain cognitive attainments seem to be associated with language acquisition. There are several important ways cognition is related to language development:

- *We Talk About Concepts*—Cognitive development has to do with the increasing ability of a child to mentally represent objects, actions, and events in the world. Most often, researchers talk about the development of concepts. For instance, we have a concept of *animal* that includes all types of species, and we can divide the concept up into domestic and wild animals. We can also divide domesticated animals into different types of pets (e.g., dogs, cats, hamsters, fish, and birds). The point here is that we have a mental construct having to do with nonhuman, animate beings. With language, we can talk about all aspects of our concept of animals using specific words and word combinations that are appropriate to that concept (e.g., jaguar, poodle, Himalayan, purr, bark). Essentially, we develop language to be able to talk about the concepts we have of the world. Without the development of concepts, we really would have nothing to talk about. So, concepts must develop prior to language (or at least simultaneously). As we develop language, our linguistic ability then helps to refine our concepts.
- *Language Is an Abstract Symbol System*—The more cognitive development a child experiences, the greater will be the ability to appreciate

abstractions. If something is abstract, it may not be totally clear to a person. For instance, a piece of abstract art depicting a man riding a bicycle may not really resemble a photograph of a man riding a bicycle. If a word is abstract, it may not be easily visualized mentally (e.g., honor, hypothesis), but if a word is concrete it can be more readily pictured in the mind (e.g., dog, sun). Language is a system of very abstract symbols. The word *dog* does not look like a canine or sound like one. Additionally, the word disappears almost as soon as it is uttered because speech is a transitory signal. Similarly, the written word *dog* is abstract and unrelated to the physical attributes of an actual dog. Because our language symbols do not represent the real world in a concrete way, it is necessary for us to develop higher or more complex brain functions. If we are incapable of abstract reasoning, we will be impaired in our ability to develop language.

- *Language Requires Minimal Levels of Cognitive Development*—The developmental psychologist Jean Piaget studied cognitive development in children and found that during the first two years of life they pass through six stages of what he called the "sensorimotor period" (Piaget, 1952; 1954; 1970). The sensorimotor period is basically a time when children physically manipulate the environment and gradually learn to manipulate reality mentally. There are tests that can locate children in the six stages of the sensorimotor period, and much research has been done to determine which stage is most associated with the onset of language. Many studies report that a child must be at least in stage 4 to use gestural communication for intentionally making needs known and must attain at least the beginning of stage 5 to use verbal language (McCormick, 1984; Owens, 2005). Thus, we can find no reports of children before stage 4 of the sensorimotor period using verbal language, and this fact suggests that at least a minimal level of cognitive development must be necessary for language to be acquired. We can also see evidence in children's behavior of post-stage 4 attainments in their play. Children who have the cognitive ability to develop language can use toys and objects appropriately, mentally represent a missing object (object permanence), use something as a means to achieve a particular end (use a stick to reach a distant object; means–end concept), and have the ability to imitate the gestures and vocalizations of a model. One of the surest indications that a child is cognitively ready to develop language is the presence of symbolic (pretend) play. If a child can pretend that a block of wood is a car, he or she is demonstrating the ability to use symbols that have some degree of abstraction, since the block does not really look like an automobile. Severely cognitively impaired children show their levels of cognitive development in their play and interaction with other objects. It is not unusual to find children below stage 4 of the sensorimotor period whose play is primarily characterized by mouthing, banging, shaking, and throwing objects. They rarely use an object or toy appropriately and may not solve problems in play involving the means–end concept or perform symbolic play. Thus, it appears that there must be a minimal level of cognitive development to understand the world, develop concepts, and to acquire abstract language symbols.

Intent to Communicate

A child will never develop language unless he or she possesses a reason or intent to use communicative symbols. In short, we talk because we have a particular goal in mind to either (1) influence the actions of a listener, or (2) influence the attention or attitude of a listener (McClean & Snyder-McClean, 1978). When you think about it, these two broad reasons to talk really can account for much of what we say during a day. Believe it or not, before a child reaches a specific point in cognitive development (stage 4), it is said that no *intentionality* exists (McCormick, 1984). That is, a child prior to stage 4 does not really *intend* to do anything, or plan it ahead of time; the behavior just occurs. As children develop cognitively, they can mentally represent objects and events to a greater extent and manipulate reality mentally instead of physically. They can actually *plan* to do something because they work it out mentally prior to doing it. Thus, at stage 4 a child can *intend* to influence the activities and attention of adults and use gestures as a *means* to accomplishing this *end* (as in the means–end concept referred to in the cognitive section). Severely cognitively impaired children may only reach stages 1–3 of sensorimotor development, and because they do not have the cognitive development to anticipate or plan an event, will not have intent to communicate. These children may never actively try to communicate with adults, even though adults often attribute communicative intent to them. For instance, a severely impaired child may produce a vocalization while clapping hands and the adult may say, "He wants me to turn on the music now." In reality, this child may just be clapping and vocalizing, and the adult treats it as a communicative intent. Also the child may have a simple association between music and clapping; however, the clapping may not be done as intent to communicate anything.

Social Abilities

There are many social abilities that are prerequisite to the acquisition of language:

- *Joint referencing*—During play, parents and children look at the same objects and events. This is called *joint referencing* because the parents and children are jointly sharing visual regard for the same object or event. It is during joint referencing that caregivers talk to children about what they are seeing and doing and provide language stimulation or language modeling. The child profits from this language stimulation in relevant interactions by learning vocabulary and the rules of language (Shulman & Haynes, in press).
- *Games and rituals*—Parents also teach language to children in the context of certain games and rituals we have all seen at family gatherings, malls, laundromats, and other places. For instance, the parent may say to a child "Say hello to Aunt Martha," "Say thank you," and "Say trick or treat." Parents also engage in routine language stimulation events such as joint book reading or naming games with their children. These activities serve to provide the child with consistent and repeated exposures to the appropriate use of language and may aid in language acquisition.
- *Turn taking*—Language is a reciprocal activity. People take turns in conversations. Children learn turn-taking skills in early play routines with parents, and these same reciprocal skills are seen in the first conversations between mothers and their children.
- *Desire to attend to and be with people*—Human communication involves wanting to interact with other people. We have a basic desire to be gregarious, and we want to influence the attitudes, attention, and activities of other people. If a child does not have a basic desire to interact with people, there is no need for language to develop. For instance, children who have been diagnosed as "autistic" are often characterized as being "in a world of their own" and may not readily develop social relationships with others (Rutter, 1978). If a child has no use for even nonverbal interaction, it is doubtful that language will be a major priority, as it is used to touch other people. Thus, children who like to be isolated, do not make eye contact with adults, or do not enjoy reciprocal play activities probably will not develop language at the appropriate age. It is easy to see that the BACIS of language can be in place when children are communicating through the use of gestures and vocalizations. The BACIS is a platform upon which verbal language is built and all BACIS elements are typically

seen in normally developing children as they approach the end of their first year of life.

Early Development of the Language Framework

We have already said that specific building blocks (BACIS) need to be in place to provide a firm foundation for the development of the complicated language rule system. If one of the building blocks is defective, the resulting linguistic framework will be distorted or at least be more difficult to erect upon the inadequate foundation. Let us say, however, that the child *has* the BACIS for language development. How do language and communication begin to emerge? This section describes communication in the nonverbal, single-word, and early multiword periods in very general terms.

The Nonverbal Period

Communication in the nonverbal period typically occurs somewhere between 7 to 14 months in normal children and consists mostly of gestures and vocalizations. There is considerable variability in the age a child begins nonverbal communication and also in the duration of the nonverbal period. In the nonverbal period, the child uses gestures of pointing and physical regulation of adults to make needs known. Toward the end of this period, the child will accompany the gestures and physical regulations with vocal productions that are not words. For instance, a child might say "ba" while he is pointing at something or "uh . . . uh" while pulling the parent toward a desired object. The major point here is that the child is expressing intent to communicate, and this intent is now coupled with vocal productions. Generally, children will communicate this way to: (1) regulate adult action (e.g., obtaining an inaccessible object using the adult as a means), or (2) regulate adult attention (e.g., obtaining adult attention using objects or sounds as a means as in banging a toy repeatedly until an adult looks or comments). Other gestures or social communications during this period involve pointing, showing, giving, and repeating an action to enlist adult attention.

The Single-Word Period

Gradually, the vocalizations seen in the nonverbal period are replaced by actual *approximations* of adult words. This can occur anywhere from 9 to 18 months in normally developing children, and there is also considerable variability in the age this stage is reached. We say the words are approximations because they may not fully resemble the productions of adults and will be missing some components. In the present chapter we discuss phonological development and the notion that early word productions may be simplified or reduced in characteristic ways. Early single words are usually consonant-vowel (CV) combinations like *ba* for ball or *da* for dog. These are regarded as approximations instead of just vocalizations because they are used in the appropriate context (e.g., when a ball or dog is around), and they resemble the adult production in terms of the initial sound. Other early words may be CVCV combinations like *dada* for daddy or *wawa* for water.

Children accumulate their early vocabulary slowly at first and then experience a vocabulary spurt or a large increase in the number of words they can say. The average age of the vocabulary spurt is around 18 months (Shulman & Haynes, in press). There is also a steady increase in the number of words these children *understand* during the single-word period. Comprehension of words is always ahead of the production of words, and research suggests that children in this period understand about four times more words than they produce (Benedict, 1979). The size of the expressive vocabulary in the single-word period increases until the vocabulary spurt; at this time the child has a vocabulary of about 50 different words. Studies have shown that these early 50-word vocabularies are primarily composed of general and specific nouns (ball, car, names of people, and such), but also include action words (go, run), personal-social words (yes, no, bye-bye), modifiers (big, dirty) and even some minimal use of function words (in, a). At the point where the child possesses the 50-word vocabulary, the first attempts at combining words begin to appear.

Early Multiword Productions

Many researchers in language acquisition have studied early word combinations produced by children, and there appears to be general agreement that specific types of combinations seem to emerge consistently, regardless of the child's culture, sometime between 15 and 30 months of age. That is, all over the world, children begin to use the same types of word combinations to talk about objects, events, and relationships in their lives. This is often cited as further evidence that children learn to talk about concepts and experiences that they have developed in the sensorimotor period of cognitive development. Some of the basic word combination types and examples of each are listed in Table 3-1.

Table 3-1 Basic Word Combination Types and Examples

Combination Type	Example
Naming (that + thing)	that doggie; that ball
Recurrence (more + thing/person)	more water; more daddy; more go
Nonexistence (no + thing/person; Thing/person + allgone)	no drink; no mommy; drink allgone
Person + action	mommy go; daddy run; doggie eat
Action + thing	hit ball; pet doggie; eat banana
Possession (person + 1 thing)	my ball; daddy sock; mommy hair
Thing/person + location	drink there; mommy outside
Modifier + thing	big drink; diaper dirty
Person + action + thing	daddy hit ball; mommy eat apple
Person + action + location	mommy go outside; daddy eat there

One can easily see that the relationships children talk about in their early word combinations are things that they have seen and participated in during the first two years of life. Also, it should be noted that most of the function words (articles, prepositions) and word endings (-ing, -ed, -s) are missing from these utterances.

The Relationship Between Age and Average Utterance Length

Research has shown that there is a strong and significant correlation between a child's chronological age and **mean length of utterance** (**MLU**) in the early stages of language development (Miller & Chapman, 1981; Scarborough, Wyckoff, & Davidson, 1986). MLU counts words as well as bound morphemes (e.g., plurals, past tense -ed, -ing, etc.) because these word endings represent important linguistic acquisitions for which a child should be given credit. It is critical to remember that these utterance lengths are averages. Thus, a 2-year-old may have some 1-word utterances, some 2-word utterances, and some 3-word productions, all which average out to two words. The relationship is especially powerful between ages 1 and 4 years. Basically, the development of utterance length and chronological age is almost linear during this period and then begins to deteriorate after age 4 years. Thus, when a child is 1 year old the utterance length is approximately one word on the average, a 2-year-old has an average length of utterance of about two words, and when the age of 3 years is reached, the average length of utterance is about three words. It is generally accurate to state that age and mean length of utterance are highly related in the early stages of language development. At the end of the early word combination period, a child should have an average length of utterance of about two words and be working on the incorporation of function words and word endings into his or her utterances.

Summary of Early Communicative Development

We now can see that the normal child by age $2^1/_2$ years should have all the building blocks of language in place (BACIS), a vocabulary of 400–500 words, and be producing word combinations consisting of two to four words, with an average utterance length of about two and a half. The 3- to 5-year-old population as well as some older cognitively impaired children in the public school system will arrive in your classroom with language abilities similar to those normally developing children exhibit in the nonverbal, single-word, or early multiword periods of language acquisition. The brief perspective provided here should orient the classroom teacher to the types of language and prelanguage abilities that must be evaluated in nonverbal to early multiword communicators. The following section will deal with language development after age 2 years.

COMMUNICATIVE REFINEMENT AFTER THE EARLY MULTIWORD PERIOD: FIVE STAGES OF DEVELOPMENT

In 1973 Roger Brown published a landmark book describing five stages of language development. To sketch the refinement of the language system as children go beyond the age of 2 years, we will follow Brown's stages and provide a general description of each. The beginning points of these stages are demarcated by mean length of utterance (MLU).

Stage I: Basic Roles and Relations in the Simple Sentence (MLU 1.75)

Thus far in the present chapter we have discussed only this first of Brown's five stages: the development of early multiword utterances. By the time a child reaches the age of 20 to 24 months he or she is constructing early multiword combinations mentioned in the previous section. These basic relationships form the critical elements of simple sentences (e.g., "Mommy run outside" and "Jimmy eat sandwich"). These basic roles and relations will be embellished by other language elements to be added in later stages.

Stage II: Modulations of Meaning in the Simple Sentence (MLU 2.25)

In Stage II, the child adds to the basic building blocks of the simple sentence by adding function words and word endings to utterances. Stage II acquisitions include function words such as *the, in, on, is,* and word endings such as *-ing, -ed,* and *-s.* There are other function words and word endings developed in Stage II; however, we will not attempt to provide an exhaustive review of this stage. It is enough to know that the child is "filling in the gaps" between the major words of sentences acquired in Stage I. Thus, a child in Stage I might say "Mommy eat," but in Stage II he or she might say "Mommy eating" and finally "Mommy is eating" near the end of Stage II. Children in Stage II are typically between 2 and 3 years of age.

Stage III: Modalities of the Simple Sentence (MLU 2.75)

In Stage III the child learns to transform basic sentence structures into different orders to make constructions such as questions and negative statements. For example, the statement "He is going" can be made into a question by inverting certain elements ("Is he going?"). The ability to move sentence elements around and transpose them is critical to making more complex syntactic utterances. Children in this stage also develop models such as "can, will, shall" and begin to use them in contractions such as "can't, don't, won't." Children in Stage III are usually about 3 years old.

Stage IV: Embedding One Sentence into Another (MLU 3.50)

When a child reaches Stage IV (usually at about age 3 or 3.5 years) he or she learns to make complex and compound sentences by embedding clauses and phrases into other sentences. For instance, a child in an earlier stage may say two simple sentences to communicate a thought ("Mommy bought me a bike. I like to ride my bike."). Embedding allows the child to construct a more adultlike sentence ("I like to eat the cookies that mommy bakes.").

Stage V: Coordination of Simple Sentences (MLU 4.0)

Stage V (typically between 3.5 and 4 years of age) involves learning how to coordinate two sentences using conjunctions. As you know there are many types of conjunctions such as *and, but, because, since, if, when,* and so on. Use of these conjunctions to join sentences allows a child to make more and more complex utterances.

As children traverse the five stages, they gain not only in their ability to produce more complex sentences, but also in their ability to process equally complex language spoken by others. One can readily see that by the time a child enters kindergarten, he or she is capable of producing and comprehending fairly sophisticated syntactic forms. But, as mentioned earlier, language development continues for the rest of our lives, although at a much slower rate. We continue to learn new vocabulary throughout life. Our grammatical structure changes very slowly between the ages of 5 and 19 years and involves the use of more subordinate clauses and some other structures in sentences. Because these syntactic changes occur slowly, they can only be detected by sensitive measures such as the subordination index (Nippold, 1988). Summarizing this period, Nippold (1988, p. 3) states:

> The research suggests that language development during the 9 through 19 years age range unfolds in a slow and protracted manner, and that change becomes obvious only when sophisticated linguistic phenomena are analyzed and nonadjacent age groups (e.g., 9-year-olds and 12-year-olds) are compared. Documenting language growth in older children and adolescents also requires that written forms of communication be scrutinized in addition to spoken forms.

Upon school entrance the acquisition of language takes on other dimensions that depend on a strong foundation in oral language development. For instance, other modalities (reading, writing), the use of figurative language (idioms, metaphors), and metalinguistic ability (analysis of language as an object of study as in spelling and language arts) are complex acquisitions for all children in the early years of education. As you will see in later chapters, children with a weak foundation in oral language development almost always have more difficulty with these later milestones in the use of their linguistic system for other purposes such as reading and writing (Catts & Kamhi, 2005).

DEVELOPMENT OF SPEECH SOUNDS AND PHONOLOGY

Children's ability to produce speech sounds and to use those sounds to make words develops over the first few years of life. Typically, children have most of their speech sound system developed by the time they begin first grade. Children begin to produce speechlike sounds in infancy. However, it is important to note that we refer to these productions as *speechlike sound* because they are occurring during a period when the child is not yet using words to communicate. They are not considered to be true speech sounds at this point. Oller (1980) has identified several stages of infant sound production prior to the use of words. These stages are presented in Table 3-2. When reviewing Table 3-2 remember that there is considerable overlap among the stages described and some variability in the ages associated with each stage. At approximately 12 months, some (but not all) children produce utterances that seem to represent a transition between babbling and true words. These utterances are known by various names, including **protowords, vocables, transitional forms**, or **phonetically consistent forms**. These are utterances that the child uses consistently to refer to objects or people, yet these utterances are not related to the adult word for that person or thing. For example, one of the author's children used the utterance *koo* to refer to yogurt. Whether he was being fed yogurt, saw it in the supermarket, or rubbed it in his hair, he always refereed to it as *koo*. This form does not appear to be a

Table 3-2 Oller's (1980) Stages of Prelinguistic Vocalizations

Prelanguage Stage and Age	*Speech Sound Activity*
Phonation stage **Birth to 1 month**	Many reflexive vocalizations such as crying; some nasal and vowellike sounds produced
Cooing stage **2 to 3 months**	Some consonant-vowellike (CV) sounds produced. Often these are back sounds such as k̲ and o̲o̲ giving this stage its name.
Expansion stage **4 to 6 months**	This is a period of vocal play. The infant begins to develop some control of the sound-producing mechanism and explores a variety of speechlike and nonspeechlike sounds including grunts, squeals, yells, and raspberries.
Canonical babbling stage **7 to 9 months**	A significant milestone in development. The child produces strings of reduplicated or repeated consonant-vowel syllables such as *bababa* or *mamama*. Parents often mistake a sequence such as *mama* or *dada* to be an attempt at naming, and report that the child said his first words at six or seven months. While babbling represents a significant milestone in speech development, the strings of CV syllables produced during this period are not attempts at meaningful speech.
Variegated babbling stage **10 to 12 months**	The child produces strings of nonreduplicated CV syllables such as *patika* or *katami*. The child also demonstrates adultlike intonation patterns causing these utterances to resemble an idiosyncratic language.

derivative of the adult word *yogurt*, but was used consistently to refer to and request that item.

At about 12 to 18 months, children begin to produce their first true words. These first words are usually not accurate reproductions of the adult form and reflect the limitations of the child's developing phonological system. First words are often single syllables such as *up* or *bye*, or reduplicated syllables such as *dada* or *baba*. Words containing initial and final consonants such as *cake* or *hat* may also occur during this early period (Stoel-Gammon & Dunn, 1985).

The phonemes that children can correctly produce during this early stage of meaningful speech are limited. Although children produce a wide range of sounds during babbling, they gradually introduce these sounds into meaningful speech. Several researchers have studied the age of acquisition of sounds in normally developing children. These studies have varied, sometimes widely, in the ages reported for acquisition of each phoneme. One reason for the variance among studies is the criteria used to determine when a sound had been acquired. For example, Table 3-3 shows the results of three studies of sound acquisition. The earliest study by Templin (1957) used a criterion of 75% of the children producing the sound correctly in initial, medial, and final position of words. Prather, Hedrick, and Kern (1975) also used the criterion of 75% but in only initial and final positions. The data of Prather and colleagues indicate an earlier age of acquisition than that of Templin. Finally, Smit, Hand, Freilinger, Bernthal, and Bird (1990) reported recommended ages of acquisition based on 90% of the children in producing the sound correctly. Smit and colleagues also reported different ages for boys and girls. Many of the ages of acquisition reported by Smit and colleagues are later because the 90% criterion is more stringent and therefore more difficult to achieve.

Although they disagree on age of acquisition, most studies of phonological development agree that children typically develop phonemes in a certain order (Poole, 1934; Prather et al., 1975; Sander, 1972; Smit et al., 1990; Templin, 1957; Wellman, Case, Mengert, & Bradbury, 1931). Stops (sounds made by stopping the flow of air then suddenly releasing it: p, b, t, d, k, and g) and nasals (consonants made by directing sound through the nose: m, n, and ng) develop early, while fricatives (sounds made with a prolonged friction noise such as f, v, s, z, and sh) and semivowels (l, r, and y) develop later.

During the period from about 18 months to 4 years, children experience a tremendous growth in vocabulary. Many new words contain phonological elements that are beyond the child's current production ability (e.g., later-

Table 3-3 Ages at Which Children Acquire Phonemes: Results of Three Studies Using Different Criteria

Phoneme	Templin et al. (1957)	Prather et al. (1975)	Smit et al. (1990)	
			Females	Males
m	3	2	3	3
n	3	2	3:6	3
h	3	2	3	3
p	3	2	3	3
f	3	2.4	3:6 (I)	3:6 (I)
			5:6 (F)	5:6 (F)
w	3	2.8	3	3
y (you)	3.5	4	4	5
b	4	2.8	3	3
k	4	2.4	3:6	3:6
g	4	2.4	3:6	4
d	4	2.4	3	3:6
r	4	3.4	8	8
s	4.5	3	7 to 9	7 to 9
ch	4.5	3.8	6	7
sh	4.5	3.8	6	7
l	6	3.4	5 (I)	6 (I)
			6 (F)	7 (F)
t	6	2.8	4	3:6
v	6	4	5:6	5:6
th (thin)	6	4	6	8
z	7	4	7 to 9	7 to 9
j (joe)	7	4	6	7
th (the)	7	4	4:6	7

developing sounds, consonant clusters, multisyllables). To use these words, it appears that children apply several simplifying processes (Ingram, 1989). These **phonological processes** simplify the adult words in several ways. Some processes simplify the syllabic structure of a word (e.g., final consonant deletion changes *hat* to *ha*). Other processes substitute an early developing class of sounds for a later developing class (e.g., stopping allows *sun* to be produced as *tun*, a stop substituted for a fricative). A third category of processes changes the manner, place, or voice characteristics of one phoneme to be consistent with another phoneme in the word (e.g., velar assimilation changes *dog* to *gog*). Not all children demonstrate the same processes. Grunwell (1987) identified the most common phonological processes in normal development. These processes, along with a brief description of each, are presented in Table 3-4.

Phonological processes are developmental devices that are usually suppressed as phonological skills improve. In normal development, most processes are suppressed by the time the child enters first grade. Stoel-Gammon and Dunn (1985) identified those phonological processes that are typically suppressed by 3 years of age and those that persist after age 3 years. A partial list of early and latter suppressed processes follow (Table 3-5).

Even those processes which persist after age 3 years are typically suppressed by the time a child enters first grade. According to Grunwell (1987)

Table 3-4 The Most Common Phonological Processes Exhibited During Normal Development

Process	Description
Weak syllable deletion	In polysyllabic words, the unstressed syllable is deleted (telephone → tephone).
Final consonant deletion	The final consonant of a word is deleted (hat → ha).
Reduplication	Two-syllable words are produced by repeating the first syllable (bottle → baba).
Harmony (This process is referred to as *assimilation* by other authors.)	The manner, place, or voice characteristics of one phoneme changes to be consistent with another phoneme in the word (dog → gog [the initial d changed to be consistent with the final g.
Cluster reduction	Consonant clusters are reduced usually to a single phoneme (stop → top).
Stopping	Continuant sounds (usually fricatives) are replaced by stops (see → tee).
Fronting	Velar sounds such as k̲ and g̲ are replaced by alveolar sounds such as t̲ and d̲ (go → do).
Gliding	Liquids such a r̲ and l̲ become glides such as w̲ and y̲ (run → wun).
Context sensitive voicing	Voiceless consonants preceding vowels are voiced, and voiced consonants at the end of words are produced as unvoiced (toe → doe and red → ret).

Note: The arrow symbol (→) should be read as *becomes* or *changes to*.
Source: Grunwell, P. (1987). *Clinical phonology* (2nd ed.). Baltimore: Williams and Wilkins.

Table 3-5 Partial List of Early and Latter Suppressed Processes

Processes That Disappear by Age 3	Processes That Persist After Age 3
Unstressed syllable deletion	Cluster reduction
Final consonant deletion	Gliding
Reduplication	Stopping
Velar fronting	Final consonant devoicing
Consonant assimilation	
Prevocalic voicing	

Source: Stoel-Gammon & Dunn (1985). *Normal and disordered phonology in children.* Austin, TX: Pro-Ed.

the only commonly occurring processes which continue in some normally developing children beyond age 5 years are gliding (run → wun) and stopping of the th sounds (think → tink and the → de). By age 5 years, children have typically completed most of their phonological development. There are still a few sounds that might need to be mastered in some positions or in some words. Yavas (1998) indicates that some children between the ages of 5 and 7 years will have difficulty with longer words such as *thermometer* and *vegetable.* Yavas also suggests that children in this age group must also learn to deal with changes in a root word when a morpheme is added. For example the i in the word *decide* is pronounced differently in the word *decision.*

Perhaps you have noticed that most of the discussion to this point has been about consonants. Reports regarding the development of vowel sounds do not occur in the literature as often as those addressing consonant development. Although there is a great deal of variability in vowel production, most studies suggest that vowels are produced reasonably accurately by age 3 years (Donegan, 2002).

Between age 4 and 7 years most children master the production of the remaining sounds of their language. During this period they also begin to correctly produce words with more complex sound structures such as multi-syllable words and words that contain consonant clusters (Ingram, 1989).

PHONOLOGICAL AWARENESS

In addition to the ability to produce sounds and use those sounds to create words, children must develop another skill called **phonological awareness**. Stackhouse (1997) defines phonological awareness as, "the ability to reflect on and manipulate the structure of an utterance (e.g., into words, syllables, or sounds) as distinct from its meaning" (p. 157). This definition identifies two aspects of phonological awareness: first, understanding that words are composed of smaller units, namely syllables and phonemes (Catts, 1991), and second, the ability to manipulate those smaller units (Cunningham, 1990). As will be discussed in Chapter 13, phonological awareness is not only related to expressive speech skills but also to reading and spelling ability. Phonological awareness is a developmental skill and therefore merits mention in the present chapter. Goldsworthy (1998) and Justice and Schuele (2004) reviewed the literature and described the phonological awareness skills of children at various age levels. The following is a summary of their findings regarding the development of phonological awareness:

- *At age 2 years*—Some children are able to detect rhyme inconsistently but at levels greater than chance. These children are able to select the word that does not rhyme from a group of three (hat, cat, boy). Tasks such as this are called rhyme oddity tasks.
- *At age 3 years*—Presented with two words, many children are able to tell if two words rhyme or not (rhyme detection). Some children are able to generate at least one word which rhymes with a target word. Many children this age can recite known rhymes such as "Jack and Jill." Many are able to identify a word in a group of words that begins with a different sound (mad, mop, cat). Tasks such as the latter are referred to as alliteration oddity tasks. Sensitivity to alliteration generally lags behind sensitivity to rhyme.
- *At age 4 years*—Children begin to exhibit awareness of syllabic distinction. For example the word *baby* can be divided into *ba* and *by*. About half of all 4-year-olds can count the number of syllables in multisyllabic words.
- *At age 5 years*—Most children can generate rhyme spontaneously during play or on demand in games. They exhibit general proficiency in rhyming detection tasks. Most 5-year-olds can count the number of syllables in multisyllabic words. Some children at this age can also count the number of phonemes in words. However, in terms of recognizing phonemes, it is more likely at age 5 years that children can separate the first sound of a single-syllable word (onset) from the rest of the word (rime) that appears to be treated as a single unit. For example, children can separate the word *top* into t (onset) and op (rime) but not into t-o-p.
- *At age 6 years*—Most children demonstrate the ability to identify phonemes as units that make up syllables. Many children can blend two to three sounds to make a word (e.g., c-a-t makes *cat*).

- *At age 7 years*—Children begin to spell phonetically. They can segment three to four phonemes in words. At this age many children can delete sounds from words (e.g., *moose* without the s̲ is *moo*).

As mentioned earlier, children who are delayed in the development of phonological awareness skills are at risk for speech, reading, and spelling problems. Speech-language pathologists, classroom teachers, and reading specialists should all work together to identify those children who appear to have delayed phonological awareness.

CONCLUSION

In this chapter we have attempted to describe how normally developing children learn to communicate. The stages of language and phonological development are relatively consistent across children; however, individual youngsters progress through these stages at different rates and with some minor variations in their acquisition patterns. An appreciation of the general progression of communication development is important because it provides a framework through which you can better understand the communicative disorders we will discuss in the remainder of the present text.

REFERENCES

Benedict, H. (1979). Early lexical development: Comprehension and production. *Journal of Child Language, 6,* 183–200.

Brown, R. (1958). *Words and things.* New York: Macmillan.

Brown, R. (1973). *A first language: The early stages.* Cambridge, MA: Harvard University Press.

Catts, H. (1991). Early identification of reading disabilities. *Topics in Language Disorders, 12,* 1–16.

Catts, H., & Kamhi, A. (2005). *Language and reading disabilities.* Boston, MA: Allyn and Bacon.

Cunningham, A. (1990). Explicit versus implicit instruction in phonemic awareness. *Journal of Experimental Psychology, 50,* 429–444.

Curtiss, S., Fromkin, V., Krashen, S., Rigler, D., & Rigler, M. (1974). The linguistic development of Genie. *Language, 50,* 528–554.

Donegan, P. (2002). Normal vowel development. In M. J. Ball & F. E. Gibbon (Eds.), *Vowel Disorders.* Boston: Butterworth-Heineman.

Goldsworthy, C. L. (1998). *Sourcebook of phonological awareness activities.* San Diego, CA: Singular.

Grunwell, P. (1987). *Clinical phonology* (2nd ed.). Baltimore: Williams and Wilkins.

Ingram, D. (1989). *Phonological disability in children* (2nd ed.). San Diego, CA: Singular.

Justice, L. M., & Schuele, C. M. (2004). Phonological awareness: Description, assessment and intervention. In J. Bernthal & N. Bankson, *Articulation and phonological disorders* (5th ed.). Boston: Allyn and Bacon.

Kretschmer, R., & Kretschmer, L. (1978). *Language development and intervention with the hearing impaired*. Baltimore: University Park Press.

McClean, J., & Snyder-McClean, L. (1978). *A transactional approach to early language training*. Columbus, OH: Merrill.

McCormick, L. (1984). Review of normal language acquisition. In L. McCormick & R. Schiefelbusch (Eds.), *Early language intervention*. Columbus, OH: Merrill.

Miller, J., & Chapman, R. (1981). The relation between age and mean length of utterance. *Journal of Speech and Hearing Research, 24*, 154–161.

Nippold, M. (1988). Later language development: Ages nine through nineteen. Boston: Little-Brown.

Oller, D. K. (1980). The emergence of the sounds of speech in infancy. In G. Yeni-Komshian, J. Kavanagh, & C. Ferguson (Eds.), *Child phonology: Vol. 1. Production*. New York: Academic Press.

Owens, R. (2005). *Language development: An introduction*. Boston: Allyn and Bacon.

Piaget, J. (1952). *The origins of intelligence in children*. New York: International Universities Press.

Piaget, J. (1954). *The construction of reality in the child*. New York: Basic Books.

Piaget, J. (1970). *Genetic epistemology*. New York: Columbia University Press.

Poole, E. (1934). Genetic development of articulation of consonant sounds in speech. *Elementary English Review, 11*, 159–161.

Prather, E., Hedrick, D., & Kern, C. (1975). Articulation development in children aged two to four years. *Journal of Speech and Hearing Disorders, 40*, 179–191.

Rutter, M. (1978). Diagnosis and definition of childhood autism. *Journal of Autism and Childhood Schizophrenia, 8*, 139–169.

Sander, E. (1972). When are speech sounds learned? *Journal of Speech and Hearing Disorders, 37*, 55–63.

Scarborough, H., Wyckoff, J., & Davidson, R. (1986). A reconsideration of the relation between age and mean utterance length. *Journal of Speech and Hearing Research, 29*, 394–399.

Shulman, B., & Haynes, W. (in press). *Language acquisition: Foundations, processes and clinical applications*. Boston: Jones & Bartlett.

Smit, A. B., Hand, L., Freilinger, J., Bernthal, J., & Bird, A. (1990). The Iowa articulation norms project and its Nebraska reduplication. *Journal of Speech and Hearing Disorders, 55*, 779–798.

Stackhouse, J. (1997). Phonological awareness: Connecting speech and literacy problems. In B.W. Hodson & M.L. Edwards (Eds.), *Perspectives in applied phonology*. Gaithersburg, MD: Aspen.

Stoel-Gammon, C., & Dunn, C. (1985) *Normal and disordered phonology in children*. Austin, TX: Pro-Ed.

Templin, M. (1957). *Certain language skills in children*. Minneapolis, MN: University of Minnesota Press.

Wellman, B., Case, I., Mengert, E., & Bradbury, D. (1931). *Speech sounds of young children*. University of Iowa Studies in Child Welfare (5th ed.). Iowa City: University of Iowa Press.

Yavas, M. (1998). *Phonology development and disorders*. San Diego, CA: Singular.

TERMS TO KNOW

BACIS

mean length of utterance (MLU)

phonetically consistent forms

phonological awareness

phonological processes

protowords

transitional forms

vocables

STUDY QUESTIONS

1. Describe the verbal behaviors that characterize each of Oller's prelanguage stages. Provide the approximate age range for each stage.

2. Identify those classes of sounds (e.g., stops, fricatives, nasals, semivowels) that typically develop early and those that typically develop late.

3. Provide examples of each of the following phonological processes:
   Stopping
   Fronting
   Cluster reduction

4. Describe the relationship between MLU and language development in Brown's five stages.

5. What kinds of behaviors would you look for in a nonverbal child that would suggest he or she is developing the BACIS for language acquisition?

6. What kind of language abilities should a normally developing child possess upon entering kindergarten?

four

chapter four

Phonological Disorders

BACKGROUND INFORMATION

Nature of the Problem

As stated in Chapter 2, speech is the process of producing sound patterns to communicate. The manner in which children develop those sound patterns was described in Chapter 3. In the present chapter we will discuss children who, for various reasons, have not mastered the sound patterns expected for children their age.

Remember that in developing their speech sound system, children must master two tasks. First they must learn to produce the various sounds of their language. Second, they must develop a system of rules for organizing and using those sounds.

Students who have problems correctly producing sounds are sometimes described as having an **articulation** problem. Those students who have not mastered the rules used to manage the sounds are described as having a **phonological** disorder. To illustrate these two types of problems, imagine a child who consistently produces the s sound as a th. This child would produce the sentence, "We went to see Aunt Sarah on Sunday," as, "We went to thee Aunt Tharah on Thunday." This child most likely demonstrates an articulation problem. He or she is unable to produce s, and instead substitutes a th for every s sound. Now imagine a child who produces the sentence, "My kitty cat climbs trees, and my dog does too," as, "My kikky cak climbs trees, and my gog does too." This child correctly produced the t in *trees* and *too* but not in *kitty* or *cat*. He or she also correctly produced the d in *does* but not in *dog*. Clearly this problem represents more than an inability to correctly produce the sounds. There appears to be some rule or pattern at work in this child's speech which allows the correct production of t and d in some words but not in others. This is an example of a phonological disorder.

The distinction between articulation and phonological disorders is not always as clear as it is in our examples. Some authors have chosen to use the term *phonology* to refer to all aspects of the study of speech sound production. In this usage, phonology can be said to include both a motor aspect (articulation) and a cognitive-linguistic aspect which deals with the rules for sound usage (Stoel-Gammon & Dunn, 1985). Because this broad definition fits well with our own view of the subject, and because the use of a single term is more convenient for purposes of this chapter, we will use *phonology* to refer broadly to all aspects of speech sound production.

Traditionally, speech sound production errors have been classified as one of three types: substitutions, distortions, or omissions.

Substitutions occur when one sound is substituted for another. For example when a child says *tan* for *can* or *wed* for *red*, sound substitutions are evident.

Distortions occur when a child attempts the appropriate phoneme but fails to produce it accurately. The "slushy" s of Sylvester the Cat is an extreme example of a distortion.

Omissions signify that a phoneme is deleted, and nothing is produced in its place. The child who says *ha* for *hat* or *baball* for *baseball* is exhibiting an omission.

Errors which affect specific sounds or classes of sounds are sometimes given a specific name. The most common example of such an error is a **lisp**. A lisp affects **sibilant** sounds. Sibilants are s, sh, ch, and their voiced cognates. There are two common types of lisps. The **central lisp** occurs when the speaker produces the sibilant sound with the tongue between the teeth resulting in a th-like sound. The child with a central lisp says *thun* for *sun* or *methy* for *messy*. A **lateral lisp** occurs when air is directed laterally around the side of the tongue rather than down the middle, resulting in air leakage between the tongue and the molars producing a "slushy" s̲ or s̲h̲ sound.

Substitutions, distortions, and omissions can occur in three positions within a word. The first sound of a word is the **initial position**, the last sound is the **final position**, and anything between initial and final is the **medial position**. In the previous example, the child who said *Thunday* for *Sunday* demonstrated a t̲h̲ for s̲ substitution in the initial position.

The system of describing phonology disorders according to substitutions, distortions, and omissions (SDO) works well when a child has few sounds in error and when the errors reflect a motoric inability to correctly produce the target sound. In the case of the t̲h̲ for s̲ substitution, we have a good idea about which sounds the child can and cannot produce. The other child in our example presents a different picture. The SDO system does not describe his or her errors as clearly as it did those of the first child. A better way to describe the second child's errors would be to identify any patterns or rules which account for the errors. One type of pattern analysis is to describe the presence of phonological processes. Phonological processes were discussed as part of normal development in Chapter 3. Some children fail to suppress these simplifying patterns at the expected age. If you closely examine the second speech sample above exhibiting the inconsistent use of t̲ and d̲ you will see a pattern to the errors. The pattern is that when the alveolar sounds t̲ or d̲ are in a word which contains the velar sounds k̲ or g̲, the t̲ and d̲ are produced as k̲ or g̲. This is a fairly common phonological process known as velar assimilation.

Prevalence

Estimates of the prevalence of articulation and phonological errors in school-age children vary because of several factors including the diagnostic criteria employed by specific investigators. However, the National Institute on Deafness and Other Communication Disorders (NIDCD) estimates that 8–9% of young children exhibit speech sound disorders (NIDCD, 2004). Because the prevalence of this type of disorder is so high, it is quite likely that all teachers will encounter students with phonological disorders.

The point needs to be made here that not all speech sound differences constitute a phonological disorder. It is important to distinguish phonological errors from pronunciation errors, normal developmental differences, and dialectal differences.

Pronunciation errors generally affect only a few words and reflect an inappropriate selection of sounds by the speaker rather than an inability to produce sounds. For example, some students may pronounce *Illinois* by including the s̲ sound at the end or refer to a photograph as a "pitcher" rather than a *picture*. Although these productions are not "correct," they are not phonological disorders. They reflect an inappropriate selection of sounds by the speaker. In most cases, when informed of the "correct" production, the child will either alter the pronunciation, or perhaps insist that it is correct because, "That is the way my Daddy says it." Also, occasionally there are specific words which children (and sometimes adults) find difficult to produce. Some children call "spaghetti" "pisghetti" or have great difficulty with the word "statistics." Again, because these are limited to specific words, such pronunciation problems are not considered phonological disorders.

Developmental differences reflect the fact that phonology, like all aspects of language, does not burst forth in its fully developed form from the time a child begins to speak. Phonological development is a gradual process; what is "normal" for a 3-year-old preschooler may not be "normal" for a 6-year-old first grader. For example, it is not unusual for a 3-year-old to say "top" for "stop" or "pin" for "spin," but a first grader who consistently deletes the s̲ from consonant clusters would be a candidate for speech intervention. It is quite helpful for teachers to know what is "normal" for children in their classes. Typical phonological development is reviewed in Chapter 3.

Dialectal differences are linguistic variations which reflect, among other factors, historical, cultural, regional, and ethnic influences (Taylor, 1986). Dialectal differences are discussed in Chapter 7, but it should be pointed out here that students who are dialectal speakers may demonstrate speech sound differences that reflect their dialect and are not considered disorders.

Causation

When teachers encounter students with severe phonological disorders, they often have questions about the cause of those disorders. Are these children cognitively impaired? Do they have some physical disorder? Are they deaf? Although these are all possibilities, in most cases, the answer to all of the above questions is no. In the following section we will discuss some of the causes of phonological disorders.

The causes of phonological disorders can be divided into two broad categories: **organic** and **functional**. Organic causes result from structural, physiological, sensory, or neurological deficits (Weiss, Gordon, & Lillywhite,

1987). Functional causes are a bit harder to identify and are usually defined by default as problems for which there are no apparent structural, physiological, sensory, or neurological deficits.

Organic Factors

There are many organic conditions that can affect the ability of a child to correctly produce speech sounds. Several of these conditions, including cleft palate, cerebral palsy, muscular dystrophy, and tracheostomy, are discussed in detail in Chapters 11 and 12. In the present chapter, we will identify and briefly describe some additional organic causes of speech sound production errors.

Malocclusion refers to the misalignment of the teeth or an improper relationship between the upper and lower teeth. Terms such as overbite, overjet, underbite, and open bite refer to different types of malocclusion. Errors on the s and z sounds are often associated with malocclusion, but not all children with malocclusions experience problems with speech sound production. Missing teeth have also been associated with speech sound production errors (Bankson & Byrne, 1962; Snow, 1961); however, most children go through the transition from primary to permanent teeth with no serious disruption of speech sound production.

Structural deviations of the tongue can result in speech sound errors. **Macroglossia** is a condition in which the tongue is larger than normal. **Microglossia** refers to a tongue that is smaller than normal. **Ankyloglossia,** or "tongue-tie," is a condition in which the flap of tissue which holds the tongue to the floor of the mouth (the lingual frenum) is too short or attached too far forward. This limits the mobility of the tongue and affects the child's ability to produce tongue-tip sounds such as t, d, l, and r. This condition is not as common as many people seem to believe. The restriction must be quite severe to interfere with speech. Many infants appear to have a short frenum at first, but after a few months of sucking and crying, the tongue becomes adequately mobile for speech. The one-time common, but mostly unnecessary, practice of surgically "clipping" the frenum in infants is now avoided by most physicians.

Another problem involving the tongue is **tongue thrust**. Tongue thrust refers to a swallowing pattern in which the tongue comes forward, pressing against the teeth and sometimes protruding between the teeth. Children with tongue thrust have a higher incidence of s and z errors than other children, but not all children with tongue thrust exhibit speech problems (Bernthal &

Bankson, 2004). There is some controversy in the field of speech-language pathology as to the role of the speech-language pathologist (SLP) in treatment. Some SLPs believe that they should treat only the speech problem associated with tongue thrust. Others feel they should attempt to alter the swallowing pattern itself. The teacher may find that different SLPs in the same school system may have different opinions on this question. Also, a school system may not consider a deviant swallowing pattern to be an educationally significant problem and therefore not an appropriate condition for a school-based speech-language pathologist to treat.

Because most children learn their phonological system through hearing, **hearing impairment** can have an effect on accuracy of speech sound production. Factors such as the degree of hearing loss, the age at onset, and the type of hearing loss determine the effect of hearing loss on phonology. Hearing loss is discussed more fully in Chapter 10.

Damage to the central or peripheral nervous system can result in a weakening, paralysis, or loss of control over the muscles of the speech mechanism; the resulting speech problem is called **dysarthria.** Many conditions, including cerebral palsy, muscular dystrophy, tumors, traumatic brain injury, and diseases such as meningitis and encephalitis, can result in dysarthria. Dysarthria is characterized by slow, effortful speech and imprecise production of speech sounds. In this condition, the speech structures, including the tongue, lips, and soft palate, cannot move fast enough to keep up with the demands of connected speech or do not have the strength to achieve the appropriate place or shape to produce the sounds accurately.

Apraxia of speech describes a condition in which the ability to program and sequence the motor movements required for the production of speech sounds is impaired as a result of brain damage. The muscles are healthy and respond to the commands from the nervous system appropriately. The problem is that the commands are incorrect. Sound substitutions and **metathetic errors** (producing sounds in an incorrect order) are common. Apraxia of speech is usually acquired as a result of injury or disease. In such situations the child had normal speech until incurring the brain damage and then loses some speech ability.

A condition known as **developmental apraxia of speech (DAS)** is believed by some to affect a child's ability to develop his or her speech sound system. DAS is a controversial diagnostic category. After reviewing the literature on DAS, Klein (1996) pointed out that there has never been total agreement on the signs and symptoms of DAS, and some lists of signs and symptoms contradict others. Davis, Jakielski, and Marquardt (1998) provided a list that includes many of the most accepted characteristics of DAS. These characteristics include the following:

- Limited number of phonemes
- Frequent omission errors
- Vowel errors
- Inconsistent errors
- More errors on longer units of speech
- Difficulty imitating words
- Use of simple syllable shapes
- Difficulty with voluntary oral movements
- Receptive skills better than expressive skills

The inconsistency of errors and the inability to imitate sounds and motor movements are just two of the factors that make children with DAS particularly challenging for SLPs.

Cognitive impairment results from a number of conditions and can affect phonological ability. There is a much higher incidence of phonological disorders among children with cognitive impairments than among their nonimpaired peers. The type and extent of the phonology disorder appears to be related to the degree and cause of impairment. For example, Wilson (1966), in a study of individuals with developmental delays, reported that lower mental age was associated with a greater number of speech sound errors. He also reported that the speech of children with developmental delays who exhibited lower mental ages was characterized by omissions, and the speech of those who exhibited higher mental ages was characterized by distortions. Dodd (1976) reported that the incidence of speech problems among children with Down syndrome is higher than among other children with similar degrees of developmental delay.

Because cognitive impairment affects both cognitive-linguistic and motor development, it is not surprising that there is a high incidence of phonological disorders among this population. It should be pointed out that, within the range of normal intelligence, intellectual functioning is not an important factor in determining phonological ability (Bernthal & Bankson, 2004; Powers, 1971).

Functional Disorders

The majority of phonological disorders are not associated with organic conditions. These disorders are termed functional and are not as easy to account for as organic disorders. In most cases, the specific factor or factors that have resulted in a particular student's phonological disorder are impossible to determine. Many factors have been investigated as they relate to functional disorders of phonology. A summary of research findings regarding some of these factors is presented in Table 4-1. It is important to keep in mind that most of the reported research is based on group data and the results may not apply to every child with a phonological disorder. A review of Table 4-1 reveals that most research has demonstrated weak relationships or no relationship at all between phonological disorders and factors many people have assumed play a large role in such disorders.

In spite of years of research and an abundance of children with phonological disorders, in most cases the specific cause of a phonological disorder in any given child is impossible to determine.

Case Examples

To provide an appreciation of the range of phonological disorders, we will present two hypothetical students, each representing opposite ends of the continuum of severity of phonological disorders. Mary and John are both in the first grade. They were referred by their teacher to the school speech-language pathologist for a speech evaluation. To obtain a sample of their spontaneous speech, the speech-language pathologist asked each child to talk about a picture of a rabbit. In response to the picture, Mary said: "That is a wabbit, a bwown wabbit. Wabbits wun fast. They eat cawots."

The same picture elicited the following response from John: "Da a bu wa. E wu pa. E ea ga. I no i pi." (Translation: That's a bunny rabbit. He runs fast. He eats grass. His nose is pink.)

Both Mary and John exhibit problems with their speech sound production system. In Mary's case, the problem appears to be limited to the r sound. Although her problem is noticeable, most people would have little difficulty understanding her. John, on the other hand, appears to have a very limited phonological system. He seems to be able to use only the earliest developing consonants (w, h and some stop consonants) In addition to the sound errors, he appears to be able to produce only single-syllable words and the syllables are very simple consonant+vowel or just a vowel. These limitations on John's phonology make his speech unintelligible. Even when the listener knows that he is talking about a rabbit, it is almost impossible to understand what he is saying.

Table 4-1 Summary of Research on Selected Factors and Articulation Ability

Factor Investigated	Relationship to Articulation Proficiency
Intelligence	Within the normal range of intelligence, a slight positive relationship exists between intelligence and articulation, however not an important consideration. Below the normal range of intelligence there is a high incidence of articulation disorders including the presence of phonological process disorders (Bernthal & Bankson, 2004; Mackay & Hodson, 1982; Moran, Money, & Leonard,1984).
Auditory discrimination	Considerable evidence exists that children with articulation disorders, as a group, perform more poorly on tests of speech sound discrimination than children without articulation disorders. However, many individuals with articulation problems show no difficulty with auditory discrimination (Bernthal & Bankson, 2004; Pena-Brooks & Hegde, 2000; Shriberg, 1980).
Motor skills	Evidence that some children with poor articulation score lower than those with normal articulation on tests of rapid alternating speech movements (e.g., rapidly repeating the syllables pu, tu, ku). There does not appear to be a relationship between articulation skill and general motor skills (Bernthal & Bankson, 2004; Pena-Brooks & Hegde, 2000; Shriberg, 1980).
Socioeconomic level	There is some evidence that proportionally more children from low socioeconomic homes have poor articulation. However this does not appear to be a significant factor (Bernthal & Bankson, 2004; Pena-Brooks & Hegde, 2000; Shriberg, 1980).
Siblings	Some evidence exists that firstborn children, only children, and children with increased spacing between siblings have better articulation at some ages (Bernthal & Bankson, 2004; Pena-Brooks & Hegde, 2000; Shriberg, 1980).
Personality and adjustment	Some evidence exists that children with severe articulation errors have a greater proportion of adjustment and behavioral problems than non-deviant children (Bernthal & Bankson, 2004; Pena-Brooks & Hegde, 2000; Shriberg, 1980).
Familial tendencies	Felsenfeld, McGue, and Broen (1995) reported that children of parents with a history of phonological/language problems were more likely to require articulation treatment than the children of parents with no history of phonological or language problems. However, the phonological errors exhibited by the children were not necessarily similar to those exhibited by the parents.

A critical first step in improving phonological problems is to describe precisely the nature of the problem. This is done by the speech-language pathologist during the assessment phase.

ASSESSMENT ISSUES IN PHONOLOGICAL DISORDERS

In a school setting, the first stage of assessment is often a **screening test**. Screening tests are usually administered shortly after the beginning of the school year. The purpose of a screening test is to determine which members of a group (e.g., all children entering kindergarten) are most likely to have a problem. Failing a screening test does not mean that the child has a disorder. It simply means that the child is a candidate for a more thorough evaluation. Screening tests must be quick and easy to administer and to score. Screening tests to assess phonology usually consist of a few minutes of connected speech during which the child may be asked to count, repeat words, name and/or describe pictures, or any other activity that will produce a sample of the child's speech. There are several published screening tests available. The speech-language pathologist may choose to use one of these published screening devices in place of, or in addition to, a less formal speech sampling technique. In most school settings, the screening test is used to assess language development as well as phonology. In addition to being quick and easy to administer, screening tests for phonological disorders, like all screening tests, must meet two other criteria. They must be able to identify a high percentage of children who have disorders (sensitivity), but must not fail too many children who do not have disorders (specificity). The SLP should monitor the screening procedure he or she uses to be sure it has high sensitivity and specificity. Teachers can provide a great deal of help in this monitoring by noting which children pass the screening but must later be referred for evaluation.

In addition to screening tests, teacher referral is another important method of identifying children with phonology problems. After a few years in the classroom, most teachers can easily identify students whose speech is markedly different from that of other students at a particular grade level. Students who are unintelligible, or who have more or different speech sound errors than other children in class (not dialectal differences) should be referred to the SLP for an opinion. When the SLP identifies a child who might have a phonological disorder, either through screening or referral, permission to evaluate is obtained from the parents and the child is given a **diagnostic evaluation**.

Standardized Methods of Assessment

The objectives of a diagnostic evaluation include: (1) determining whether the child has a phonological disorder; (2) determining the nature and extent of the disorder; and (3) suggesting methods which might be effective in remediating that disorder. To meet these objectives, the SLP has three basic types of assessments: **speech sound inventories, contextual tests,** and **pattern analyses**. Depending on the speech pattern exhibited by the child, the SLP may choose to administer one, two, or all three of these assessments.

Speech Sound Inventories

A speech sound inventory is a test of each phoneme in the context of a word. Each consonant is generally tested in each word position (initial, medial, final) in which it occurs. Consonant clusters are usually tested in at least the initial position. Some, but not all, inventories also test vowels. Speech sound inventories usually require a child to name pictures which contain one or more target phonemes. For example, a picture of a foot may be used to assess f̱ in the initial position and ṯ in the final position. Picture naming is preferable to reading because it allows the examiner to test students who cannot read and avoids possible confusion of a reading problem with a phonology problem. Having the child repeat words might be easier and faster than picture naming, but there is research which indicates that spontaneous picture naming provides a more accurate sample of phonological ability (Carter & Buck, 1958; Kresheck & Sokolofsky, 1972; Smith & Ainsworth, 1967; Snow & Milisen, 1954). There are many published speech sound inventories. Some of the more commonly used include the following:

- The *Goldman-Fristoe Test of Articulation* provides color pictures to elicit single-word responses and a story retelling section to elicit a connected speech sample (Goldman & Fristoe, 2000).
- The *Photo Articulation Test* uses photographs of objects to elicit single-word responses and a set of sequential photos to elicit a connected speech sample (Lippke, Dickey, Selmar, & Soder, 1997).
- *The Arizona Articulation Proficiency Scale* provides a weighting of each sound in order to provide an intelligibility rating (Fudala, 2001).

Speech sound inventories are quick and easy to administer. Therefore, they are quite popular with most school speech-language pathologists who have large caseloads and a minimum of time available for diagnostic testing.

Although they provide some helpful information, speech sound inventories are quite limited. Testing each phoneme once in each position of a word does not, in most cases, adequately define the child's ability to produce that sound. Because a child says s̲ correctly in *scissors, pencil*, and *house*, does not mean that the child can produce s̲ correctly in all words in all situations. On the other hand, because a child cannot produce s̲ in *scissors, pencil*, or *house*, does not mean that he or she cannot produce the sound correctly in any word under any circumstances. For example, the second month of the year has an r̲ in the second syllable, but most people omit the r̲ and pronounce the word as *Febuary*. Does this mean that most Americans cannot produce a medial r̲? Of course not. The r̲ in February is omitted because its presence makes for a rather difficult sequence of articulatory movements. (Also, most people learn the names of the months in sequence. The pronunciation of January suggests a similar pronunciation for the second month). If you listen closely, you will hear that most people do not produce a t̲ in words like *butter* or *water*; rather, they substitute a d̲. The d̲ occurs because it is more efficient to continue voicing from the first vowel to the second vowel than to interrupt it for the few milliseconds required to produce t̲. In each of these words, the sounds around the target sound referred to as the **phonetic environment** or the **phonetic context** affect production of that sound. Speech sound inventories do not sample enough words to assess the effects of phonetic context. To assess such effects, an SLP may elect to use a contextual test.

Contextual Tests

The first widely used contextual test was the *Deep Test of Articulation* (McDonald, 1964). Subsequent tests employing a variety of phonetic contexts are sometimes referred to as deep-type tests. In the original *Deep Test of Articulation* a picture containing the error sound in the initial position is preceded by a series of 30 pictures ending with a different sound. For each picture pair, the student is instructed to say the two words together, so they sound like one big word. For example, if s̲ was the error phoneme, a picture of *sun* would be preceded by pictures such as *cup, tub, kite*, and so on. The child would then produce words such as *cups̲un, tubs̲un* and *kites̲un*. The procedure is then repeated with the error sound in the final position, for example *house* followed by a series of words resulting in productions such as *hous̲epipe, hous̲ebell* and *hous̲etie*. When the test is complete, the examiner has a sample of the error sound as it is preceded and followed by many different phonemes. By using this deep test, the SLP will frequently identify one or more contexts in which the error sound is produced correctly. Although the McDonald Deep Test is the most widely known, there are other published deep-type tests including *Clinical Probes of Articulation Consistency* (C-PAC) (Secord, 1981) and a portion of the *Test of Articulation Performance* (TAP) (Bryant & Bryant, 1983). Whether one of the published deep-type tests are administered or not, the SLP will probably want to assess troublesome phonemes in several different contexts to determine the effect of phonetic context.

Pattern Analyses

Speech sound inventories and deep tests assess individual sound errors. In many cases, the SLP wants to determine the presence of patterns that may underlie multiple sound errors. There are several types of patterns for which an SLP may search, including distinctive feature patterns or patterns of phonological rules. However, SLPs frequently search for phonological processes that may account for the errors heard in a child's speech. We have discussed the concept of phonological processes in Chapter 3 as part of phonological development. Some children fail to suppress these normal processes at the expected age. Other children develop and maintain unusual processes that are not part of normal development. If the SLP can identify one or more processes affecting a number of phonemes in the speech of a child, the intervention that follows is much more efficient than working on each individual error sound. Two of the more frequently used tests of phonological process are the *Hodson Assessment of Phonological Patterns* (HAPP-3) (Hodson, 2004) and the *Kahn-Lewis Phonological Analysis-2* (KLPA-2) (Kahn & Lewis, 2002). The HAPP-3 uses spontaneous naming of objects, body parts, and colors to assess numerous processes and patterns. The KLPA-2 uses the words from the sounds-in-words section of the *Goldman-Fristoe Test of Articulation* as its speech sample.

Combination Tests

Some recently developed tests are designed to allow the speech-language pathologist to perform more than one kind of analysis. An example of this kind of test is the *Clinical Assessment of Articulation and Phonology* (CAAP) (Secord & Donohue, 2002), which includes an "articulation inventory" and two "phonological process checklists."

Also popular, because of the large amount of data that can be provided in a small amount of time, are computer-based analyses such as the PROPH+ program of *Computerized Profiling* (Long, 2004). Once the child's utterances are typed, this program provides an analysis of several phonological processes plus a great deal of additional information about the child's phonological inventory, in a matter of seconds.

Type of Speech Sample

Speech sound inventories, deep tests, and many of the published pattern analysis tests elicit speech one word at a time. Several studies have demonstrated that children exhibit more sound errors on words in connected speech than on those same words in isolation (DuBoise & Bernthal, 1978; Faircloth & Faircloth, 1970; Haynes, Haynes, & Jackson, 1982; Panagos, Klich, & Quine, 1979; Panagos, Klich, & Schmauch, 1978). Several factors may account for this variability. The production of a sound may be influenced by other sounds in the utterance. For example, notice the lip rounding on the s sound in the word *stew* (due to the influence of the w) and retraction of the lips on the s in the word *steam* (due to the vowel sound). This influence of one sound on another is known as **coarticulation**. Coarticulation can exert an influence across word boundaries (Daniloff & Moll, 1968). The opportunities for coarticulation to affect a sound are greater in connected speech than in single words. Another factor is linguistic complexity. Connected speech involves sentences. Sentences require the child to be concerned with tense constructions, subject–predicate agreement, and a myriad of other syntax considerations not involved in the production of single words. Connected speech is a more complex linguistic task than producing single words. As with most tasks, complexity increases the chance of error. Because of this, a speech-language pathologist will most likely want a sample of the child's connected speech.

Although there are no hard and fast rules about how extensive a connected speech sample should be, an often sited minimum is 80 to 100 different words, which usually requires a total sample of about 200 to 250 words (Shriberg & Kwiatkowski, 1980). Obtaining such a connected speech sample can be challenging. Some children are shy with nonfamiliar adults and speak only in 1- or 2-word utterances if at all. Even with a talkative child, it might take a very long time before he or she uses all the sounds in all of the contexts we wish to examine. Some children may avoid words containing sounds which are difficult for them to produce. Further complicating matters, when a child is unintelligible, it is difficult or impossible to determine the error patterns, because the listener does not know what the child intended to say.

Faced with these problems, an SLP will often use some structured task to maintain control over the content in eliciting a connected speech sample. Having the child describe a picture is one way to elicit connected speech. By carefully selecting the pictures, the SLP samples a variety of sounds in different contexts, and has some idea of the topic. Another frequently used technique is story retelling. In this procedure, a child is shown pictures and told a story, then shown the pictures again and asked to repeat the story. This technique is used in published test instruments such as the sounds-in-sentences subtest of the *Goldman-Fristoe Test of Articulation-2*.

How Teachers Can Help in Assessment

Teachers can be an important source of diagnostic information. Next to parents, it is teachers who have the most opportunity to observe their students' communicative behavior. Teachers can provide a great deal of assistance by answering the following questions:

1. With which sounds or words does the child seem to have difficulty?
2. Does the child ever produce any of the error sounds correctly?
3. Do you have trouble understanding the child?
4. Do other students have trouble understanding the child?
5. Are other students aware of the child's speech problem? How do they react?
6. How does the child get along with classmates?
7. Does the child talk as much as most students in the class?
8. Is the child's vocabulary and grammar appropriate for grade level?·
9. How well does the child follow directions?
10. How is the child performing academically?

DIRECT TREATMENT OF PHONOLOGICAL DISORDERS

When the assessment is completed, the SLP makes a recommendation to the eligibility committee. If the student is to receive treatment, a schedule must be worked out between the SLP and the teacher. Scheduling procedures vary from school to school and reflect the individual student's needs. A typical schedule for a child with a phonological disorder is twice each week for 30 minutes. The child may be seen alone or in a small group. In many places, the SLP must divide time among several schools. In this itinerant situation, scheduling can become a problem, but a collaborative effort by the SLP, teacher, and administrators can solve most such problems.

There are many therapy techniques and procedures that can be employed to remediate a phonological disorder. While it is not the purpose of this text to teach specific therapy techniques, we do feel that it would be helpful for teachers to have some understanding of what the SLP does in attempting to improve a student's production of speech sounds.

Common Techniques Used by the SLP

Throughout this chapter we have made the point that phonology problems may occur on two different levels: a motor level, in which the child is unable to correctly produce the sound, and a cognitive-linguistic level, in which the child may be able to produce sounds but does not use them appropriately. Because there are two levels of phonological problems, there are two types of treatment to remediate these problems. Motor-based treatments are designed to teach the student to correctly produce a target sound; to transfer the correct production of that sound to all positions, contexts, linguistic units, and situations; and to maintain the correct production of that sound in habitual speech. Cognitive-linguistic approaches are designed to teach patterns that affect entire classes of sounds. The theory is that by selecting certain sounds (exemplars) that can be used to teach the new pattern, the pattern will generalize to the untreated sounds saving a considerable amount of treatment time. Sometimes children exhibit phonological problems on both levels. In such cases, both motor-based and cognitive-linguistic approaches might be incorporated into the therapy program.

Motor-Based Treatment

Bernthal and Bankson (2004) suggest that most articulation–phonology treatment programs can be divided into three major stages: **establishment**, **generalization**, and **maintenance**. During the establishment phase, the sound or sound pattern to be taught is elicited and stabilized. During the generalization stage, correct production of the target sound or sound pattern spreads to additional words, linguistic units, and situations. During maintenance, the student retains the correct production with decreasing support from the SLP. Although important at all stages, it is probably during generalization and maintenance that the cooperation of the teacher is most critical. We can refer to John and Mary, the hypothetical children described earlier in this chapter, to illustrate the type of activity that might occur at each stage of a therapy program.

Establishment

Recall that Mary had difficulty with the r̲ sound. During the establishment phase Mary would be taught to produce the r̲ either in isolation or in a syllable such as *ro, ri, ray* and so on. Whether the sound is first taught in isolation, syllables, or words depends on the nature of the problem and the philosophy of the SLP. In addition to the context in which the sound is introduced, the specific techniques for teaching the sound will vary from child to child and from clinician to clinician. With young children, it is often helpful to give the target sound a name. For Mary, the r̲ might be called the "growling tiger" sound. In other cases f might be called the "angry kitty" sound or z̲ the "buzzing bee" sound. In some cases treatment might begin with **ear training**, in which the student is taught to identify the sound when it is heard and to discriminate the correct production of the target sound from an incorrect production (Van Riper & Emerick, 1984). After ear training, the treatment shifts to production training. It is in production training where the student is first taught to produce the sound correctly. There are a number of techniques that may be used to achieve this first correct production. Sometimes the sound can be produced correctly in a particular phonetic context (word or syllable). In that case, it is a matter of expanding the contexts in which the sound can be produced correctly. If the sound is not correctly produced in any context, the child must be taught to produce the troublesome phoneme.

One technique frequently used to teach a sound is **auditory stimulation**. Children with normal hearing appear to learn the sound system of their language through hearing. There is a mechanism in each of our brains that allows us to match sounds that we hear. Sometimes this takes practice and may be easier for some children than for others. Many people who study foreign languages that contain phonemes not found in English know that it takes a great deal of practice before we can come close to correctly producing some German or French phonemes. For some children, the structured practice of trying to match the sound they hear results in correct production. Another technique is **phonetic placement**, in which the child is instructed where to place the articulators to correctly produce the target sound. Phonetic placement is often easier with visible sounds, such as t̲h̲ or f̲, when a mirror can be used to aid in proper placement. A third technique that may be used to teach a sound is **successive approximation**. In successive approximation, the child moves in small steps from a sound that can be produced correctly to the target sound. A child who can correctly produce the s̲h̲ sound but cannot produce the s̲ might be told to make the s̲h̲, then gradually move the tongue closer and closer to the alveolar ridge until a correct s̲ is produced. In Mary's case, an attempt might be made to achieve correct production of the r̲ from the production of a closely related sound such as the l̲. When a sound is first produced correctly, it is often with much effort and inconsistency. The final stage of the establishment phase involves working toward an effortless and consistent production of the sound. It is only when the sound is produced in this manner that the child can move on to the generalization phase of therapy.

Generalization

Some SLPs refer to this phase as *transfer*, or *carry-over*. Regardless of the label, the goal of this phase is to enable the child to use the behavior learned in the establishment phase in all words and speaking situations.

Bernthal and Bankson (2004) describe five types of generalization which are of concern in articulation therapy. The first type of generalization is **position generalization**. Here, the student must generalize the correct production of the target sound from the position in which it was established (initial, medial, or final) to other positions in words. In the case of Mary, if we established the r̲ sound in the initial position in a word such as *run*, we must now generalize that correct production to words such as *carrot* and *car*. The second type of generalization is **context generalization**. Here we are concerned with extending the correct production of a sound to all phonetic environments. If Mary could say r̲ when it occurred with back vowels such as in the words *root*, *rope*, and *rot*, we must extend her production to front vowel contexts such as *read*, *rich*, and *ran*. She must also produce the sound in clusters such as *brown* and *price*. **Linguistic unit generalization** involves maintenance of the correct production of a sound or sound pattern in increasingly more complex utterances. Typically, the progression goes from isolation, to syllables, to words (if the sound is first established at the word level, isolation and syllables are omitted), to phrases and sentences, then to connected speech. This progression would be appropriate for both Mary and John. **Sound and feature generalization** is especially important when the SLP is working with a cognitive-linguistic phonological disorder. The goal in this type of therapy is to teach a pattern using a few sounds and encourage the child to generalize the pattern to the entire class of sounds affected. Once again, let us use John as an example. To teach him to eliminate final consonant deletion, we may provide practice on words that end in p̲, s̲, and g̲. Once he learns to use these three sounds appropriately in the final position and recognizes the pattern of using final consonants, the behavior should generalize to all consonants, even though we have only taught p̲, s̲, and g̲. The last type of generalization to be discussed is **situation generalization**. The child must learn that "good speech" is expected in all speaking situations, not just in therapy or school, but on the playground, at home, at summer camp, and in all other speaking situations.

Maintenance

The goal of the maintenance phase is for the newly acquired sound or pattern to be incorporated as a natural part of the child's everyday speech. Maintenance usually involves a reduction in the frequency of therapy sessions. The child may go from two sessions a week, to one session each week, to one every two weeks, and so on. Many of the activities used during maintenance will be similar to those used during the generalization phase, but with less frequent reinforcement. Some SLPs use **negative practice** during the maintenance phase. In this technique, the child is asked to intentionally produce the error sound or sound pattern in order to sharpen the contrast between the "old" and "new" productions. Using negative practice, Mary might say, "I used to call a rabbit a wabbit, and I used to say bwown for brown. But I don't say that anymore."

The teacher can probably expect consistently correct use of the target at this stage. When an error does occur, a raised eyebrow or a request to "Say that again please" will usually be sufficient stimulation to elicit a correct production. Since the SLP sees the child less frequently during this stage, feedback from the teacher is critical. Any apparent regression should be reported as soon as it is noted. Reports that the child is maintaining good speech are also important, as they allow the SLP to determine which techniques have proven successful.

Oral-Motor Exercises

Recently, some speech-language pathologists have begun to employ oral-motor exercises to strengthen and improve muscle function before teaching specific sounds. Actually, this trend represents the most recent revival of a controversial approach to articulation disorders that goes back more than 50 years. The controversy revolves around the use of oral-motor training techniques even in cases where there is no obvious physical cause for the disorder. The assumption is that many so-called functional articulation–phonological disorders have underlying neuromuscular coordination or muscle strength problems as a contributing factor. These are not the severe motor problems exhibited by students with cerebral palsy or other clinically identifiable neuromuscular disorders or even those exhibited by children with the label of developmental apraxia of speech. Rather, these oral-motor problems are much more subtle and become noticeable only under the demands of complicated coordinated activities such as those required for speech production.

Oral-motor techniques generally involve separating and simplifying the complex coordinated movements involved in speech production so that these simpler activities can be mastered before they are combined with other movements to produce speech. A wide variety of techniques are used to accomplish this purpose including flexibility and strength drills for individual articulators, sucking and blowing activities to facilitate coordination of oral and respiratory muscles, and sensory stimulation to improve the sensory abilities of the muscles of speech (Boshart, 2004). In some cases these activities are presented to the child as oral exercises or oral "gymnastics." In some cases a variety of devices are used to shape, stimulate, and stabilize the various oral structures. Teachers of students enrolled in speech intervention programs using an oral-motor approach may be asked to help monitor homework assignments that require the children to "spear" Cheerios with their tongue, lick peanut butter from around their mouth, suck on straws which have the other end covered by a finger, blow horns or bubbles, or many other activities that involve the speech mechanism but not during speech activities.

Although many SLPs who use oral-motor techniques attribute excellent results to these activities, there is very little empirical evidence to support their use. Forrest (2002) reviewed the existing literature that examined the use of oral-motor techniques in the treatment of articulation–phonological disorders. She concluded that, "Based on currently available resources, oral-motor exercises cannot be considered to be a legitimate treatment protocol for children with phonological–articulatory disorders" (p. 22). The use of such techniques remains a very controversial subject.

Cognitive-Linguistic Approaches

For children who exhibit problems of a cognitive-linguistic nature the treatment program is somewhat different. In this case, the SLP most likely targets a pattern rather than a specific sound. The patterns most frequently targeted in such approaches are distinctive feature patterns or phonological processes (Stoel-Gammon, Stone-Goldman, & Glaspey, 2002). Stoel-Gammon and Dunn (1985) identified three characteristics of the approaches that we will describe as cognitive-linguistic:

1. These approaches are based on the systematic nature of phonology. This means that no matter how unusual a child's phonology may be, it has *some* organization. The job of the SLP is to discover how the child's phonology is organized and reorganize it in a more typical fashion. That is one reason that patterns rather than individual sounds are targeted. For example, with the child who substitutes p̲ for f̲, b̲ for v̲, t̲ for s̲, and d̲ for z̲, rather than teach four different sounds, a cognitive-linguistic approach targets the elimination of the process known as stopping.
2. These approaches use conceptual rather than motor activities. An excellent example of a conceptual approach was provided by Weiner and Bankson (1978). To eliminate the process of stopping on fricatives, they associated stop consonants with dripping water and fricatives with flowing water, complete with pictures of a dripping and flowing faucet. The child was then taught to make flowing sounds in contrast to dripping sounds.
3. These approaches have generalization as their ultimate goal. By teaching the appropriate concept with a few phonemes, that concept will generalize to the entire class of phonemes. For example, an SLP might be able to get a child to make all fricatives into "flowing" sounds, based on work with s̲ and v̲.

In the case of the second child described, John, the SLP might want to teach him to eliminate or suppress the process of final consonant deletion. Just as the motor-based therapy began with ear training, the cognitive-linguistic approach might begin by teaching the student awareness of the pattern to be targeted through a process called **conceptualization** (Weiner & Bankson, 1978; Winitz, 1975). Conceptualization is a more cognitive process than auditory discrimination. It is not enough that the child is able to hear the difference between *boat* and *bo* (discrimination); it must be recognized that *boat* has a sound on the end that makes it a different word than *bo*. Often the student demonstrates understanding of the concept through some sorting task where pictures of words that end in a consonant are put in one pile and pictures of words that lack a final consonant are put in another pile. Words such as *bo* (possibly pictured as a bow) and *boat*, which differ in only one aspect, are called **minimal pairs**. Minimal pairs can be used to contrast a number of features. For example, *pie* and *bye* differ only in the voicing of the initial consonant. *See* and *tea* differ only in that *see* begins with a voiceless alveolar fricative and *tea* begins with a voiceless alveolar stop. Because the presence or absence of a feature changes the meaning of the word, minimal pairs constitute a powerful tool in the remediation of cognitive-linguistic phonology problems and can be applied to phonological disorders in several different ways (Barlow & Gierut, 2002).

A minimal pairs technique could be used in the production stage of John's therapy. An example of how minimal pairs might be applied to John's problem of final consonant deletion was provided by Weiner (1981). In this approach, the SLP placed five pictures of a boat and four pictures of a bow on a table in front of the child. The child was told that every time he said *boat*, the SLP would pick up a picture of boat. When the SLP had all five pictures, the child received a star. Weiner reported very rapid success in establishing the presence of final consonants using this minimal pairs technique.

One problem which is often encountered in cognitive-linguistic approaches is that, since a pattern is targeted rather than a specific sound, the early stages of treatment might require reinforcement of an incorrect sound. For example, if John, our final consonant deleter, learned to say *boat* and *seat* rather than *bo* and *see*, we would say, "Great!" But what if he said *gat* for *gas* and *bat* for *bath*? The SLP might say, "Great!" Teachers and parents might say, "Isn't it still wrong?" From a traditional motor-based view, it is just another error. However, in a cognitive-linguistic approach, we are trying to establish the pattern of placing a final consonant at the end of words. John has established that pattern. John will work on getting the appropriate sound in the generalization stage of therapy.

How Teachers Can Help with Direct Treatment

The point cannot be made too strongly that the effectiveness of speech and language treatment is greatly enhanced by the active participation of parents and teachers. However, teachers clearly have their hands full with their required classroom work. Therefore, as Mowrer (1971) suggested, classroom teachers should be asked to perform only activities that are compatible with normal classroom activities. As the SLP relates the goals and progress of the child, the teacher may be able to suggest classroom activities which fit into generalization goals for the student. An effective means of communication between the SLP and the teacher is the **speech notebook**. This can be an inexpensive spiral notebook or even a folder with brads and pockets. Speech goals, activities, exercises, progress charts, instructions, and comments can all be placed in the notebook by the SLP. Teachers and parents can check the notebook after each session or at the end of each week to find out what the child is doing in speech and how they can assist in the remediation program. Although specific activities must be determined on an individual basis for each student, the following represents a broad outline of the information that a teacher should have regarding students enrolled in therapy for phonological disorders:

1. The teacher should know the goals of the student's treatment program. Which sound errors are being targeted? Is the child working on one sound or on a class of sounds such as voiceless consonants? The teacher will probably be aware of long-term goals from the IEP, but short-term goals may change frequently during a school year.
2. The teacher should be aware of progress toward the treatment goals. What kind of speech production can be expected? Is the child working toward correct production via a sequence of closer and closer approximations of the target sound? Does a change in the sound a child substitutes for the target sound represent progress?
3. Perhaps most important of all, the teacher needs to know how to help in achieving the speech goals. Should a certain level of performance be demanded? What kind of feedback should be provided to the SLP? How can everyday teaching activities be used to reinforce treatment and enhance the student's success? Weiss, Gordon, and Lillywhite (1987) identify some activities teachers may perform to help the student generalize new skills from the treatment room to the classroom:
   a. Help the student carry out speech assignments. The assignments may involve repeating a word list, using "good speech" during a particular classroom activity, or demonstrating a newly learned ability to a variety of people. The assignments are often described in the student's speech notebook.
   b. Monitor the student's speech during certain activities. The SLP should keep the teacher informed as to what the student should and should

not be able to do. The teacher may use the speech notebook to report to the SLP.

c. Provide the SLP with classroom materials to be used during the treatment session. This allows for relevance of the speech activity; also, the classroom activities and speech activities reinforce each other.

d. Monitor the student's error productions. Is the sound being used correctly in more words? Are other sounds improving? Is the improved production being maintained in all speaking situations?

e. Reinforce correct sound productions when appropriate, and remind the child to use the target sound or sound pattern. The SLP should clearly communicate to the teacher what feedback or correction technique should be used with the student. A student should never be made to feel embarrassed or "picked on."

INDIRECT TREATMENT OF PHONOLOGICAL DISORDERS

The treatment methods just described all incorporate a very direct approach to remediation. Those methods target specific sounds or error patterns usually in a drill or drill–play format. The efforts of the SLP are focused on achieving a specified criteria at various levels of linguistic complexity (i.e., words, sentences, conversation). Typically the direct methods involve removing the child from the classroom for approximately 30 minutes at a time in what has come to be known as a "pullout" approach. Recently, some authors have suggested that intervention for phonological problems, in some cases, might be more effective using a less direct model. Because many of these less direct approaches to phonological problems incorporate realistic communication activities in natural language environments, the classroom becomes an important site for intervention. As a result, the opportunity for involvement on the part of the teacher is much greater. Many of these less direct treatment methods are referred to as *language-based* models. Most teachers are familiar with such language-based approaches to reading, sometimes called *whole language* approaches. Our use of the term language-based in this chapter is from the perspective of speech-language pathologists. A brief explanation of how we are using the term may be helpful. In recent years there has been a tendency to view the various components of language (e.g., semantics, syntax, phonology, pragmatics, etc.) as interdependent and interactive (Camarata & Schwartz, 1985; Campbell & Shriberg, 1982; Panagos & Prelock, 1982; Panagos, Quine, & Klich, 1979; Paul & Shriberg, 1982; Weiner & Ostrowski, 1979). Therefore, performance on any one component of language would likely benefit from improvement in another component. As a result of this thinking, several authors have suggested that for some children phonological problems may be improved by intervention in a broader language-based context (Christensen & Luckett, 1990; Hoffman, Norris, & Monjure, 1990; Low, Newman, & Ravsten, 1989; Norris & Hoffman, 1990; Tyler, Lewis, Haskill, & Tolbert, 2002). The various approaches described by these authors fall along a continuum of directness within the language-based context. We will present here a few selected intervention techniques to illustrate this type of approach.

Christensen and Luckett (1990) described a procedure which combines the direct pullout-type approach with a less directive in-class approach, referred to as a **whole-class language experience.** In this approach, the speech-language pathologist designs procedures that will enrich the language skills of an entire classroom of children but still allow for the targeting of specific skills for students with phonological disorders. Using this procedure, the child is seen twice each week, once in a traditional session, and once as part of the whole class language experience. Specific skills for students with phonological problems are targeted in the traditional treatment session. Then, responses emphasizing that skill are incorporated into the weekly whole class language experience.

For example, a student who has difficulty producing the s̲ sound may work on s̲ in the initial position of words during a traditional pullout therapy session once each week. Later in the week, the student may be asked questions during the whole-class language experience that require the use of words which contain s̲ in the initial position. Involvement of the classroom teacher in the whole-class language experience is critical. If the teacher clearly understands the goals and objectives for the phonologically impaired child, he or she will be better able to monitor the child's speech during other class activities. The teacher may also be able to help monitor the child's responses during the whole-class activity for IEP purposes. The teacher can be helpful to the SLP in terms of sharing knowledge of classroom management and working together with the SLP to develop whole-class activities that are consistent with the curriculum.

A method in which all work is done in a natural language environment was described by Low and colleagues (1989). They refer to this method as **Communication-Centered Instruction (CCI).** CCI consists of "practicing speech sounds in prosocial communicative activities in which correct responses are reinforced by natural consequences" (Low et al., 1989, p. 217). Because of the emphasis on communication, CCI is ideally suited for group activities. CCI differs from the traditional approaches described earlier in this chapter in that it never focuses on sounds in isolation and does not involve drills on individual words outside of a communicative context. Instead, the target sounds are always in words that are part of longer meaningful and relevant utterances. In this approach then, generalization is not held for a later phase of intervention but rather becomes a part of each session and of the conversations engaged in by the child between sessions. Low and colleagues provide principles for the stimulus conditions, response conditions, and reinforcement in CCI. A review of those principles, presented in Table 4-2, may help you to better understand the communicative nature of this approach.

Hoffman, Norris, and Monjure (1990) described an experimental procedure in which phonological errors were not specifically targeted, but other

Table 4-2 Principles of Stimulus, Response, and Reinforcement in the CCI Method

Stimulus
The practice situation should be similar to the performance situation.
The ultimate goal of treatment is the correct use of the sounds of the language in meaningful communication. Therefore, the practice required to achieve the goal should be in the context of communication with other people for a specific purpose rather than artificial, meaningless drill activities.

Response
The response should:
Include the target phoneme in a communicative utterance.
Target words should be used in meaningful communication and not in activities incorporating the production of lists of words devoid of context.
Be at the level of the child's functioning.
Productions do not have to be completely correct from the start. As long as productions are moving toward a more correct production, they can be accepted.
Be useful for the child and occur frequently in his or her daily communication.
Words that the child uses and has a need for in his or her environment will facilitate learning of the target sounds.
Be powerful in controlling the environment.
The response should be one that achieves a desirable result for the speaker.

Reinforcement
Communicative reinforcement is the fulfillment of the communicative response.
The best way to reinforce communication is to make it successful in terms of accomplishing its purpose. If the child asks for a truck, giving him the truck is more reinforcing than giving him a token or a check on a graph.

Source: Low, G., Newman, P., & Ravsten, M. (1989). Pragmatic considerations in treatment: Communication centered instruction. In N. Creaghead, P. Newman, & W. Secord (Eds.), *Assessment and remediation of articulation and phonological disorders.* Columbus, OH: Merrill.

language components, particularly syntax, were the primary focus. An interesting aspect of this study was that the subjects were two 4-year-old brothers from a set of identical triplets. The brothers exhibited delays in phonology as well as in other language components. One child was enrolled in an intervention program targeting his specific phonological disorder. The second child was enrolled in a whole language program that involved having the child retell stories to a puppet. In this whole language program the child was encouraged through questions and modeling to make revisions, additions, and increases in sentence complexity. No particular attention was paid to the phonological errors of the second child. Results indicated that both children made about the same improvement in phonology, but the child enrolled in the whole language approach made greater improvement in expressive language. This study suggested that reorganization of language on one level, such as syntax, may result in reorganization at other levels, such as phonology.

Intervention programs for children with phonological disorders that do not direct at least some attention to phonology must, however, be viewed with caution. Fey and colleagues (1994) and Tyler and Sandoval (1994) both reported carefully controlled experimental studies in which treatment directed primarily toward other aspects of language had negligible effects on phonology. Tyler (2002) indicated that a language-based approach is not appropriate for all children with phonological impairments and when such an approach is chosen, the clinician must monitor progress closely to ensure its effectiveness. Of course, one of the ways in which an SLP could monitor progress in a language-based approach would be through feedback from classroom teachers.

HOW TEACHERS CAN HELP WITH INDIRECT TREATMENT

From the examples of indirect treatment programs discussed above, it can be seen that meaningful language activities in a natural language environment are at the heart of most such approaches. Because the classroom, playground, and cafeteria are common natural language environments for children, these situations provide ideal intervention opportunities. Some of the following opportunities for intervention involve the presence of the SLP, and some do not.

1. Inform the SLP of the topic, objectives, and materials used in class so that any intervention activities can be designed to fit with the teacher's lesson plan.

2. Provide suggestions to the SLP for classroom management. Remember that most SLPs are more accustomed to working with individuals or small groups. The skill of an experienced teacher in classroom management could be very valuable to the success of indirect intervention programs.

3. Work with the SLP to understand the kinds of communication situations that will facilitate speech goals, and attempt to create such situations in the classroom and other settings.

4. Be flexible in planning activities (e.g., in classes with large numbers of students, the teacher may work with one group during a class period while the SLP works with another group that includes the student[s] with phonological problems).

5. Be able to monitor the child's speech so that appropriate feedback and reinforcement may be provided when the SLP is not present, and so that the SLP may be kept apprised of how well newly learned phonological skills are generalizing to the classroom setting.

CONCLUSION

In this chapter we presented two children with phonological disorders. Many people think that speech like Mary's is "cute," and that children will grow out of it "in their own time." Children who speak like John are often assumed to be cognitively impaired or to have some neurological disorder. Some people believe that it is normal for children of ages 6, 7, 8 years, or older to use "baby talk." All of these assumptions are incorrect. Although they may not produce all sounds correctly in all situations, children should have a fairly good mastery of their phonology by the time they are in kindergarten. Phonological disorders can be associated with delayed language development and problems in educational achievement. Early identification and intervention can reduce the potential for any associated problems.

REFERENCES

Bankson, N., & Byrne, M. (1962). The relationship between missing teeth and selected consonant sounds. *Journal of Speech and Hearing Disorders, 24,* 341–348.

Barlow, J., & Gierut, J. (2002). Minimal pair approaches to phonological remediation. *Seminars in Speech and Language, 23,* 57–68.

Bernthal, J., & Bankson, N. (2004). *Articulation and phonological disorders* (5th ed.). Boston: Allyn and Bacon.

Boshart, C. A. (2004). *Practical procedures to generate speech development* [Seminar series]. Temecula, CA: Speech Dynamics.

Bryant, B., & Bryant, D. (1983). *Test of articulation performance-diagnostic.* Austin, TX: Pro-Ed.

Camarata, S., & Schwartz, R. (1985). Production of object words and action words: Evidence for a relationship between phonology and semantics. *Journal of Speech and Hearing Research, 28,* 323–330.

Campbell, T., & Shriberg, L. (1982). Associations among pragmatic functions, linguistic stress and natural phonological processes in speech-delayed children. *Journal of Speech and Hearing Research, 25,* 547–553.

Carter, E. T., & Buck, M. W. (1958). Prognostic testing for functional articulation disorders among children in the first grade. *Journal of Speech and Hearing Disorders, 23,* 124–133.

Christensen, S., & Luckett, C. (1990). Getting into the classroom and making it work. *Language, Speech and Hearing Services in Schools, 21,* 110–113.

Daniloff, R. G., & Moll, K. L. (1968). Coarticulation of lip rounding. *Journal of Speech and Hearing Research, 11,* 707–721.

Davis, B. L., Jakielski, K. J., & Marquardt, T. M. (1998). Developmental apraxia of speech: Determiners of differential diagnosis. *Clinical Linguistics and Phonetics, 12*(43), 25–45.

Dodd, B. (1976). A matched comparison of the phonological systems of mental age matched, normal, severely sub-normal, and Down's disorders. *British Journal of Communication Disorders, 11,* 27–42.

DuBoise, E., & Bernthal, J. (1978). A comparison of three methods for obtaining articulatory responses. *Journal of Speech and Hearing Disorders, 43,* 295–305.

Faircloth, M., & Faircloth, S. (1970). An analysis of the articulatory behavior of a speech-defective child in connected speech and in isolated-word responses. *Journal of Speech and Hearing Disorders, 35,* 51–61.

Felsenfeld, S., McGue, M., & Broen, P. (1995). Familial aggregation of phonological disorders: Results from a 28-year follow-up. *Journal of Speech and Hearing Research, 38,* 1091–1107.

Fey, M., Cleave, P., Ravida, A., Long, S., Dejmal, A., & Easton, D. (1994). Effects of grammar facilitation on the phonological performance of children with speech and language impairments. *Journal of Speech and Hearing Research, 37,* 594–607.

Forrest, K. (2002). Are oral-motor exercises useful in the treatment of phonological/articulatory disorders? *Seminars in Speech and Language, 23,* 15–26.

Fudala, J. B. (2001). *Arizona articulation proficiency scale* (3rd rev.). Los Angeles: Western Psychological Services.

Goldman, R., & Fristoe, M. (2000). *Goldman-Fristoe test of articulation* (2nd ed.). Circle Pines, MN: American Guidance Service.

Haynes, W., Haynes, M., & Jackson, J. (1982). The effects of phonetic context and linguistic complexity on /s/ misarticulation in children. *Journal of Communication Disorders, 15,* 287–297.

Hodson, B. W. (2004). Hodson assessment of phonological patterns (3rd ed.). Austin, TX: Pro-Ed.

Hoffman, P., Norris, J., & Monjure, J. (1990). Comparison of process targeting and whole language treatments for phonologically delayed preschool children. *Language, Speech and Hearing Services in Schools, 21,* 102–109.

Kahn, L., & Lewis, N. (2002). *Kahn-Lewis phonological analysis* (2nd ed.). Circle Pines, MN: American Guidance Service.

Klein, E. S. (1996). *Clinical phonology: Assessment and treatment of articulation disorders in children and adults.* San Diego, CA: Singular.

Kresheck, J., & Sokolofsky, G. (1972). Imitative and spontaneous articulatory assessment of four-year-old children. *Journal of Speech and Hearing Research, 15,* 729–732.

Lippke, B., Dickey, S., Selmar, J., & Soder, A. (1997). *Photo articulation test* (3rd ed.). Austin, TX: Pro-Ed.

Long, S. (2004). *Computerized profiling.* Retrieved from www.computerizedprofiling.org

Low, G., Newman, P., & Ravsten, M. (1989). Pragmatic considerations in treatment: Communication centered instruction. In N. Creaghead, P. Newman, & W. Secord (Eds.),

Assessment and remediation of articulation and phonological disorders. Columbus, OH: Merrill.

Mackay, L., & Hodson, B. (1982). Phonological process identification of misarticulation of mentally retarded children. *Journal of Communication Disorders, 12,* 243–250.

McDonald, E. T. (1964). *A deep test of articulation.* Pittsburgh, PA: Stanwix House.

Moran, M. J., Money, S., & Leonard, D. (1984). Phonological process analysis of the speech of mentally retarded adults. *American Journal of Mental Deficiency, 89,* 304–306.

Mowrer, D. (1971). Transfer of training in articulation therapy. *Journal of Speech and Hearing Disorders, 36,* 427–446.

National Institute on Deafness and Other Communication Disorders (NIDCD) Web site. Retrieved 2004 from http://www.nidcd.nih.gov

Norris, J., & Hoffman, P. (1990). Language intervention within naturalistic environments. *Language, Speech and Hearing Services in Schools, 21,* 72–84.

Panagos, J., & Prelock, P. (1982). Phonological constraints on the sentence productions of language-disordered children. *Journal of Speech and Hearing Research, 25,* 171–177.

Panagos, J., Quine, H., & Klich, R. (1979). Syntactic and phonological influences in children's articulations. *Journal of Speech and Hearing Research, 22,* 841–848.

Paul, R., & Shriberg, L. (1982). Associations between phonology and syntax in speech-delayed children. *Journal of Speech and Hearing Research, 25,* 536–547.

Pena-Brooks, A., & Hegde, M. N. (2000). *Assessment and treatment of articulation and phonological disorders in children.* Austin, TX: Pro-Ed.

Powers, M. J. (1971). Clinical and educational procedures in functional disorders of articulation. In L. Travis (Ed.), *Handbook of speech pathology and audiology.* Englewood Cliffs, NJ: Prentice-Hall.

Schmauch, V., Panagos, J., & Klich, R. (1978). Syntax influences and accuracy of consonant production in language disordered children. *Journal of Communication Disorders, 11,* 315–323.

Secord, W. (1981). *C-PAC: Clinical probes of articulation consistency.* Columbus, OH: Merrill.

Secord, W., & Donohue, J. (2002). *Clinical assessment of articulation and phonology.* Greenville, SC: Super Duper.

Shriberg, L. D. (1980). Developmental phonological disorders. In T. Hixon, L. Shriberg, & J. Saxman (Eds.), *Introduction to communication disorders.* Englewood Cliffs, NJ: Prentice-Hall.

Shriberg, L., & Kwiatkowski, J. (1980). *Natural process analysis.* New York: Wiley.

Smith, M. W., & Ainsworth, S. (1967). The effect of three types of stimulation on articulatory responses of speech defective children. *Journal of Speech and Hearing Research, 10,* 333–338.

Snow, K. (1961). Articulation proficiency in relation to certain dental abnormalities. *Journal of Speech and Hearing Disorders, 26,* 209–212.

Snow, J., & Milisen, R. (1954). The influence of oral versus pictorial representation upon articulation testing results. *Journal of Speech and Hearing Disorders, 4,* monograph supplement, 29–36.

Stoel-Gammon, C., & Dunn, C. (1985). *Normal and disordered phonology in children.* Austin, TX: Pro-Ed.

Stoel-Gammon, C., Stone-Goldman, J., & Glaspey, A. (2002). Pattern-based approaches to phonological therapy. *Seminars in Speech and Language, 23,* 3–13.

Taylor, O. (1986). Language differences. In G. Shames & E. Wiig (Eds.), *Human communication disorders* (2nd ed.). Columbus, OH: Merrill.

Tyler, A. (2002). Language-based intervention for phonological disorders. *Seminars in Speech and Language, 23,* 69–81.

Tyler, A., Lewis, K., Haskill, A., & Tolbert, L. (2002). Efficacy and cross-domain effects of a morphosyntax and a phonology intervention. *Language, Speech and Hearing Services in Schools, 33,* 52–66.

Tyler, A., & Sandoval, K. (1994). Preschoolers with phonological and language disorders: Treating different linguistic domains. *Language, Speech and Hearing Services in Schools, 25*, 215–234.

Van Riper, C., & Emerick, L. (1984). *Speech correction: An introduction to speech pathology and audiology* (7th ed.). Englewood Cliffs, NJ: Prentice-Hall.

Weiss, C., Gordon, M., & Lillywhite, H. (1987). *Clinical management of articulatory and phonologic disorders* (2nd ed.). Baltimore: Williams and Wilkins.

Weiner, F. (1981). Treatment of phonological disability using the method of meaningful minimal contrast: Two case studies. *Journal of Speech and Hearing Disorders, 46*, 97–103.

Weiner, F., & Bankson, N. (1978). Teaching features. *Language, Speech and Hearing Services in the Schools, 9*, 29–34.

Weiner, F., & Ostrowski, A. (1979). Effects of listener uncertainty on articulation inconsistency. *Journal of Speech and Hearing Disorders, 44*, 487–493.

Wilson, F. (1966). Efficacy of speech therapy with educable mentally retarded children. *Journal of Speech and Hearing Research, 9*, 423–433.

Winitz, H. (1975). *From syllable to conversation*. Baltimore: University Park Press.

TERMS TO KNOW

ankyloglossia
apraxia of speech
articulation
auditory stimulation
central lisp
coarticulation
communication-centered instruction (CCI)
conceptualization
context generalization
contextual tests
coarticulation
developmental apraxia of speech (DAS)
diagnostic evaluation
distortion
dysarthria
ear training
establishment stage
final position
functional disorder
generalization stage
hearing impairment
initial position
lateral lisp
linguistic unit generalization
lisp
macroglossia

maintenance stage
malocclusion
medial position
metathetic errors
microglossia
minimal pairs
negative practice
omission
organic disorder
pattern analyses
phonetic context
phonetic environment
phonetic placement
phonological
position generalization
screening test
sibilant
situation generalization
sound and feature generalization
speech notebook
speech sound inventories
substitution
successive approximation
tongue thrust
whole-class language experience

STUDY QUESTIONS

1. Discuss the relationship between phonological disorders and each of the following:

   intelligence   language development
   reading   malocclusion
   spelling   siblings

2. Briefly describe the differences between a speech sound inventory, a deep test, and a pattern analysis.

3. Identify the three major phases of therapy for phonological disorders, describe the goals of each phase, and provide specific suggestions as to what teachers can do to support each phase of therapy.

4. Identify and provide examples of the five types of generalization that are of concern in the treatment of phonological disorders.

5. Discuss specific activities that a classroom teacher can use to assist in communication-centered treatment for a student with a phonological disorder.

chapter *five*

Children with Limited Language

EPISODE 1

Arnold Stephens was 3-years-old and he could not talk. One might assume that this would make his existence quite difficult, but actually, Arnold's life was fairly uncomplicated. He had no consistent playmates, received the full attention of his parents, and was catered to around the clock. At noon, soup and sandwiches magically appeared on the kitchen table. At 3:00 P.M., it was "juice time" and mother opened the refrigerator and poured juice into his Mickey Mouse cup. Arnold rarely had to ask for anything; it was always there, because his needs were anticipated. After all, he couldn't talk, although his parents desperately wanted him to. Mom and Dad often tried to make Arnold talk by encouraging him to imitate. He watched these adults with fascination, and a certain sense of amusement, but he did not imitate. One time the parents went too far and tried to get Arnold to imitate "juice." They said he couldn't have the drink unless he tried to say the word. Arnold threw a tantrum that registered about a seven on the Richter scale, and the parents knew never to do *that* again. As time went by the mother talked less and less to Arnold. After all, if no one answers, you tend to give up. Arnold's favorite activity was to play outside in the fenced backyard in his sandbox. One day on a talk show, Mrs. Stephens learned that the local public school system would be providing a preschool program for 3- to 5-year-old children with disabilities (including speech and language). She was elated that finally someone was going to do something about Arnold's problem.

EPISODE 2

Max Metcalf could only produce utterances consisting of a single word. This meant that he could make simple requests quite efficiently. When he wanted some milk he could say "milk" and it would be provided. But, when Max wanted to explain something more complicated, it was quite difficult to communicate this in a few single words. For instance, one time his family was at the mall and Max wanted to go home. He did not have the words to explain this to his mother. Ultimately, he became so frustrated that he threw himself onto the carpet in the wide, central hallway of the mall and propelled himself around in a small circle, screaming like one of the Three Stooges used to do in the movies. Max's mom hated his tantrums, especially when they occurred in public, so she scooped him up and the family terminated their shopping. The mother always felt guilty giving in to these behavioral displays, which were quite frequent both at home and in public, but sometimes it was the only way to make it through the day. The parents spent many hours arguing about Max and how to deal with his lack of communication and behavior problems, because it was having a negative impact on both the child and the family.

BACKGROUND INFORMATION

Episode 1 illustrates several interesting aspects about some children with **limited language**. It could just as easily have been about a special education teacher with a child in the classroom who did not talk, or a kindergarten teacher who had a nonverbal child in the classroom for part of each day. The tendencies are the same; if a child does not talk, we often tend to address less language to that child and to anticipate his or her needs. We sometimes do these things because we know the child cannot communicate effectively in gestures or words. This is especially true if the teacher is responsible for many other children in the same room or if a parent has several children in the family to care for.

One important point to realize about children with limited language is that their problem often involves a number of participants. Parents, teachers, siblings, and peers become unwitting confederates and integral parts of the disorder. In the case of Arnold Stephens, he could not talk, and his parents learned to lower their expectations for communication. He could not ask for things, so people anticipated his needs and provided items before they were even requested. Life became a series of episodes that almost automatically unfolded without a real need to communicate. Soon, a comfortable medium was reached in which the child's life ran effectively without much communication. Does this mean that parents and teachers *caused* the child's language delay? Certainly not. The reactions of the parents and teachers are most likely the *result* of the child's language delay and not the cause. But these reactions do serve to *maintain* the problem.

Episode 2 illustrates another common scenario involving children with language disorders. In this situation, unlike the one with Arnold Stephens, life is *not* going along smoothly for the child and his parents. In fact, there is frustration, guilt, and behavior problems. Baltaxe (2001) reported that around 50% of children with communication disorders exhibit significant behavior problems. Some authorities attribute at least a portion of these difficulties to the communication disorder itself. When a child cannot communicate needs with gestures or language, acting out behaviorally is often quite effective, as illustrated in episode 2. Just as in episode 1, however, people in Max's environment are playing a role in his disorder by reinforcing tantrums as an effective method of communication. Fortunately, most studies generally support the finding that as children learn to communicate more effectively, behavior problems tend to decrease (Silverman, 1989).

Another curious aspect about dealing with limited-language children is that some parents and teachers may expect the speech-language pathologist (SLP) to remediate the problem single-handedly, shrouded in a small treatment room away from all legitimate needs to communicate in daily life. If the SLP does try to work with the child in isolation, situations that mimic real activities are constructed, and it is hoped that these artificial circumstances will generalize to the complex world of the classroom and home. An illogical and impossible task, you say? We agree!

The child with no language or limited language may not learn to communicate effectively unless at some point, the treatment is conducted in the real world, with real people in legitimate interactions. Throughout the day, good language models must be provided and cues must be given at opportune times so the child can produce target utterances. The child's life must be made a little more difficult by people failing to anticipate his needs and requiring the best communicative attempt the child is capable of producing during interactions. The reader can already see that we are going to push very hard in this chapter to make the case that *the child with limited language is part of a working system of people and events.* The implication of this is that assessment and treatment *must* include as much of the child's natural system as possible. This is not to say that individual treatment is not necessary, because it certainly is in many cases. However, as stated in Chapter 1, at some point a team approach is necessary if the child has any hope of generalizing communication into natural environments. Teachers and parents should *expect* the SLP to encourage their involvement in both assessment and treatment because of the vast amount of information they possess and the significant number of hours they spend with the child.

Chapter 3 established that language is the system of rules and symbols that we use to communicate. It is rather like language is the music, and speech is the instrument that produces the song. Without the music, you would have just random notes played by the instrument. So, children must learn word meanings and how to combine words to make their needs known to others in the environment. In the space of only 3 to 4 years, a normal child must learn both the language and how to produce it intelligibly for communication. The typical child often receives little direct help in acquiring language, and sometimes even develops language in spite of a good deal of interference.

Two Major Divisions of Language Impairment

Child language disorders may be divided, for our purposes, into two major groups that represent children who are in two different phases of linguistic development. Dividing children by language level rather than by etiology or disorder makes understanding language impairment a bit easier and has been commonly done in textbooks on the subject (Haynes & Pindzola, 2004; Paul, 2001). The first group of children exhibits primitive communication most often seen in the beginning stages of language development. The communication of these children may range from exclusive use of gestures to the possible combination of 2 to 3 words in an utterance. Throughout this chapter we will refer to these children as having "limited language." Notice that we have not mentioned a child's chronological age as a requirement for having limited language. This is because a child, or an adult for that matter, can be communicating at this level regardless of age. A severely cognitively impaired person can be a single-word or early multiword communicator for an entire lifetime.

The second group of children with language disorders communicates in full sentences and may very well be capable of constructing utterances that are very long and complex. However, these children may exhibit more subtle disorders of language involving use of word endings, construction of certain complex sentences, or comprehension of elaborate utterances. These children often have difficulty making their language appropriate for the variety of changing social and educational circumstances in daily life. In the present text, we will refer to this second group of children as "syntax-level" youngsters. The present chapter deals with children who have "limited language"; youngsters talking at the sentence level will be discussed in Chapter 6.

Who Encounters Students with Limited Language?

This textbook is intended for teachers in regular as well as special education classrooms. With the advent of **PL 99-457** the public school systems of America were required to provide services for children with disabilities between the ages of 3 and 5 years. Early childhood special education teachers will have the primary responsibility for dealing with this population of children and perhaps will benefit the most from this particular chapter. The bulk of the preschool children seen by the early childhood special education teacher will have language delays.

The literature is clear on the point that, regardless of the category in which a child is placed (e.g., autism spectrum disorders, cerebral palsy, cleft palate, developmentally delayed, hearing impaired, visually, or cognitively impaired) a significant deficit *will* be communication (Haynes & Pindzola, 2004). Regardless of what kind of biological, behavioral, or psychological disorder a child has, language development always seems to be one of the primary areas affected. This is because, as mentioned in Chapter 3, language depends on a firm foundation of adequate neurological, motor, cognitive, social, and sensory development. If *any* of these areas are affected, language will be delayed. This is especially true in the high-risk populations of children who begin their lives with poor nutrition, low birth weight, early respiratory distress, abusive home environments, or a wide variety of "syndromes" (Fox, Long & Langlois, 1988; Hubatch, Johnson, Kistler, Burns, & Moneka, 1985; Paul, 2001). Thus, whatever handicapping condition makes a 3- to 5-year-old child developmentally delayed, we can be certain that communication will probably be a major goal on the individualized educational program (IEP). Early childhood special education teachers need to know about the kinds of language impairments observed in the preschool population, about the speech-language pathologist's functions as a team member in assessment and treatment, and about the way(s) to make a contribution to the intervention process during day-to-day classroom interactions. This also applies to kindergarten teachers and those who teach developmental kindergarten or prekindergarten classes.

Those regular classroom teachers who are preparing to deal with normally developing children may be reading this and saying to themselves, "This doesn't apply to me." However, as we indicated in an earlier chapter, the current trend is toward more *inclusion* of children with disabilities in the normal classroom, not *exclusion*. The movement toward inclusion seems to be gaining momentum among professionals, and we should not expect it to diminish any time soon; on the contrary, we should anticipate *increased* integration of children with disabilities into classroom environments. The idea of incorporating children with disabilities into typical classrooms is consistently supported by legal decisions going back three decades. It is not unusual for a visitor to a "normal classroom" to see children with electronic communicators, wheelchairs, auditory trainers, or a child with an aide to assist him or her in basic daily tasks. Even teachers who conduct classes in music, physical education, or art will teach children with disabilities who are integrated into regular classrooms for all or part of their day. All of these regular education teachers, as mentioned in Chapter 1, *will* be asked to become part of the intervention team.

The Symptoms Seen in Children with Limited Language

Children with limited language comprise three basic subgroups that are based on the length of utterance in their verbal communication. First, there are **nonverbal communicators** who, by definition, are not using verbal language. They may be communicating with gestures or a combination of gesture and vocalization; however, they never say identifiable words. It should also be noted that the nonverbal child is not a child with an articulation disorder (see Chapter 4) who *has* language and is just unintelligible due to problems with sound production. Nonverbal children are nonverbal because they *have* no words. It is important to emphasize that these children may be *nonverbal*, but they are by no means *noncommunicative*. As stated above, they may be quite adept at communicating their needs through a combination of gestures and/or vocalizations. Many of these children understand some language, but just cannot produce it.

The second subgroup of limited-language children is those youngsters who speak primarily in 1-word utterances. These are called **single-word communicators**, and they seem to be unable to produce word combinations. Thus, a single-word communicator may say "up" when trying to get the mother to lift him, "drink," when requesting a drink, or "horsie" when the car passes a pasture filled with horses. The parents of single-word communicators will attest to the fact that their child talks in 1-word utterances. When asked if the child has ever produced a 2-word combination, the parents will probably say "no." A child communicating at the single-word level is not necessarily using words produced verbally. The child can be on the single-word level if he or she is using some sort of **alternative/augmentative communication (AAC)** device such as a communication board or electronic communicator. The point here is that most communications may be limited to the single-word level regardless of how the words are produced. We will discuss AAC in more detail in Chapter 12.

The third subgroup of limited-language children is **early multiword communicators**. They are called early multiword communicators because they are producing the most primitive and earliest developing combinations of words that have been reported in the language development literature. For instance, an early multiword communicator may produce utterances such as "more milk," "daddy run," "mommy shoe," "juice allgone," "big doggie," "eat more cracker," "mommy fix car," "me drink more milk," "daddy garage." Note that some of these verbalizations are 2 words in length and some are 3 and 4. Another item to notice is that most of the "little words" used in adult sentences such as *is*, *the*, *a*, and *in* are missing. Also omitted are word endings such as *-ing* and *-ed*. Just as children who use AAC devices can be at the single-word level as described above, they can also be producing early multiword combinations. Thus, these utterances do not have to be produced verbally, but can be produced by an AAC device.

As you can see, one way to characterize the primary "symptoms" seen in children with limited language is to describe the type of communication they produce. Note that we have not mentioned age, syndromes, or diagnostic labels here. A nonverbal client can be a preschooler, a school-age child, an adolescent, or even an adult. The same goes for single-word and early multiword clients. Children representing all diagnostic labels (e.g., mental retardation, autism, fragile X syndrome, hearing impairment, etc.) can be performing at any level of limited language described above. The task of the speech-language pathologist is to focus on and describe the communication of any child in assessment, and move that child to the next higher level in treatment.

Children with Limited Language Who Have Different Labels

Some readers may be curious as to why we have not organized the language disorders section of this book by the type of disability a child represents. For example, we could have had a chapter on autism, one on mental retardation, and one on learning disabilities. One reason we did not organize the text in this manner is that the book is about communication disorders and not about the nature of these various conditions. There are some other important reasons as well. As most of you know, people in psychology and education have a history of labeling children as representing certain types of disorders. For instance, a child with an IQ below 70 may have formerly been labeled as *mentally retarded*. This term has fallen out of favor and is gradually being replaced by *cognitively impaired* or some other term, depending on geographical and professional preferences. There are many labels from which to choose, and interestingly many children have several of them (e.g. a single child could be labeled *cognitively impaired, hearing impaired*, and *language delayed*). Also, professionals may not always agree on a particular label for a certain child. Unfortunately, labeling is not yet an exact science. As we stated earlier, children with a variety of labels will have limited language. These children may or may not exhibit delays in domains other than communication such as motor skills, self-help abilities, social skills, or intelligence. In fact, a child with limited language may be perfectly normal in all of these abilities with communication as the primary developmental deficiency. These children are sometimes called **specifically language impaired (SLI)** (Watkins & Rice, 1994). Of course, language delay is seen in almost every type of condition affecting young children, including: cognitive impairment, developmental delay, autism, hearing impairment, cleft palate, cerebral palsy, high-risk populations (due to respiratory distress or low birth weight), and other syndromes. The interesting point, however, is that there are no particular types of language symptoms associated with various congenital or developmental conditions in children that significantly differentiate one group from another. In other words, there is no specific profile of language errors associated exclusively with a particular population. This in part is due to the heterogeneity of the disorders found in a particular diagnostic group. For example, children with autism can range from those with severe cognitive and linguistic disabilities involved, to those with complex language and literacy abilities. The diagnostic label of *autism* tells us very little in terms of what to expect with regard to language. Also, if you group children with different diagnostic labels by their language level (e.g., nonverbal, single-word, early multiword, syntax-level) you will probably find that the types of language errors they make are similar whether they are children who are autistic, mentally retarded, hearing impaired, learning disabled, or SLI. There certainly may be big differences in the way these groups respond to intervention or perhaps in the ways tests are administered to them, but the specific deficiencies in communication are often far more similar than different. The implication here is that when the SLP evaluates a child the focus is on *communication ability and the level of language development attained by the child,* as opposed to what label he or she has been given. The other implication is that regardless of label, children who have language disorders are treated using the same basic set of techniques. So, when a teacher is trying to help a child with autism, mental retardation, or specific language impairment learn communication skills, she will use the same basic techniques for all of these children. The fact that you will not have to learn many different techniques to help children with communication in your classroom should be *good news* for teachers.

Why Not Have a Chapter for Each Type of Language Disorder? Autism As a Case Example

Earlier we made the point of saying that certain etiological groups or labels of children who have language disorders are not particularly useful in assessment and treatment. Even though we make this statement, some people still seem to be "hung up" on labels for children with language disorders. For instance, in the past, readers of this textbook and some reviewers of new editions have asked why we do not have a major section or a whole chapter on autism spectrum disorders. Others have expressed concern about the lack of individual chapters on language disorders in children with mental retardation, hearing impairment, psychological disorders, and all sorts of various "syndromes" that affect language. However, we feel it is important to remember that terms such as autism, mental retardation, hearing impairment, and learning disability are not descriptions of language disorder. These terms refer to much broader conditions with many developmental domains that can be potentially affected, but in which language impairment may play a large or small role. A focus on a generic "label" such as autism or mental retardation says little about language and communication challenges for a particular child. It is only when we specifically examine communication that we can develop individual goals for a child with any condition. The challenges of the SLP and teacher in dealing with a child who has autism epitomizes why a particular label is not necessarily helpful. While we are using autism as a case example for purposes of this chapter, the same issues can be illustrated with any diagnostic group. Here is the scenario. You are a first-grade teacher, and a new child has transferred from another school system into your classroom. You have not yet met this new addition to your classroom, but your special education coordinator has received some paperwork from the child's old school system. According to the previous IEP, the student has been diagnosed with autism. In many cases, even though it may seem redundant, your school will want to reassess the child to determine if he meets eligibility criteria for your school system and determine if the former IEP goals are appropriate. Unfortunately, assessment methods and eligibility criteria vary considerably from state to state, and in some cases from system to system. So, how helpful is the fact that the child has been diagnosed with autism?

Do We Know What to Expect?

Actually, we do not know much at all if we look at the diagnosis. We have already stated that a child with autism can vary significantly in terms of cognitive, social, emotional, behavioral, and linguistic skills. If there ever was a disorder that exemplifies the BACIS of communication development, autism is very high on the list. We know that children with autism vary considerably in cognitive ability ranging from significant mental retardation to high-level children with Asperger's syndrome who are capable of abstract thought, complex language, and literacy skills. Thus, the diagnosis of autism tells us nothing about the child's cognitive status. Socially, children with autism vary from those who will not even make eye contact with others to those who frequently demonstrate affection by hugging and who enjoy the company of others. Some children with autism exhibit frequent negative emotion while others seem devoid of emotional reactions. Behavioral symptoms are highly variable in children with autism and can include self-stimulation, self-injury, obsession, insistence on sameness, vestibular stimulation (spinning), and many other manifestations. The particular pattern exhibited by an individual student, however, is highly variable across children. Many children with autism seem similar in some respects, yet each one is quite different. Regarding language symptoms, a child with autism can be communicating with gestures, single words, early word combinations, simple sentences, or complex sentences. Some children with autism who are higher level can read and write. So, what have the teacher and the SLP learned from the fact that this new student has autism? The answer is very little. This student can come in talking and carrying his or her favorite reading book, or he or she could require assistance in every aspect of activities in the normal classroom.

Does Knowledge of the Diagnosis Help Us to Design Our Assessment?

The answer is probably not. It would be handy if there was a particular test of autism that focused on communication skill, but there is no such thing that is universally accepted. Basically, the IEP team will have to do assessments of the child and focus on individual areas of cognition, social interaction, temperament, behavior, and language. We have already said that a child with autism can have differing strengths and concerns in all areas and there is no profile that we should expect. Speaking for the SLP, the assessment will focus on play, **communicative intent**, social interaction, analysis of language comprehension, inventory of phonology, gestural communication, and language production among other things. The only way to find out how a child communicates is to focus on communication, not the label. So when someone tells the SLP that a child has a particular condition, it always goes back to analyzing how the child communicates. This is often true whether the child has been diagnosed with autism, mental retardation, learning disabilities, hearing impairment, or any other syndrome. We have to inventory the strengths and limitations of expressive and receptive communication.

Does Knowledge of the Diagnosis Tell Us Which Therapy Technique to Use?

This would only be true if there was a specific type of treatment that just applied to autism. Unfortunately, there is no single treatment that has been universally effective with children diagnosed as autistic. For example, you will see some children with autism in your classroom who are being treated by the SLP and school psychologist using highly behavioral techniques applied intensively to increase language and alter specific behaviors. On the other hand, some approaches focus on the BACIS of communication and incorporate most of the child's goals in play, social interaction, and functional communication. Finally, you will see other children with autism who are using some sort of nonverbal response mode such as sign language, communication boards, electronic communicators, and the Picture Exchange Communication System (PECS). The point is that the diagnosis of autism does not dictate the type of treatment a child receives. What dictates the treatment mode is a thorough assessment, trial therapy to determine if goals can be accomplished, and altering the treatment approach if the child is not making progress using a particular regime.

So, why do we not have separate chapters on the different general conditions that may result in language disorder? The answer is that a focus on the general condition does not tell us much about the nature of the communication disorder we are likely to see, and does not necessarily have implications for assessment or the type of treatment that will be prescribed.

ASSESSMENT ISSUES

Evaluation of Children with Limited-Language Abilities

A very important point to make at the outset of discussing the assessment of a child with limited language is the necessity of a multidisciplinary evaluation. In almost every case, the child with limited language is at high risk for a wide variety of developmental disabilities. Because of the complexity in making a correct diagnosis, the involvement of a variety of professionals from audiology, the field of communication disorders, education, psychology, special education, and a variety of other allied health disciplines is required. The first thing to understand about evaluation of the child with limited language is that no single professional should ever do it alone. This is not only against federal laws, but it is at best foolhardy, and at worst unethical. When the speech-language pathologist is faced with a child who has limited language abilities, regardless of the youngster's chronological age, a primary consideration is always to ask the question *why*. If a child is 4-years-old and should be speaking in 4-word utterances but is still a non-verbal communicator, there must be some reason for this. If a child is 3-years-old and still communicating in single-word utterances when the mean length of utterance should be near three words, we must be curious about what has happened to the child. Unfortunately, we are not always able to answer the question of why a child has not developed normally with regard to communication. It is the ethical responsibility of the SLP, however, to at least examine potential reasons for the language delay. In examining these potential reasons for language impairment, we often *do* find at least a partial explanation for the child's communication problem. But, where would we look? What abilities would possibly be involved if a child's linguistic framework is inadequate, distorted, or nonexistent? As we have stated previously in Chapter 3, the linguistic framework is built on the foundation of **BACIS**, and it is possible that the language is impaired because of problems with these building blocks.

Thus, the SLP will examine in detail, the *biological* bases of language, the *access* to a good language model, the *cognitive* abilities related to language, the presence of communicative *intent*, and the child's *social* behaviors. If any of these areas shows a deficit, then we might begin to understand why a child has a language impairment. It is important for the teacher to know that in the assessment of these building blocks of language, there are precious few standardized tests. The SLP must, therefore, rely on a combination of formal and informal assessment measures if information relevant to treatment is to be gathered. There is no test for access to a good language model, communicative intent, social behavior, or many cognitive and biological bases of language. Much of what the SLP will want to do involves observation of relevant play and interactions in natural settings such as the classroom and home. Recent research has confirmed that variables such as the following are predictive of success in language development over a period of months in prelinguistic children (Calandrella & Wilcox, 2000):

- Language comprehension ability
- Level of play development
- Use of sounds in vocalizing
- Evidence of an intent to regulate adult behavior or attention
- Use of communicative gestures

Thus, as a classroom teacher, you should be aware that the SLP will appreciate spending a significant amount of observation time, and perhaps interaction time, in your classroom to develop treatment goals for the child with limited language. Any cooperation that you can give in terms of allowing these observations and providing the SLP with the benefit of *your own* longstanding observations will be greatly appreciated. We will briefly profile some assessment examples in each area below.

Biological

The assessment of the biological prerequisites to language is very important and includes several areas.

Sensory Abilities

One of the first things that the SLP will require in the evaluation of a child with limited language is an audiometric (hearing) evaluation. It is very important to determine if the child can hear adequately because it is *essential* to early language development. Also, performance in the assessment and treatment processes depends upon the child being able to hear language presented by the teachers, parents, and other team members. If the child does have a significant hearing loss, some sort of amplification such as a hearing aid or FM system may be recommended. In this case, the classroom teacher will want to become familiar with some information on types of hearing loss and amplification (see Chapter 10). Children with significant visual problems may need to be examined by an ophthalmologist and fitted with corrective lenses.

Motor Abilities and Neurological Status

If the child appears to have significant motor difficulties, it may be recommended that a neurologist be contacted for a consultation. A physical therapist may also be consulted regarding improvement of motor skills, and an occupational therapist may give input about adapting various objects (e.g., spoons, pencils, clothing) so the child will have less difficulty in the activities of daily living. Chapter 12 deals with communication disorders that have specific neurological causes.

Anatomical Structure

In most cases, children with significant anatomical problems already will have been treated surgically or with some sort of prosthetic device by the time they are seen in the school setting. If, however, an anatomical problem is discovered that may relate to speech and language production, this must be attended to if at all possible. Chapter 11 discusses craniofacial anomalies and communication disorders. One can see that in the biological area, the SLP is interested in determining if the mechanisms used for speech and language are operating at their highest level. Without adequate biological support, the language framework will not develop appropriately.

Access to a Language Model

One of the most important aspects of learning language is the presence of a model or models that present examples of communication in relevant situations. The child listens to these models and incorporates them into the developing language system. The major way that the SLP gains insight into the language model is to observe the caretaker–child interaction. This may be done by placing the parent and child in a playroom and taking note of the types of communication modeled during play. Appendix A lists important social and linguistic characteristics of the language model presented to a child and is based on hundreds of studies of interactions of parents and normally developing children. In the school setting, the SLP is also interested in the language presented to the child by the teacher and others in the classroom setting. Often the SLP will ask to sit in the classroom and observe the language-limited child, the teacher, aides, and other children in the classroom to determine the frequency, type, and quality of interactions. Clinical observations and recent research have shown that some classroom environments are not particularly facilitative of interactions involving children with communication impairments. Specifically, Rhyner, Lehr, and Pudlas (1990, p. 95) found the following:

> Teachers did not provide a responsive classroom communicative environment for young, developmentally delayed children in either child-directed or teacher-directed activities. In fact, the teachers often were either nonresponsive or responsive in a limited way to the children's attempts to initiate communicative interactions in both activities. There were few instances in which the teacher contingently responded to the child's communicative initiations in ways that led to maintenance of the interactions.

These results are especially interesting as the teachers involved in the research had stated that their specific intent during interactions was to "facilitate the children's communication and language learning." Prospective teachers reading the present book should not view this as an indictment of *all* teachers who deal with language-impaired children. There certainly are many teachers who *do* provide good environments for communication development. The point here is that in most cases the SLP simply does not know what kind of classroom environment a particular language-impaired child is experiencing. We also realize that it is extremely difficult to remember the needs of a few language-impaired children when the teacher has 18 or so other children whose communication abilities are within normal limits. Most children in a classroom covet attention and verbal interaction, and it is difficult to take the extra time needed to provide specialized stimulation to a child with a communication impairment. An important part of the assessment process for children with limited language is a thorough evaluation of the classroom communication environment and an analysis of communicative demands of the curriculum. Teachers also vary considerably in their speech rate, language complexity, use of figurative language, and frequency of interaction with specific students. This will let the SLP know if a particular child is exposed to the type of language models needed for development or not. If more or different types of models are required, the SLP can either train the teachers and aides to provide such cues during normal interactions or the SLP can arrange specific times to enter the classroom and provide increased models during certain prescribed activities suggested through collaboration with the teacher.

Another important provider of a language model is the parent. A routine part of assessing a child with a language disorder is to examine caretaker–child interaction strategies during free play and other activities (Haynes & Pindzola, 2004). A popular parent–child literacy activity is joint book reading, and the SLP may want to observe parents and children sharing books together to see the types of **language stimulation** or **modeling** provided by the parent (Kaderavek & Sulzby, 1998; Rabidoux & Macdonald, 2000).

Cognitive Ability

As we stated previously, language rests on a cognitive base. Thus, children who are diagnosed as cognitively impaired are at risk for language delay. It is probable that the cognitive deficits are the cause of the language problem in such youngsters. If the child with limited language is nonverbal, whether of normal or below normal intelligence, the SLP will attempt to examine the cognitive abilities most associated with language development. There are several ways to gain insight into a child's cognitive abilities associated with language. First, the SLP may simply want to watch the child play. We mentioned in an earlier chapter that children with cognitive deficits often play in a very primitive manner. For instance, they may throw, bang, or shake objects instead of using them appropriately. They may show little evidence of functional object use, object permanence, or means–end concepts discussed earlier. Thus, one level of cognitive assessment is to examine a child's free play and make some inferences about knowledge of concepts associated with language (Westby, 1980). This will most likely involve a visit by the SLP to your classroom. We would like to emphasize here that while research has shown certain cognitive abilities to be associated with language development, these abilities are not necessary for learning communication skills (National Joint Committee for the Communication Needs of Persons with

Severe Disabilities, 2002). Often, cognitive goals are worked on concurrently with communication, and children have been shown to benefit from such services (Brady & McLean, 2000; McCathren, 2000). On a general level, however, a child must have some basic understanding of objects, events, and relationships in the world before he or she will be able to communicate about them.

Intent to Communicate

Without a reason to talk, a child will never develop language. There are at least two important aspects the SLP will want to gather data on. First, the SLP will be interested in determining why the child does or does not make communicative attempts using gestures and or vocal behaviors. We know that gestural communication develops prior to verbal communication and that there is a fairly predictable order to gestural development (Crais, Douglas, & Campbell, 2004). Most reasons for communication involve either regulating the attention of other people or regulating the activity or behavior of other people. At the very least, the SLP will want to see if the child regulates the attention and activity of others in natural situations. The SLP may also set up some particular situations in which the child might respond. For instance, the SLP would be greatly interested in finding out if the child asks for adult assistance to accomplish some task in the classroom environment (e.g., pulls an adult to a shelf to obtain a toy) or tries to direct an adult's attention to a novel activity (e.g., points to a puddle of spilled paint and looks at adult). If a child has these two types of intent to communicate he or she is well on the way to making progress in language treatment.

The second aspect the SLP will want to note about communicative intent is the *level* on which the intent is realized. For instance, a child can regulate adult attention in a totally nonverbal manner, simply by physically pulling the adult around. On the other hand, a child can pull an adult around and accompany the pulling with a vocalization. Finally, the child can regulate the adult behavior with words (*want*, *up*). Thus, the SLP will want to gather data on the types of communicative intents shown by the child with limited language and the levels on which these intents are demonstrated. This can be done using a variety of tasks and systems (Coggins, Olswang, & Guthrie, 1987; Snyder, 1981; Wetherby, Prizant, 1993; 2002). Brunson and Haynes (1991) and Rice, Sell, and Hadley (1990) provide concrete and practical examples of how communication intent can be evaluated in a classroom context by the SLP. Also included in the assessment of communicative intent will be the influence of the environment on the child's reasons to talk. Does the child have *opportunities* to communicate, or does the teacher anticipate all needs? Are peers or teachers talking for the child, eliminating the need to communicate? The SLP should do a careful analysis of the classroom and home environments.

Social Abilities

The SLP will want to determine if the child possesses the social abilities mentioned in Chapter 3, namely: joint referencing, turn-taking, and the desire to interact with others. In an evaluation context the SLP will observe the child in play routines with peers and significant adults to find out if the child has a preference for playing with others and focusing jointly on objects and activities. It is during these joint referencing routines that language can be stimulated by the SLP, teacher, and parents, and much learning could potentially occur in this context.

Evaluation of Verbal/Nonverbal Communication

Perhaps the easiest task the speech-language pathologist has with limited-language children is the assessment of their verbal communication. This, of course, is because such children typically do not talk a great deal (especially if they are nonverbal), and there is little to actually assess. The greatest difficulty in assessing language productions of these children is to obtain a **representative language sample**. It is often the case that a child will talk more in the classroom and at home than in a testing situation where the SLP takes the child off to a small room and tries to talk one on one. Therefore, the classroom teacher should expect the SLP to ask permission to observe the child in the classroom setting, and the parents may be asked about home visits. In the case of a nonverbal child, the SLP will take a complete inventory of gestures and vocalizations produced by a child who is not yet producing words. This can tell the SLP what sounds the child is capable of making even if he or she is not using real words. Research has shown that some of the areas of BACIS are strong predictive variables for determining language growth in prelinguistic children. For instance, children who were assessed as having more sophisticated play (cognitive), clear communicative intent shown in gestures, good language comprehension, and the ability to make a variety of speech sounds have the best prognosis to develop language one year later (Calandrella & Wilcox, 2000; McCathren, Warren, & Yoder, 1996;

Yoder, Warren, & McCathren, 1998). The SLP also will ask teachers and parents many questions regarding particular utterances they have heard the child produce in the classroom and home environments. There are some subtle differences in assessment of verbal productions depending on the child's level of language development. These will be briefly discussed.

The Single-Word Child

If the child is talking in single words, the SLP will want to gain insight into the number and types of words in the child's expressive vocabulary. It is unrealistic to expect that the SLP could possibly take such a large sample of language that every word the child knows would be captured. Probably the best way to obtain this type of information is to use the parents and teachers who have spent the most time with the child. In many cases, the SLP will ask these informants to either write down words the child says consistently or to complete a vocabulary checklist on which many words are listed that are often seen in the single-word period. Such checklists are typically arranged in categories such as foods, toys, people, etc. The teacher or parent simply checks the words that the child typically produces in each environment. Similar information can also be gathered on language comprehension. Also, using informants in the single-word period has been shown to be quite valid and reliable in studies of this issue (Fenson et al., 1993; Klee, Pearch, Carson, 2000; Rescorla & Alley, 2001; Rescorla, Alley, & Christine, 2001).

The Early Multiword Child

When the child begins to combine words, it becomes quite a bit more cumbersome to ask teachers and parents to remember the types of word combinations produced by the child. While these informants can easily recognize single words on a checklist that the child may have produced at a given time, there is much less reliability in asking parents and teachers to remember specific word combinations. This is not to say that parents and teachers should not be asked about word combinations, because they often can reliably report specific utterances by the child in question (e.g., "I remember he said 'want book'"). Most SLPs rely to a larger extent on language sampling for the analysis of early multiword utterances. This can be done by visiting the classroom and taking notes on what the child says or by videotaping or audiotaping a play session and later transcribing the child's utterances.

Whatever the child's level of language development, the SLP will want to pinpoint the types of utterances the youngster can produce and compute the mean length of utterance (MLU) in order to select target therapy goals and monitor future progress. In Chapter 3 we provided a list of common multi-word utterances that are produced by children. The SLP will want to take an inventory of the specific types of multiword utterances produced by the child to determine if he or she has a good variety of multiword combinations.

DIRECT AND INDIRECT TREATMENT FOR CHILDREN WITH LIMITED LANGUAGE

There are three areas we want to emphasize that deal with increasing the communication abilities in children with limited language. First, the types of treatment for these children will vary on a continuum from structured to more child directed. This same continuum can be viewed as artificial on one end and **naturalistic** on the other. Doing drill work with a child in a small treatment room is artificial, and performing treatment tasks in the classroom during normal activities would be regarded as more naturalistic.

A second area of importance is the targets worked on by the SLP in treatment. Often, the SLP will not just focus on language, but also on some of the components (e.g., BACIS) that underlie linguistic acquisition. Thus, the SLP may be targeting biological, access to model, cognitive, intent, or social goals exclusively or in addition to the language objectives.

Finally, the mode of communication chosen for specific children may or may not involve exclusively using speech. The SLP may work with other team members and determine that it is unrealistic for certain children to express themselves using the speech mechanism due to motor, structural, cognitive, or other obstacles. In these cases the child may have a gesture system, communication board, a picture exchange system for requesting things, or an electronic assistive (augmentative) device prescribed to use in communicative interchanges. We will briefly expand on each of these three areas.

Structured Versus Naturalistic Treatment

As we mentioned, a continuum of services is available from the SLP. On one end of the continuum is direct service provision in which the SLP takes the child out of the classroom and typically performs drill work activities calculated to increase the child's communicative ability. Basically, these sessions involve training the child to pay attention to language models and imitate words or word combinations to gradually encourage the child's spontaneous productions in more natural situations.

The number and length of sessions per week will be determined jointly by members of the intervention team. The **structured treatment** format is best for teaching particular skills that may require massed practice, such as motor production of speech sounds or early establishment of imitative responses. This format is also used in cases of highly distractible children or those who may not benefit from treatment cues presented in more natural contexts. One can easily see that highly structured treatment is only a temporary method used at the beginning of some treatment cases. It is unlikely that the language trained in a drill procedure in an unnatural setting would generalize well to the natural environment. Thus, children receiving structured treatment must finally be dealt with using a more naturalistic approach. In most cases, the highly structured therapies in the school setting will not be exclusively used over long periods of time with a child. The SLP may also use a structured approach coupled with a more naturalistic classroom intervention approach. It would not be unusual, for example, for a child to be seen by the SLP for individual structured treatment, and again in the classroom setting during more natural activities.

Naturalistic approaches to treatment of the child with limited language are conducted in the classroom and home environments by a variety of members of the intervention team. The SLP may want to come into the classroom to conduct activities that the teacher has planned and provide language stimulation, models, and cues to facilitate language production in the limited-language child. On the other hand, the SLP may feel that the stimulation, models, and cues provided by the teacher or parent will be enough to result in adequate progress. In this case, the SLP will act mainly as a consultant and assist the teacher in making routine classroom activities more easily facilitate language development for a particular child. The SLP will be active in periodically assessing the child's progress and acting as a resource for the teacher. For instance, the SLP might inform the teacher that the goal has changed to include additional types of word combinations, or that a particular cue seems to work extremely well to elicit a correct response from a child. The SLP will be in close contact with the teacher if a consultative or collaborative model is used.

Most naturalistic approaches to language have the following elements in common:

- Use of people, objects, and events in the natural environment
- Modification of daily routines so that they are facilitative of language development

- Provision of a greater number of opportunities for communication
- Presenting many models of appropriate language in real situations using teachers, parents, and peers
- Presentation of specific cues to the limited-language child that are designed to elicit correct and more high-level language productions in real contexts

The keys then, are *use of the natural environment, modification of daily routines, increased opportunity to communicate, provision of models in natural situations*, and *provision of specific cues the child can use to communicate at a higher level*. There are many ways to provide increased opportunity in the classroom. Appendix A illustrates seven principles that any teacher could easily incorporate into the daily routine. Appendix B provides 19 characteristics of a good language model for limited-language children. Any parent or teacher who talks to language-impaired children should bear in mind that every interaction is a potential opportunity for the child to learn about the structure and use of language from a model. The more of these characteristics that can be incorporated, the greater the chance that the limited-language child will learn something about more advanced communication. Appendix C and Appendix D illustrate two popular approaches to naturalistic language training that can easily be adapted to the classroom environment. The incidental teaching or milieu approach has decades of classroom research attesting to its efficacy (Warren & Kaiser, 1986; Warren, Yoder, Gazdag, Kim, & Jones, 1993). There is no question that language treatment conducted in classroom environments is effective with a wide variety of children representing different language levels and etiologies. There is also ample evidence that classroom teachers can effectively learn and implement these principles in classroom environments (Warren, McQuarter, & Rogers-Warren, 1984). Appendix E shows the most popular methods of stimulating language (providing models) that have been used with limited-language children. These techniques are applicable to the classroom and can be used in a variety of activities. Finally, Appendix F illustrates the steps a teacher or parent can go through to make *any* activity a language-learning experience for a limited-language child. The key is to *think language and communication* in every activity with these children. It is very easy to forget that a particular child has communication goals, especially when the teacher has other children in the classroom to deal with, and sometimes timing makes it impractical to provide extra stimulation to the child with limited language. However, if the teacher can incorporate communication and language into even half of the interactions with the limited-language child, it will go a long way toward creating progress in treatment, as well as progress in the classroom.

Judicious use of more advanced peers and aides also will facilitate the process. The SLP will want to work with the child in activities the teacher has planned that will demonstrate the language stimulation and cueing techniques and provide added practice for the child. Take time now to read Appendices A–F so you will have a good idea about providing opportunities for communication, giving good language models, stimulating specific types of language, and creating classroom activities that facilitate communication goals.

Work on the BACIS of Language

We have made it clear in prior sections that the language framework will not develop normally without a strong BACIS. In some cases, a child with limited language may have to work on some of these building blocks in treatment along with language goals. Two foundation blocks that often are incorporated into treatment programs are cognitive and social skills. For instance, a cognitively impaired child who lacks some of the cognitive abilities associated with language development may need some treatment designed to improve these concepts. A child may have primitive play behavior and not even understand the functional use of objects. Clearly, such a child will not talk about things if they are not understood to some degree. For example, a child will never say "push car" if all he ever does with cars is to chew on them or throw them. Some research has shown that training of cognitive abilities (e.g., object permanence, means–end, functional object use) may facilitate the acquisition of language (Kahn, 1984). The reader should recall, however, that there is not strong support for viewing such cognitive attainments as a *prerequisite* for language training (Brady & McLean, 2000; McCathren, 2000). Cognitive and social skills can be targeted concurrently with language goals. For example, a child with autism may lack social prerequisites or the intent to communicate. Such children often need assistance with eye contact, joint referencing, reciprocal play, turntaking, and imitating adult models. An important point to make here is that teaching a child to play more appropriately and engage socially will also facilitate the development of peer interactions, which are critical to learning language as well as many other skills. These examples all illustrate that the SLP may be involved in more than merely teaching language, but also in training the BACIS for language in some cases. Teachers and parents may incorporate activities in the classroom or home dedicated to the advancement of various social, cognitive, intent, and language goals. Appendix G shows some routine things teachers can do to facilitate the social requisites for linguistic acquisition. Some suggestions for the cognitive area are in Appendix H. It should be noted that most of these suggestions would benefit all children in a classroom, not only the child with limited language. Take some time to read these suggestions now.

Verbal and Augmentative Modes in Treatment

Most children with limited language can learn to talk. We must always remember, however, that language is the "music" and speech is the "instrument." A composer can write a beautiful song only to have it rendered dissonant by an untuned instrument. The major goal of the SLP is to facilitate *communication*, and this is not done exclusively through the speech mode. It is altogether possible for a child with language-impairment to understand and even use the rules of language given the appropriate response mode. Communication using gestural or electronic assistance is called *augmentative/ alternative communication (AAC)*. For instance, a child with cerebral palsy who has immense difficulty coordinating the speech mechanism may be able to communicate complex ideas using an electronic device with a keyboard or a pointing device. Much research has shown that many children with severe mental retardation or autism tend to be able to learn a sign language, picture communication system, or other augmentative systems more easily than speech (Silverman, 1989). Further, once an augmentative mode is introduced to a child, the research is clear that as communication increases, speech attempts increase, and negative aspects, such as behavior problems, decrease (Silverman, 1989). The bottom line is that the SLP will want the child to have *some* way to communicate at the earliest possible age. Introduction of an augmentative system does not preclude working on speech and language at the same time, and research shows that children using augmentative devices usually use a combination of gesture, speech, and whatever system they have. Much research has demonstrated that after an augmentative system is introduced, speech attempts tend to increase as opposed to decrease. Chapter 12 discusses augmentative devices in more detail.

Determining the Success of Treatment

Some people think of evaluation and treatment as two separate components of working with children with communication disorders. This, however, is an unfortunate misconception. Evaluation is an ongoing process that begins when a child is first diagnosed with a particular problem and ends when he or she is finally dismissed from treatment (Haynes & Pindzola, 2004). Evaluation and treatment must be intimately linked because we must constantly gather assessment data to determine if the child is making progress. With the advent of accountability and efficacy studies, both teachers and SLPs must not only be able to claim progress in their work, but they must also be able to *prove* it. Thus, the SLP who is working with a limited-language case in the classroom environment will not only be designing treatment programs in collaboration with the teacher, but he or she will also be building in methods of determining if the therapy is successful. In most cases, spontaneous interactions in the classroom will be the best barometer of progress. For example, a 4-year-old child begins the year with an MLU of 1.0 in classroom activities. His treatment goals include increasing MLU with the typical types of early word combinations seen in normally developing children. The treatment involves the teacher modeling specific words and word combinations, expanding the child's 1-word utterances into multiword combinations and reinforcing attempts and multiword communications. Every two weeks, the SLP takes a 30-minute sample of the child's utterances in the classroom during similar activities. She sits on the periphery of the room and writes down what the child says on a clipboard. As the 10-week period progresses, the MLU data look like this:

- First sample: MLU = 1.0
- Second sample: MLU = 1.3
- Third sample: MLU = 1.9
- Fourth sample: MLU = 2.3
- Fifth sample: MLU = 2.4

Clearly, the child is increasing his utterance length under the treatment being provided by the SLP and teacher. The data show improvement on the goals stated on the child's IEP. There are many measurements that could be taken by the SLP to monitor progress, and as the treatment continues, the measurements will change. For instance, in the child mentioned above, work may now be started on increasing the variety (number of different types) of his multiword utterances or introducing some function words to place between the multiword combinations. Whatever the new treatment goal, there must be a valid and reliable way of measuring it. If the evaluation data show that the child is making progress, this will be reinforcing to the SLP and teacher and impressive to parents and administrators. If the data show that the child is not progressing, this is a valuable cue to the SLP and teacher to make either alterations in the treatment approach so that progress *can* occur, or to consider an alternative assessment method which will allow documentation of growth. Nothing is sadder than to have continued an unsuccessful treatment program for the entire school year without any attempt at systematic modification of the approach. Every child should be able to make progress at *something!* Perhaps the treatment goals need to be less ambitious, the tasks simplified, the therapy more intensive, the stimuli more interesting, the reinforcer more reinforcing, or increases need to be made on parent involvement. None of these modifications would be attempted without accurate data on treatment progress to justify trying them. Teachers should *expect and demand* to see evaluation data on treatment progress from the SLP. The common phrase, "He's getting better," is no substitute for objective clinical documentation.

Suggestions for Teachers

The appendices at the end of this chapter provide numerous suggestions for teachers and parents of children with limited language, and we will not reiterate them here. These specific suggestions on providing a good language model, language stimulation, and activities for treatment are easily incorporated into an academic or a home setting.

CONCLUSION

We began this chapter by indicating that children with limited language need to have treatment that extends beyond the therapy room and into the classroom. If you reflect on all of the suggestions provided in this chapter, you will find that *no* suggestion was made that would require a teacher to do special activities with a limited-language child. All of our suggestions involved slight modification of interaction style, language models, and use of *existing* activities that the teacher has planned for use in the classroom. This is the way it should be in a consultative approach to language treatment. We hope that most of you will have the opportunity to participate in the treatment of a child with limited language, because what this youngster learns from you will make possible any further social or academic achievements. It is gratifying, indeed, to play such a pivotal role in the life of a child.

REFERENCES

Baltaxe, C. (2001). Emotional, behavioral, and other psychiatric disorders of childhood associated with communication disorders. In T. Layton, E. Crais, & L. Watson. *Handbook of early language impairment in children: Nature.* Albany, NY: Delmar.

Brady, N., & McLean, L. (2000). Emergent symbolic relations in speakers and nonspeakers. *Research in Developmental Disabilities, 21,* 197–214.

Brunson, K., & Haynes, W. (1991). Profiling teacher/child communication: Reliability of an alternating time sampling procedure. *Child Language Teaching and Therapy, 7,* 192–211.

Calandrella, A., & Wilcox, M. (2000). Predicting language outcomes for young prelinguistic children with developmental delay. *Journal of Speech, Language, and Hearing Research, 43,* 1061–1071.

Coggins, T., Olswang, L., & Guthrie, J. (1987). Assessing communicative intents in young children: Low structured observation or elicitation tasks? *Journal of Speech and Hearing Disorders, 52,* 44–49.

Crais, E., Douglas, D., & Campbell, C. (2004). The intersection of the development of gestures and intentionality. *Journal of Speech, Language, and Hearing Research, 47,* 678–694.

Fenson, L., Dale, P., Reznick, S., Thal, D., Bates, E., Hartung, J., et al. (1993). *MacArthur communicative development inventories,* San Diego, CA.

Fox, L., Long, S., & Langlois, A. (1988). Patterns of language comprehension deficit in abused and neglected children. *Journal of Speech and Hearing Disorders, 53,* 239–244.

Hart, B., & Rogers-Warren, A. (1978). A milieu approach to teaching language. In R. Schiefelbusch (Ed.) *Language intervention strategies.* Baltimore: University Park Press.

Haynes, W., & Pindzola, R. (2004). *Diagnosis and evaluation in speech pathology,* Boston: Allyn and Bacon.

Hubatch, L., Johnson, C., Kistler, D., Burns, W., & Moneka, W. (1985). Early language abilities of high-risk infants. *Journal of Speech and Hearing Disorders, 50,* 195–206.

Kaderavek, J., & Sulzby, E. (1998). Parent-child joint book reading: An observational protocol for young children. *American Journal of Speech-Language Pathology, 8*(3), 261–272.

Kahn, J. (1984). Cognitive training and initial use of referential speech. *Topics in Language Disorders, 5,* 14–28.

Klee, T., Pearch, K., & Carson, D. (2000). Improving the positive predictive value of screening for developmental language disorder. *Journal of Speech, Language, and Hearing Research, 43,* 821–833.

Lucas, E. (1980). *Semantic and pragmatic language disorders.* Rockville, MD: Aspen.

McCathren, R. (2000). Teacher-implemented prelinguistic communication intervention. *Focus on Autism and Other Developmental Disabilities, 15*(1), 21–29.

McCathren, R., Warren, S., & Yoder, P., (1996). Prelinguistic predictors of later language development. In K. Cole, P. Dale, & D. Thal (Eds.), *Assessment of communication and language.* Baltimore: Paul H. Brookes.

National Joint Committee for the Communication Needs of Persons with Severe Disabilities (2002). *American Speech-Language-Hearing Association Technical Report IV,* 59–68.

Paul, R. (2001). *Language disorders from infancy through adolescence: Assessment and intervention* (2nd ed.). St. Louis, MO: Mosby.

Rabidoux, P., & Macdonald, J. (2000). An interactive taxonomy of mothers and children during storybook interactions. *American Journal of Speech-Language Pathology, 9,* 331–344.

Rescorla, L., & Alley, A. (2001). Validation of the language development survey (LDS): A parent report tool for identifying language delay in toddlers. *Journal of Speech, Language, and Hearing Research, 44,* 434–445.

Rescorla, L., Alley, A., & Christine, J. (2001). Word frequencies in toddlers' lexicons. *Journal of Speech, Language, and Hearing Research, 44,* 598–609.

Rhyner, P., Lehr, D., & Pudlas, K. (1990). An analysis of teacher responsiveness to communicative initiations of preschool children with handicaps. *Language, Speech, and Hearing Services in Schools, 21*(2), 91–97.

Rice, M., Sell, M., & Hadley, P. (1990). The social interactive coding system (SICS): An on-line, clinically relevant descriptive tool. *Language, Speech, and Hearing Services in Schools, 21*, 1, 2–14.

Silverman, F. (1989). *Communication for the speechless.* Englewood-Cliffs, NJ: Prentice-Hall.

Snyder, L. (1981). Assessing communicative abilities in the sensorimotor period: Content and context. *Topics In Language Disorders, 1*, 31–46.

Warren, S., & Kaiser, A. (1986). Incidental language teaching: A critical review. *Journal of Speech and Hearing Disorders, 51*, 291–299.

Warren, S., McQuarter, R., & Rogers-Warren, A. (1984). The effects of mands and models on the speech of unresponsive language-delayed preschool children. *Journal of Speech and Hearing Disorders, 49*, 43–52.

Warren, S., Yoder, P., Gazdag, G., Kim, K., & Jones, H. (1993). Facilitating prelinguistic communication skills in young children with developmental delay. *Journal of Speech and Hearing Research, 36*, 83–97.

Watkins, R., & Rice, M. (1994). *Specific language impairment in children.* Baltimore: Paul H. Brookes.

Westby, C. (1980). Assessment of cognitive and language abilities through play. *Language, Speech, and Hearing Services in Schools, 11*, 154–168.

Wetherby, A., & Prizant, B. (1993). *Communication and symbolic behavior scales.* Chicago: Riverside.

Wetherby, A., & Prizant, B. (2002). *Communication and symbolic behavior scales: Developmental profile.* Baltimore: Paul H. Brookes.

Yoder, P., Warren, S., & McCathren, R. (1998). Determining spoken language prognosis in children with developmental disabilities. *American Journal of Speech-Language Pathology, 7*, 77–87.

TERMS TO KNOW

alternative/augmentative communication (AAC)

BACIS

communicative intent

early multiword communicators

language stimulation or modeling

limited language

naturalistic treatment

nonverbal communicators

PL 99-457

representative language sample

single-word communicators

specifically language impaired (SLI)

structured treatment

TOPICS FOR DISCUSSION

1. Make a list of activities that preschool or kindergarten children perform in the classroom setting.

2. For each of the activities listed above, rank them in terms of the teacher's opportunity to stimulate language during performance of the task.

3. Discuss the positive and negative effects of the SLP assisting the teacher in conducting certain classroom activities in order to stimulate language.

4. Discuss the advantages and disadvantages of the SLP removing a child with limited language from the classroom for treatment.

5. How could the teacher and SLP work together to gain cooperation of a parent in treatment of a limited-language child?

Appendix A

Creating Communicative Opportunities

Whatever the language-impaired child's level of communication (gesture, single word, word combinations), one of the most important parts of therapy is giving him or her the opportunity to communicate. Creating opportunity for the language-impaired child involves providing him/her with many chances to use language appropriately. The ideal setting for facilitating a child's use of language is the natural environment (e.g., home, classroom). Following are some specific ways to create communicative opportunities:

Do Not Anticipate the Child's Needs

Expect the child to perform necessary tasks independently rather than doing them for him or her. Do not anticipate the child's needs; wait for him or her to verbalize a request. For example, if the child knows you will automatically provide juice and cookies at snack time, he or she will not verbalize a request for these. When snack time comes, do not give the child refreshments until he or she asks for them (or tries to). If you see the child struggling with a jar lid screwed on too tightly, do not quickly offer assistance. Wait for the child to ask for your help.

Withhold Access to Objects and Events

Withholding the child's participation in a desired task or withholding a desired object provides the opportunity for more language use. The language-limited child should not get a chance to participate or obtain an object until a verbal, vocal, or gestural attempt is made. For example, you might say, "Who wants to play ball?" Withhold the child's participation in this task until he or she responds to you.

Use Sabotage

Set up a situation in which the child needs to ask for your assistance. This can be done by providing objects that do not work correctly or omitting a familiar step in a routine activity.

Use Cues That Provide Opportunities to Elaborate

Make open-ended statements and ask questions that require more than single-word answers (Lucas, 1980).

Examples: "What do you want?" "Ask Mike to play with us." "Tell me about that." "Tell me more."

Let the Child Speak for Him- or Herself

When a child is not a good communicator parents and teachers sometimes let a sibling or friend talk for him or her. This reduces the opportunities for communication and should not be encouraged.

Pause Time

Use pause time when interacting with the child. After asking a question or making a statement, do not immediately provide an answer or reply for the child. Wait for the child to respond. Open-ended utterances such as, "Who wants to help?" "Who can tell me?" "What do you want?" followed by a pause are ideal ways to provide language opportunities because these leave an opening for the child to respond verbally.

Limit Your Talking Time

Reduce your utterances when interacting with the child. By reducing your utterances you are providing more opportunities for the child to initiate and use language.

Appendix B

Characteristics of a Good Language Model and Interaction

- Encourage and respond to communication—Whenever possible, talk to the child about things that are happening at that moment. Whenever possible, answer the child's verbalizations with what you think is an appropriate response at the child's level. You can also imitate the child's speech and try to have him or her imitate you.
- Alternate your emphasis between directing the child and following his or her lead—Do not always direct the child by trying to get him or her to talk about and pay attention to things *you* are interested in. About 50% of the time talk about and pay attention to the things that *the child* is interested in.
- Always talk about objects that are present and events that are currently happening—Do not talk about things in another room or things that have happened in the past or will happen in the future. Language is learned first in talking about objects in the "here and now."
- Reduce your sentence length—Your sentence length should be one or two steps ahead of the child. If the child is nonverbal you can use 1-word to 3-word utterances. If the child is at the 1-word to 2-word stage, you should use 3-word to 5-word utterances.

- Reduce your sentence complexity—Do not use complex sentences. Simplify your sentences, and when possible avoid connecting two thoughts together or using many modifiers.
- Paraphrase and repeat a lot—Repeat your sentences a few times in a conversation with the child. Sometimes, say the same statement in a few different ways ("Want a cookie? Want one? Does Johnny want a cookie? Want it?" etc.).
- Exaggerate your intonation and put stress on important words—Emphasize important words and concepts by the way you say words. For example, "This is a *big* ball."
- Use simple, concrete vocabulary—Do not use big words for things. For instance, call a car *car*, not *Chevrolet*.
- Use "broad-based" words—Choose words that can be used over and over again for many objects and events. For instance, *go* can be used for cars, people, walking, running, swinging, and so forth. On the other hand *spin* can only be used for objects that twirl.
- Stimulate the language forms that are the next ones the child will develop—Use language models that are 1 step ahead of the child's. For example, if the child uses mostly 1-word utterances, you should model 2-word to 3-word utterances.
- Talk at eye-level with the child—Speaking to your child at his or her eye level may mean kneeling, sitting on the floor, or sitting across the table. Such a position not only secures the child's attention, but also helps the child understand the meaning of the message from your facial expression and eyes.
- Create communication opportunities—Encourage the child to become more mature by urging him or her to do more activities independently. Do not anticipate the child's wishes. The child has fewer reasons to talk if needs are fulfilled before there is an opportunity to use language. You might even arrange situations so that the child must use language to get a desired object, food, information, and such.
- Avoid baby talk—Permit the child to grow up. Avoid using baby talk when talking to the child. If the child hears baby talk, he or she will talk baby talk.
- Do not talk too much—Try to avoid overwhelming the child by providing so many verbal models that there is no time left for him or her to respond or contribute to the conversation. It is acceptable and even desirable for periods of silence to occur in conversation. This gives the child the opportunity to initiate new utterances.

- Avoid too many questions and commands—Model good conversation and language but do not *command it*. Avoid commands and asking too many questions such as: "Say this," "What's this?"
- Demonstrate your expectations—Show the child that you expect him or her to communicate. For example, after you provide a model, pause and show the child that you expect a response. Do this by maintaining eye contact and looking at the child expectantly.
- Try to figure out what your child means—Interpret the child's utterances as meaningful. When the child attempts to communicate, interpret the utterances as important and communicative.
- Enthusiasm—Be enthusiastic. Let your face and voice show the child that what you are doing is interesting and fun. Let the child actively participate. Language is best learned while doing.
- Slow down and pause—Reduce your rate of talking and use natural pauses to highlight the main idea of your utterances.

Appendix C

Suggestions by Lucas for Naturalistic Language Treatment

Two overriding aspects that Lucas (1980) emphasizes are the treatment must not be dominated by the adult (it should be child directed), and the child will benefit most by observing peer models performing legitimate speech acts. The suggestions are in several areas:

1. Providing opportunity—This can be done in several ways. First, the adult should *stop anticipating the child's needs*. A number of studies have recommended incorporating *pause time* into interactions with these children. One group of researchers found that teachers in a preschool handicapped class frequently provided materials, treats, and opportunities for activities before the children had the opportunity to make a verbal request. When these researchers asked teachers to *wait 5 seconds* before providing things, the children's rate of spontaneous verbal responses increased dramatically. One key to establishing opportunity for speech acts is to make as many problems as possible for the child to solve verbally (Lucas, 1980, p. 213):

Taped together scissors, plugged glue bottles, empty or dried-up pens, broken pencil leads, coat sleeves turned inside-out by the morning aide when the children aren't watching, not enough chairs, not enough snacks, cups with holes in the bottom, missing toys, flat balls, short jump ropes, missing colors or paints, not enough paper, no tacks for hanging pictures, tables with missing legs, water faucets turned off tightly, baseballs without bats or bats without baseballs, etc. The problem-solving tasks require more than the performance of speech acts; the tasks necessitate better attending to the environmental cues and thus more discrimination and sorting of the features that lead to knowledge development.

Opportunity is important in classroom environments and in home situations as well!

2. Models—The child needs to see and hear other children using language to accomplish various purposes. The more variety in models the better in terms of varying the forms (gimme *x*, I want the *x*, can I have the *x*, want *x*, etc.).
3. Direct cues or prompts—For some children the opportunity and a chance to see models is not enough. There are a variety of cueing systems to be used in language training. We should provide the cue that gives the *least amount of information first*. Lucas gives examples like, "If you want the ball you can get it from me," "You can ask me for the ball," and so on.
4. Utterance act imitation—This should be a last resort, to imitate an utterance after the clinician. The one saving grace of this procedure is that the imitation takes place *in context*; it is at least done in a real communication situation.

Picture the above four steps as part of a continuum. Some children will respond by developing communication skills only when you provide opportunity. Others need many models to finally develop. Others require prompts and imitations. The point here is that the treatment is being done in the natural environment, and the clinician is not being intrusive.

Appendix D

Incidental Teaching Suggestions

This is sometimes called the *milieu* approach, but has more recently been referred to as *incidental teaching* (Hart & Rogers-Warren, 1978). There has been an increasing amount of research on this type of intervention and it has been shown to be effective with a variety of types of language cases. It is also adaptable in that the SLP can use it for nonverbal, single-word cases, and early multiword cases. The basic model assumes that language will be taught in functional ways. The training is carried out in the place where the child spends the most time (classroom, home). All waking hours are infested with training opportunities. The settings can be arranged to learn language and reinforcers are natural consequences of communication acts.

1. Arranging the environment—You must have a variety of attractive materials and activities (child should be the judge, not the clinician). Certain materials should be accessible to the child, while other materials can only be obtained on request. The adult mediates the materials and you make this a *rule* (that all materials must be asked for). If a child doesn't ask put your hand over his or hers and say, "You need to ask for that."

2. Building rate—You respond to the child's highest level of communication (gestural, vocal, verbal, single-word, early multiword). Thus, any level child or a mixture of children can be incorporated into this type of treatment. The teacher's response should be immediate, consistent, and strong when a child makes a request (that is, give the child what is asked for, attend to what he or she wants you to look at). Note that a child must be able to initiate requests at some level, be able to imitate, and the environment must be controlled.

3. Building requesting—A version of the specific procedure is as follows:
   a. Focus attention on the child when he or she initiates.
   b. Allow time for the child to make a request at his or her level.
   c. If the child can't request, ask a question: "What is this?"
   d. If the response is incorrect, provide a model of the language expected from the child (want ball). Listen for a correct imitation or approximation.
   e. Confirm the behavior of the child ("OK, you can have the ball.")

4. Building commenting—A version of the specific procedure is as follows:
   a. Teacher focuses full attention on the child who initiates a statement.
   b. Adult confirms and repeats all or some of what the child says; take a guess if you don't understand (e.g., "That *is* a big horsie.")
   c. Adult can model a statement in appropriate context if child is not talking and thus can hope for imitation.

Appendix E

Language Stimulation Techniques

The following techniques give a child an example of a higher level of language complexity than he or she is presently using. The techniques can be administered while the child plays or in response to a verbal turn in a conversation.

Self-Talk

Verbalize what *you* are seeing, hearing, doing, and feeling. This type of speech is useful for children who are reluctant to interact because it provides some model of speaking while making no demands on the child.

> *Examples:* "I am washing my hands."
> "The water is warm."
> "I dropped the soap."

Parallel Talk

Talk about what *the child* sees, hears, does, and feels. The adult producing utterances that are related to what the child is experiencing demonstrates possible utterances the child may say.

Examples: "You're petting the dog."
"Johnny is pushing the car."
"That feels hot."

Expansions

Take the child's utterance and expand it into a closer approximation of a grammatically correct utterance. This shows the child that you are interested and listening to what he or she says. Young children are likely to imitate expansions of their own utterances.

Examples: The child might say "eat." The adult would say:
"Eat banana."
The child might say "baby sleep." The adult would say:
"The baby is sleeping,"
The child might say "want ball." The adult would say:
"I want the ball."

Expatiation

Take the child's utterance, expand it, and add something new to the child's meaning. Make sure to keep your expatiations in a simple sentence format.

Examples: The child might say "want milk." The adult would say:
"The milk is cold."
The child might say "eat." The adult would say:
"Eat more cereal."

Buildups and Breakdowns

The adult takes the child's utterance, expands it, breaks it down into sentence components and then builds it up again using all components that were modeled.

Examples: Child: *"Baby sleep."*
Adult: "Yeah, the *baby* is *sleeping."* (breakdown) *"Sleeping* in the *bed."* (breakdown) "The *baby* is *sleeping* in the *bed."* (buildup)
Child: "Baby sleep bed."

Recast Sentences

This is a specific type of expansion where the language model does not change the child's meaning but only adds grammatical information. For example, if the child says, "The doll is sick," the language model may respond by saying, "She is sick." In this example, the adult has shown the child how pronouns can be used to substitute for nouns.

Appendix F

Incorporation of Language Goals in Classroom and Home Activities

The speech-language pathologist does not necessarily want you to do specific language activities in the classroom or the home. Typical home and classroom activities can be adapted to include language goals. For instance, in the classroom, the following activities can be easily used for language development: snack time, music time, motor skills, play time, story time, nap time, arts and crafts, show and tell, and so on.

In the home environment, the following activities can be easily used for language development: bath time, meal time, dressing, changing, play time, traveling, playing outside, helping, preparing for bed, book reading, and so on.

Thus, it can be seen that special activities do not need to be devised for language training; language can be easily incorporated into the classroom and home daily routines. Incorporating language into the daily routine requires only that the parent or teacher think about these daily activities in a particular way. The following steps may be helpful:

1. Decide on a normal daily activity that you are willing to use for language training.

2. Remind yourself of the child's specific language goal, for example: producing single words, producing certain word combinations, initiating more utterances, use of prepositions, etc.
3. Mentally rehearse steps in the activity, and consider the objects and actions involved in the activity.
4. Pinpoint where the specific language goal can be included in an activity step, object, or action. For example, during bath time, the target might be action+object utterances. The parent will stimulate action+object and encourage the child to produce action+object utterances. The activity allows for some of the following action+object utterances: turn water, splash water, drink water, push boat, wash face, wash hair, throw soap, dry hair, pull plug. Other specific bath routines may provide additional opportunities for action+object combinations. What are some classroom activities that could be used to stimulate action+object word combinations?
5. Recycle steps 1–4 in other activities throughout the day.

It can be seen from the above example that if parents or teachers simply think of routine activities in terms of language, the daily routine is saturated with opportunities to stimulate and encourage language use.

Appendix G

Social Aspects Related to Communication

Social interaction is the basis of communication. Before children will communicate, they must first have the desire to interact socially with others; they express this desire through many different social behaviors. The child's communication does not necessarily require the use of verbal language, but the acquisition of language is associated with the development of these social behaviors. These behaviors include:

Joint Referencing

This refers to both you and the child focusing your attention on the same thing at the same time. It is important for you to allow the child to direct your attention about half of the time. Encourage the child's direction of joint referencing. The adult should direct joint referencing about half of the time. Encourage the child to become interested in objects and events focused on by the adult. For example, when looking at a book together, name the pictures the child is looking at. Show the child how a toy works, but be sure he or she is looking at it and sharing reference on it while you demonstrate. When talking together, if the child says "car," do not begin talking about crayons; share something about the car with him such as, "Yes, the car is red."

Encourage Social Play

You should encourage the child to participate in activities that include other children. The child's social behavior will improve when playing with others because he learns to cooperate, participate, and share, and also to respect other people's feelings. Because communication is social, encouraging the child to participate in social play will stimulate his communication behaviors. Parents and teachers should discourage isolated play in language-delayed children.

Eliminate Antisocial Behavior

You should try to eliminate any antisocial behaviors the child might have (e.g., biting, spitting, hitting, kicking, etc.). These behaviors will decrease the child's opportunity for social interaction and communication.

Turn-Taking

Develop routines or games which contain pauses for the child to respond. The child's turn does not necessarily have to be verbal; a gaze, facial expression, body movement, or vocalization can fill the child's turn. This teaches the child to wait for another person's action and to take his or her own turn in response. It also teaches the child to assume responsibility for his or her turn. You can encourage the development of this skill by playing games such as peek-a-boo or rolling a ball back and forth with the child.

Games and Rituals

Establish games and rituals with the child that have assigned roles and predictable events (who does what and what comes next). Repeat them over and over again so that the child becomes familiar with the games and language associated with them. Choose a few common games such as: give-and-take (objects), peek-a-boo, horsie, pat-a-cake, bye-bye, roll a ball back and forth, build and knock down blocks, no-no, point and name, put on/take off, open/shut, joint book reading, question/answer, verbal imitation.

Appendix H

Cognitive Skills Related to Language Development

Research in language development has shown that certain concepts relate to a child's ability to communicate. These important concepts are learned from frequent interactions with people, objects, and events in the environment. There is recent support in the literature for encouraging language-impaired children to learn these communication-related concepts. The activities listed below will facilitate the development of these concepts in the classroom and home environments. Teachers and parents should think of specific activities that can foster these concepts. Throughout these activities, teachers and parents should talk about important aspects of these events.

Categorization

Children should learn to put similar things in categories. For example, children should eventually be able to group objects by shape, color, size, and class (foods, transportation, and animals). Practice in pointing out similarities and differences among objects will facilitate this skill.

Means–End

The concept of means–end has to do with the child knowing how to make things happen. For instance, a toy that is out of reach (end) can be obtained by using a large stick (means). If a child does not know how to turn on the television (end), mother (means) can be used to achieve this. Ultimately, speech is used as a means to acquire a variety of ends (attention, objects, and such), and a basic understanding of this concept is essential to good communication.

Using Objects Appropriately

A child needs to know what an object is and what to do with it before he or she can talk about it. Show the child how to use objects correctly. Do not allow him or her to throw objects, bang them, or put them in the mouth.

Concepts of Objects

A child needs to be able to hold a picture of something in his or her mind. If a child is playing with a toy and it suddenly rolls under the couch, the child should realize that the toy still exists but cannot be seen. If a child does not have this skill, play games such as hide-and-seek. Leave part of the object showing so that the child can see it; then gradually hide the whole object and see if the child can find it.

Immediate Imitation

A child needs to be able to imitate things you do right after you do them. Do things with the child that would be easy for him to imitate. Games such as pat-a-cake and peek-a-boo are good to keep a child's attention and teach this skill.

Delayed Imitation

A child also needs to be able to imitate things you do at a later time. Perform different activities with the child such as putting a puzzle together or putting rings on a stick. See if the child can later play these games without a model.

Symbolic (Pretend) Play

A child needs to be able to use pretend play. One of the earliest kinds of pretending is using one's own body in play (pretending to eat, sleep). Later, see if the child can pretend to feed a doll or pretend to be talking to someone on the phone. If a child is able to do these activities, see if he or she can pretend without having appropriate objects to help (e.g., use a block of wood as a car). Finally, a child can pretend with no objects at all. This could include pretending to be a cowboy by using the fingers for a gun or pretending to drive a car with no steering wheel.

Combining Two or More Objects in Play

See if the child can combine objects in play. For example, see if the child can put a doll in a toy car or hammer pegs in a pegboard.

Separating and Combining Objects

A child needs to be able to take things apart such as stacked rings, blocks, or nesting cups. A child will usually be able to take things apart before he or she can put them together. A child then needs to be able to put these things together again.

chapter six

School-Age and Adolescent Language Disorders

Answer given by a pragmatically disordered 8-year-old:

> SLP: "Tell me what your favorite toy is, Calvin."
> Calvin: "An orange, because a motorcycle doesn't have doors."

An adolescent explains a basic process (Chappell, 1985, p. 226):

> Well . . . to fix a tire . . . or your wheel . . . you gotta take the tire off.
> You gotta lift up . . . you jack up the car and use this thing . . . its
> square metal wrench . . . to loosen the bolts . . . you know the nuts
> . . . then you take the wheel off the axes. First you ask the guy at the
> garage if he will fix the tire. You lock up the car so it won't . . . you
> put the car in gear so it stays put.

BACKGROUND INFORMATION

The examples mentioned above are the utterances of students and adolescents
that have trouble expressing themselves. Often their sentences are well formed
from a grammatical point of view, but the students struggle to make themselves

understood and frustrate their listeners. They have trouble finding the right words to explain even the simplest events. They do not tell their story in the correct order and/or leave out important elements of their explanation. They have difficulty in staying on a conversational topic. Often these students will pass language tests and screenings given by the speech-language pathologist, but their problems will be quite evident to the people who interact with them frequently in conversations or classroom work. Students who have conversational abilities like those just mentioned also may have trouble with other language skills such as reading and writing. They may have difficulty following directions and comprehending concepts taught in the classroom. This chapter is about these students who have trouble with the more subtle aspects of language and, as a result, may have academic problems as well.

When children are first learning to talk, the importance of language in their lives is relatively simple to understand. In essence, very young children use language for two major purposes: (1) speaking to others in their environment, and (2) listening and understanding others in their environment. When a child enters school, however, the importance of language becomes quite a bit more complex. In addition to speaking and listening, children are taught to use language for purposes of reading and writing. Laymen often consider these later skills taught in school to be radically different from the language used in speaking and listening; however, *all* of these operations involve the use of the basic language rules that are learned in the preschool years. That is, a student must have a basic grasp of the rules of language to be able to read, write, speak, and listen because all of these skills have these basic rules in common.

You will recall from Chapter 3 that language has a number of components that must be mastered in order to have linguistic competence. We will mention these areas again, just to refresh your memory. **Semantics** are the rules for word meaning that we associate with vocabulary. Thus, a child is applying semantic rules whenever a word is selected and placed in an utterance. Children with small vocabularies have underdeveloped semantic systems. **Syntax** refers to rules that we use to combine words into the variety of types of sentences in a language. There are acceptable ways to string words together (e.g., The boy hit the ball) and there are also unacceptable ways of doing this (e.g., Boy the ball hit the). Children who leave out words in a sentence (e.g., My car in garage) or misuse words in a sentence (e.g., Her is my sister) are said to have problems with syntax. **Morphology** refers to the attachment of certain endings to words to refine and add additional meaning (e.g., cat*s*, runn*ing*, Mary'*s* car, walk*ed*,). Children who omit these endings from words (e.g., Yesterday I walk), or misuse them (e.g., He gotted the bike) are said to have morphological problems. **Phonology** or the sound system of our language, also has rules for sound selection and combination. Children who misuse sounds in systematic ways (e.g., *tat* for *cat*) are said to have phonological problems. **Pragmatics** refers to the rules we have for the use of language in a particular communicative context. The context can take into account different types of listeners (adults, children, cognitively impaired, deaf, socially prestigious, principal, teacher) to whom we would talk differently because of their various characteristics or positions. The context also can take into account the physical arrangement in which the communication takes place. For instance, we can point to a chair and say "I like this one," and not have to use the word *chair*. If, however, a chair is not present in the communicative context, we would have to use the word *chair* and probably also spend some time describing the type of chair we like best. Another pragmatic area concerns the rules we use to carry on conversations and involves how to introduce, maintain, and change different topics of conversation and take turns with a conversational partner. Pragmatics also includes the ability to generate an utterance that is clear (not ambiguous) and that is presented in a well-ordered sequence, so the listener will have no trouble understanding the contribution to the conversation. If someone tries to give directions to another person on how to fix something and the directions are unclear or the steps are out of order, a pragmatic failure has occurred. The sentences may be well formed from semantic, syntactic, and morphological points of view, but if they do not communicate accurately, a pragmatic problem exists. The area of pragmatics is quite complex, but it is enough to say that it concerns the use of language in real communication situations that take into account the context, the clarity, and the accuracy of the message generated.

One basic message of this section is that the language rules a child learns before age 5 years underlie all functions in which linguistic symbols are used, including speaking, listening, reading, and writing (Catts & Kamhi, 2005). The implication of this is that if a child has a difficulty with language, *all* of the language-dependent functions could be affected. That is, a child who makes errors in spoken language also may make mistakes in written language or have trouble reading and understanding the spoken utterances of others. It is common for laymen not to see the intimate relationships among all of the language activities of reading, writing, speaking, and listening, but to view all of these as separate skills. In reality, there is a common bond among all of these functions, and it depends on a thorough understanding and facility with language. These issues will be addressed more fully in Chapter 13.

A second aspect emphasized earlier was the fact that language is made up of a number of components that one must learn and use together to be a competent language user. The implication of this is that a language disorder can occur in one or all of these component areas. That is, a language disorder can have a variety of "faces." One student may have obvious problems with omission or misuse of words in sentences. Another may have all of the language elements correct, but because of sequencing problems and an inability to take into account the listener's perspective, simply cannot describe how to get downtown. Thus, the "territory" to be covered when we are talking about older students and their disorders of language includes all the components of language and all of the potential uses of language between early elementary school years and adolescence.

Symptoms Reported in Students with Language Problems

It has often been said that as students with language impairments get older their problems become more subtle in nature. In fact, it is not unusual for a language-impaired student to be rediagnosed several times during school. For instance, a child may begin with a preschool language delay and enter kindergarten with the remnants of this disorder. It is hoped this child would be enrolled in language treatment, and the speech-language pathologist (SLP) would eliminate all major residual symptoms of the problem. When the student begins learning to read, he or she may have difficulty and be diagnosed as exhibiting a reading problem (Catts, Fey, Tomblin, & Zhang, 2001). Later, as the content of the academic program becomes more complex, the student may be diagnosed as having a specific learning disability. It is altogether possible that most of the student's problems may represent a broad, underlying difficulty with learning language and using it effectively to solve problems, even though the student may *speak* clearly. Thus, the high-risk groups for language disorder in older children are as follows:

1. Students with a history of late talking or language delay as a preschooler (Johnson, et al., 1999; Rescorla, 2002)
2. Students who score low on standardized reading tests or struggle with learning to read (Catts, 1997)
3. Students diagnosed with language-based learning disabilities
4. Students who are struggling academically.

Table 6-1 lists some linguistic symptoms reported in the literature by researchers and clinicians who work with older students diagnosed as

Table 6-1 Common Symptoms of Language Disorder in Older Students

Semantics
- Word finding/retrieval deficits
- Use of a large number of words in an attempt to explain a concept because the name escapes them (circumlocutions)
- Overuse of limited vocabulary
- Difficulty recalling names of items in categories (e.g., animals, foods)
- Difficulty retrieving verbal opposites
- Small vocabulary
- Use of words lacking specificity (thing, junk, stuff, etc.)
- Inappropriate use of words (selection of wrong word)
- Difficulty defining words
- Less comprehension of complex words
- Failure to grasp double word meanings (e.g. can, file, etc.)

Syntax/Morphology
- Use of grammatically incorrect sentence structures
- Simple, as opposed to complex, sentences
- Less comprehension of complex grammatical structures
- Prolonged pauses while constructing sentences
- Semantically empty placeholders (e.g., filled pauses, "uh," "er," "um")
- Use of many stereotyped phrases that do not require much language skill
- Use of "starters" (e.g. "you know")

Pragmatics
- Use of redundant expressions and information the listener has already heard
- Use of nonspecific vocabulary (e.g., thing, stuff) and the listener cannot tell from prior conversation or physical context what is referred to
- Less skill in giving explanations clearly to a listener (lack of detail)
- Less skill in explaining something in a proper sequence
- Less conversational control in terms of introducing, maintaining, and changing topics (may get off the track in conversation and introduce new topics awkwardly)
- Rare use of clarification questions (e.g., "I don't understand," "You did what?")
- Difficulty shifting conversational style in different social situations (e.g., peer to teacher; child to adult)
- Difficulty grasping the main idea of a story or lecture (preoccupation with irrelevant details)
- Trouble making inferences from material not explicitly stated (e.g., "Sally went outside. She had to put up her umbrella." The inference is that it was raining)
- Difficulties comprehending and using slang
- Difficulties in deriving meaning from vocal inflection and prosodic cues (e.g., sarcasm)

language impaired or learning disabled. Some of these behaviors also may be found in academically low-achieving students who are ineligible for special education services. If a teacher notes students from the high-risk categories mentioned in this chapter who exhibit some of these symptoms, a referral to the SLP is suggested. Note that the behaviors cross *all* areas of language (semantics, syntax, and pragmatics); that they can be manifested in speaking, reading, or writing; and that they can be present in production *or* comprehension of language. The list is certainly *not* all-inclusive and should not be viewed as exhaustive.

ASSESSMENT ISSUES

One of the most important aspects in dealing with older language-disordered students is the initial detection of these youngsters. An equally critical process involves the thorough evaluation of their language-based competencies. This section describes the importance of these processes.

The Importance of Teacher Referral

In most school systems, the SLP does not engage in screening large numbers of older students for communication problems. If a student is observed to be experiencing a communication difficulty, the classroom teacher is often the first one to note its occurrence. It is relatively obvious when a student has a problem with articulation, stuttering, severe hoarseness, or some language problem where an element of language is omitted or clearly misused. On the other hand, it is sometimes quite difficult for teachers to discriminate the more subtle disorders of pragmatics and **metalinguistics** that plague the older student with a language disorder. Also, it is not always clear that the academic problems exhibited by a particular student may have a partial basis in a subtle language difficulty. What the teacher sees is a student who is performing poorly on an academic level, and it may not seem that a referral to the SLP might be indicated. We would suggest that teachers make *routine referrals* for a language screening or evaluation in the following cases:

1. Any student who is experiencing sustained academic problems (consistent below-average grades, retention in a grade)
2. Students who have been diagnosed as learning disabled and are experiencing academic difficulty
3. Students who exhibit obvious problems with reading (either orally or reading comprehension)

4. Any student who appears to have trouble with communication in spoken language. More specifically, the teacher should watch for the following symptoms:
   a. Inability to explain something clearly and concisely
   b. Problems with sequencing information appropriately
   c. Problems staying on the topic of conversation
   d. Problems understanding or giving directions
   e. Evidence of retrials, hesitations, filled pauses, and such
   f. Word-finding problems
   g. Inappropriate use of words
   h. Grammatically incorrect sentence structures

It is *only* through teacher referral that these students will be detected in most school systems, so this role of the classroom teacher is extremely important and cannot be overemphasized. Many SLPs will conduct brief in-service training presentations to school faculty on the symptoms that indicate the appropriate referral for screening or evaluation (McKinley & Larson, 1985).

Evaluation

If a student is referred to the SLP for testing, there are several areas that need to be explored; these will be tapped by both formal as well as informal assessment techniques. By formal testing, we refer to standardized examinations that have been given to large groups of normally developing students that provide norms for performance on the measure. Through formal testing, we can determine how the student is performing compared to same-age peers in areas of language comprehension and production. There are literally hundreds of standardized tests of language ability, and providing all the names and references for these examinations is beyond the scope of this text. It is enough to say that a large variety of formal tests exist for evaluating all aspects of language ability, and the SLP will be using these for part of the assessment. Specific tests used by SLPs vary with their background, training, and professional preferences, thus the examinations would change from one school system to another. No doubt, the SLP will consult with the classroom teacher and with other school personnel regarding the types of tests that have been used in a student's evaluation, the results, interpretation, and classroom application of the findings.

The use of informal evaluation tasks is another way to gain insight into a student's language and communication ability. Many authorities suggest that using informal, more descriptive methods in evaluation actually provides more information that is directly relevant to treatment and academic performance (Haynes & Pindzola, 2004; Paul, 2001).

Since the biggest concern of the SLP is language and communication, most of the formal test instruments and nonstandardized evaluation tasks focus on a number of areas. As mentioned earlier, language may be divided into components of semantics, syntax, morphology, phonology, and pragmatics. All of these components are used in both input (language comprehension) and output (language production). Thus, for a thorough evaluation, the SLP will want to test the student's facility with vocabulary, sentence structure, word endings, and the use of language in various contexts. For instance, standardized tests and informal tasks will be directed toward assessing the student's understanding of semantic elements (vocabulary) as well as the ability to produce or retrieve words given a specific cue. Syntax ability is tapped by having a student follow directions that vary in their grammatical complexity (syntactic comprehension). The production of syntax is evaluated by having the student engage in conversation or description tasks, and then taking an inventory of the sentence types constructed and any grammatical errors produced by the student. Morphological ability in comprehension is assessed in a similar manner through asking a student to point to pictures illustrating a particular word ending (e.g., asking the student to point to a picture of cats when one picture contains only one cat and the other has two). Production of morphemes can be evaluated best by noting morphological errors in spontaneous conversation (e.g., "I goes to the store") and the use of other specific elicitation tasks (Balason & Dollaghan, 2002). Phonological ability can be evaluated through a variety of articulation tests (see Chapter 4). Finally, since there are no widely accepted standardized tests of pragmatics, these skills are best assessed in spontaneous conversation using a series of specific tasks that require the student to carefully describe pictures or provide particular information to a listener. Another popular task is to have the student produce a narrative about a favorite book, movie, or event such as a vacation. Students with pragmatic disorders often produce narratives that have sequence problems, shorter length, less syntactic complexity, less story grammar elements, and have more problems taking into account the listener's perspective (Haynes & Pindzola, 2004). Pragmatic disorders are often associated with social difficulties in children with language impairment (Fujiki, Brinton, Isaacson, & Summers, 2001; Fujiki, Brinton, & Todd, 1996). This again illustrates how the SLP should extend assessment beyond formal testing and determine environmental effects of the communication disorder using teachers and peers as informants. After the evaluation, the SLP should know if the student is performing within normal limits in all areas of language and in the use of language to solve problems.

Since reading and writing are language-based activities (Catts & Kamhi, 2005) these areas represent another assessment concern for the SLP. Apel (1999, p. 229) states that "Speech-language pathologists should assess and facilitate reading, and writing skills, in addition to oral language skills, if they have been identified as areas of concern." Specific skills such as decoding, spelling, reading, and writing not only can be assessed by the SLP, but integrated into treatment activities as well (Apel & Swank, 1999; Graham & Harris, 1999; Masterson & Crede, 1999).

A final assessment area involves the student's environment. The SLP may be interested in visiting the student's classroom(s) to gain an idea about the teaching styles that he or she encounters in different classes. The SLP needs to determine if aspects of a teacher's presentation (e.g., speech rate, use of complex or **figurative language**) could interfere with the processing of information by the language-impaired student. The SLP also needs to determine what types of teaching aids (e.g., media, study guides, outlines, etc.) are used by different teachers. Such aids are very helpful to all students in the class, but especially the student with a language impairment. The curriculum is also a target of evaluation by the SLP. She will ask about textbooks and the order of teaching material in a particular class. Many SLPs have incorporated "portfolio evaluation" into their assessment of students with language problems (Kratcoski, 1998). Thus, samples of a student's written work, classroom tests, and projects can be incorporated into the assessment. Many times linguistic problems surface across the different modalities of reading, writing, and speaking, and use of portfolio materials can provide a broader evaluation of a student's language ability. In this way, the SLP will also find out what kinds of subject matter the student should be able to talk about and explain. Often, the treatment sessions will center on academic subjects and classroom work.

DIRECT AND INDIRECT TREATMENT FOR STUDENTS WITH LANGUAGE IMPAIRMENT

It should be noted here that many of the ideas that follow are not merely suggestions. Children with disabilities such as language impairment are protected under several federal laws that *require* teachers and school systems to make appropriate accommodations in the classroom (see Chapter 1 for further details). Adjustments such as extended time on exams, permission to tape-record lectures, use books on tape, use of FM amplification systems, preferential seating, and many other accommodations are reasonable and appropriate for students with disabilities. It is a sad commentary that some students receive their first classroom accommodations when they begin their university careers and learn about their rights when they report to the office for students with disabilities their first week at college. We can only speculate about the quality of learning that could have occurred if such students had received appropriate classroom accommodations in elementary, junior, and senior high school.

Treatment goals generally are drawn from a number of areas when dealing with school-age children with language disorders (Boley, Larson, & McKinley, 1993; Butler & Wallach, 1994; Larson & McKinley, 1995; McKinley & Larson, 1985; McKinley & Schwartz, 1984; Miller, 1989;):

- Academic organization—Students with language disorders often have difficulty with time management, study skills, and the ability to perform critical thinking activities. These are compounded if the student has attention deficit disorder (ADD) or a learning disability on top of the difficulties with language. The SLP can work with the student on these academic organizational issues in concert with other professionals and try to develop strategies that will allow the student to succeed in the school culture. Often, teachers do not perceive the need or make the time to work with students who have language disorders on academic organization. While the SLP can do this, it must be recommended by others as a valid need or goal. The SLP can integrate these goals into the treatment plan, which both justifies and necessitates providing time and resources to accomplish these additional objectives.
- Listening/comprehension—As mentioned previously, students with language disorders will often have difficulty comprehending classroom language because of the interaction of their language disorder with the complexities of teacher utterances. If the student has difficulty comprehending instructions, academic information, or even social interaction language there will be communication failure that has academic as well as social consequences. Thus, the SLP often has listening and comprehension goals for the student with language disorders.
- Oral language production—Table 6-1 listed a number of symptoms of language disorder in older students. Some of the most frequent language pro-

duction goals include maintaining a conversational topic, taking into account the listener's perspective, providing adequate detail, and putting information in a correct sequence. Some of these students also need assistance in producing more syntactically complex utterances and correcting errors in sentence formulation.

- Written language and reading—It was noted earlier in this chapter that language-based activities such as speaking, writing, reading, and spelling are most often affected as a group in a student with a language disorder. The SLP will often incorporate reading and writing goals into the language work and use written language as stimuli in treatment (Fleming & Forester, 1997).

Four General Guidelines in Designing Treatment

No matter what mode of treatment is used (direct or indirect), four guidelines for the conduct of language therapy with older students should be considered.

Teach Strategies, Not Just Memorization

Older students tend to require strategies for academic, social, and communicative success, rather than learning a series of rote behaviors for each difficult situation they encounter. That is, these students need to learn methods to increase their organization, comprehension, memory, test-taking skills, oral communication, and reading and writing abilities that will apply to a broad range of circumstances. We do not just want to help the student get through only one problem situation. The notion of *strategy* implies that they will learn ways of dealing successfully with a variety of circumstances that are similar. For example, teaching a study skill for certain types of information will be applicable on other occasions when similar material will have to be learned by the student. Teaching a social interaction strategy (stay on the conversational topic) will be applicable to all of the student's conversations.

Design Activities Appropriate to Age or Cognitive Level

This guideline should be obvious; however, sometimes we forget. Dealing with teenagers or preteen students is a slippery slope. Sometimes a teacher or clinician may forget that certain materials that have been designed for younger children may not be appropriate for older students. By the same token, we do not want to use materials that are significantly above the student's level of performance.

Make Activities Relevant

It is especially important when dealing with older students that they see the relevance of treatment activities. Topics such as getting a driver's license, dating, getting a part-time job, improving study skills, understanding politics, and so on may be great activities to use in language treatment because the language trained can be generalized to other important situations. It is a great waste of time for the SLP to center treatment sessions around talking about what the student did on the weekend and exclude academic and social issues. One of the most important facets of language treatment is to include "survival language." Survival language is the type of communication we use to be successful in everyday life. If we teach a student language used in a successful job interview, or how to take accurate telephone messages or tell a story or joke correctly, then we have trained a basic life skill. If we focus on teaching vocabulary associated with specific survival areas such as cooking, transportation, label warnings, health issues, and so on, we have increased the student's ability to more easily communicate about activities of daily living. This is much more important than teaching arbitrary vocabulary words that might not relate to the student's ultimate success in society.

The Triple Payoff

Any language treatment activity should be considered in light of whether it has a triple payoff in communication, social, and academic areas. It is easy to design an activity to enhance a student's language abilities (e.g., using more complex sentences). It is more difficult to make that activity communicatively, socially, and academically relevant. For example, the SLP can work on production of more complex sentences while talking about the federal government, which is the topic of concern in the student's political science class. Talking about how the government is organized is just as easy as talking about what the student did at the beach last summer, but it has an academic payoff. If the SLP uses the student's textbook as a springboard for conversations about classroom material, there is an academic as well as a communication payoff. If the SLP works on production of more complex sentences while teaching the student to produce oral narratives, the telling of personal experiences and humorous stories will be enhanced. This constitutes a social payoff. Ideally, the SLP should be seeking activities that have this triple payoff instead of just working on communication.

Lasky (1985) provides some of the most useful suggestions we have found for classroom teachers and SLPs who deal with language-learning-disabled students. The suggestions fall into several areas and will be discussed next.

The Information to Be Communicated

While it is not recommended that the SLP perform tutoring of classroom material, some academic content can certainly be used to teach strategies that could apply across classes. For example, in teaching a student a strategy for how to retrieve new vocabulary, the SLP could use words peculiar to a certain class to illustrate the concept. This is certainly preferable to teaching a retrieval strategy using vocabulary that is unrelated to the student's academic work. Some specific suggestions about modifying information follow:

1. Let the SLP check comprehension and expression of specific concepts taught in the classroom (social studies, science, reading, and so on). In this way it can be determined if the student really understands and can explain concepts learned in class. The teacher does not have time to routinely check the understanding or speaking facility of individual students until it is time for a test. This, of course, is too late for a student with language-learning problems.
2. If there are new vocabulary words associated with a chapter, the teacher and SLP could put these in a handout to emphasize their importance. As part of a larger process to teach vocabulary learning strategies, the SLP could work directly on tasks that require the student to explain or comprehend these new vocabulary items.
3. If the student has difficulty comprehending complex sentences, the SLP could explain new classroom concepts in simpler grammatical sentences and then gradually increase the syntactic complexity when he or she talks about the new concept. Thus, the student may be better able to grasp the material in classroom presentations where the teacher is likely to use more complex language.
4. Again, as part of an overall program to increase vocabulary size, new semantic concepts could be taught by the SLP in advance of the teacher's classroom presentation. This could enhance the student's ability to clearly understand the material when it is presented later by the teacher.

5. If there are specific tasks that involve use of metalinguistic ability, complex language, or nonliteral meanings (e.g., figurative language), the SLP could drill the student on these types of skills prior to or concurrently with their use in the classroom.

Modifying the Presentation

Lasky (1985, p. 119) indicates that another important aspect of helping the language-learning-disabled student is to present material in such a way as to facilitate comprehension:

> Clinicians and teachers need to work as a team not only to present contextual cues but also to help the child recognize *when* contextual cues are presented. Types of contextual cues include (1) stating the topic to be discussed; (2) providing specific verbal instructions to guide the listener; (3) supplying a prepared outline; (4) using slides, charts, pictures, graphs, diagrams, or a film; and (5) presenting directed questions. These cues trigger listeners' expectations, help focus their attention on critical points, and aid listeners to anticipate information, see relationships, and organize and remember information.

Other suggestions for modifying the presentation involve the following:

1. Redundancy—The more the teacher can repeat a particular concept in a number of different ways, the greater the chance that the student will understand it. This aid will not just be important or helpful for the language-learning-disabled student, but for everyone in the class.
2. Slower rate—Many investigations have shown that language-impaired children and adults are more likely to comprehend utterances that are presented at slower speech rates. The teacher who has a language-impaired student in her class should try to use a slower rate, especially when explaining important and abstract concepts.
3. Students with language disorders and learning problems can also be encouraged to tape-record lectures, so they can repeat them as often as needed at home to fill in gaps in class notes.

Modifying the Environment

A potential problem for language-learning-disabled students in the classroom is paying attention. We know that many studies have shown this population to exhibit attentional difficulties. The classroom is especially susceptible to ambient noise and distractions from a variety of sources. Some studies have shown that, while most classrooms have varying degrees of environmental noise (e.g., traffic, hallway noise, and sounds from fans) the conversations of others provide the most distracting type of noise (Lasky & Tobin, 1973). This is especially true if the language-impaired student is listening to a small number of talkers seated nearby as opposed to large numbers of talkers in, for instance, a lunchroom (Miller, 1947). When students with language impairments listen to small numbers of talkers they hear certain words and phrases, and this is more distracting than listening to a large group of talkers, where particular parts of the conversation cannot be deciphered. At any rate, the teacher must be aware that both environmental noise and classroom talking and whispering can and do affect the attention of students with language impairments. Perhaps preferential seating in the front of the room would enhance listening and could be coupled with cautions to the class members against talking when they should be listening. Also, several study carrels or isolated work areas can be made available for use by these students to enhance their attention and concentration on assignments.

Modifying the Response

Sometimes in teaching a particular concept, we tend to demand responses from students that are relatively shallow activities requiring little processing of information. For instance, when we have students imitate, point to pictures, or memorize lists of information, they may not truly learn the essence of the concept or how it may be applied in a variety of contexts. Some students with language impairments may have more difficulty memorizing material if they do not see its application in meaningful contexts. The SLP and teacher can work with such students on meaningful application of material that may facilitate understanding and memory, instead of using shallower and less meaningful response modes. For students who have particular difficulty with written language, the teacher might consider allowing the use of a computer for written assignments. Computers add the advantages of spell-checking, thesauruses, and word-prediction software that could be valuable to the student with a language disorder. When the student's writing is very poor, perhaps orally taping a book report that the rest of the class is writing would be a reasonable alternative. This, of course, must be decided on an individual basis for each student and assignment.

Modifying Learning Strategies

Students develop strategies for processing information in the early elementary school years that are modified as grade levels and teacher expectations change over time (Naus & Halasz, 1979). Several researchers have pointed out that language-impaired students are not as adept as normally achieving students at developing specific strategies for organizing material and devising overt methods for learning it (Kavale, 1980; Lasky, 1985; Schworm & Abelseth, 1981). Among the typical strategies used by normally achieving children are verbal mediation, rehearsal, paraphrasing, visual imagery, analysis of key ideas, networking, use of systematic retrieval strategies (Lasky, 1985). Research has shown that these strategies can be overtly taught to students, and this training is effective, retained over long periods of time, and generalized to different situations (Kestner & Borkowski, 1979). The teacher and SLP could actively teach the student with a language disability to use specific strategies to enhance the understanding, recognition, recall, and application of concepts taught in the classroom. While normally developing students evidently need little overt assistance in developing study skills and learning strategies, the student with a language learning disability may not spontaneously generate such abilities. Direct teaching would be of help not only for the understanding of material, but also for methods to demonstrate such knowledge on the quizzes and tests upon which course grades depend. The teacher and SLP will no doubt need to experiment with a variety of methods for each language-impaired student to determine the optimal strategies for learning particular material presented in the classroom. In the ideal scenario, the particular learning style of the language-impaired student would be matched with a teacher having a compatible teaching style. While this is not always feasible, it is possible to consider such a match when there is flexibility in which classroom to assign a student with language impairment.

What Type of Treatment Format Is Best?

In the suggestions included earlier, it is implied that the classroom teacher and SLP work together in facilitating the language-disordered student's linguistic, communicative, and academic performance. Some of this work can be accomplished through individual sessions with the SLP, but much work can be done with these students in groups. In fact, many authorities recommend group treatment in preference to individual treatment for the majority of students (McKinley & Larson, 1985; Simon, 1987). Many strategies for learning, memory, and retrieval that benefit most language-impaired students could be taught and practiced in group work. Even listening skills, study skills, organizational skills, and strategies for more effective expression can be taught in a group environment. McKinley and Larson (1985, p. 8) also recommend the following, especially for the adolescent with a language disorder:

1. Use existing time modules. Removing students from classes twice a week for 20 minutes is token service and can cause serious disruption academically and socially.
2. Use supportive labels for services. *Speech therapy* and *language therapy* may be poor labels for adolescents with language disorders trying to appear similar to their peers. Better labels might be *individualized language skills* or *oral communication strategies*.
3. Recognize students' efforts. Offering language intervention as a course for credit (e.g., one fourth credit per semester) is more appropriate than not offering any credit at all. Students invest at least as much time and energy working on their communication skills as they do on other skills taught as courses for credit.
4. Use group settings. Intervention with adolescents requires much more grouping of students into classes than does intervention with younger students. Students need to be grouped to facilitate interaction, as a major goal for many language-disordered adolescents is appropriate and effective communication (i.e., having pragmatic skills).

Many SLPs in elementary grades conduct group units in communication for English classes or other related subjects (Simon, 1987). Such group (class) instruction can benefit large numbers of students, often without the formal process of IEP writing, unending meetings, or the reams of paperwork required to formally add the child to the SLP's caseload. The students receive additional services focusing on communication skills, study skills, and "playing the school game," and they are not singled out as "disordered." While most students can benefit greatly from such group sessions, some require the individual attention of the SLP to work on specific language disorders and would be formally evaluated and added to the caseload. The most current recommendations suggest that the SLP offer a variety of treatment options for the older language-impaired student (Larson et al., 1993).

The child with language impairment may also benefit from additional tutoring, both within and outside of the school setting. Some students may enjoy peer tutoring, if it proves practical and effective. Finally, there is a need to recognize that a child with a language disorder may never fully develop a normal ability to deal with linguistic material in reading, writing, speaking, or listening. These children can especially benefit from career testing and vocational counseling early on in their secondary school years. They need to know which types of jobs require complex language and communication skills to perform successfully. In fact, school systems are required by federal law to provide a transition plan for students with disabilities by age 16 years or younger, if appropriate (Prendeville & Ross-Allen, 2002). If university training is required, students need to be directed to campuses that offer services for language- and learning-disabled students.

CONCLUSION

There is a large group of students struggling in the academic setting who could benefit from the combined assistance of the classroom teacher and the speech-language pathologist. Through a true collaborative effort, teachers and SLPs can save these students from falling between the cracks of our educational system and give them a better chance to succeed academically.

REFERENCES

Apel, K. (1999). An introduction to assessment and intervention with older students with language-learning impairments: Bridges from research to clinical practice. *Language, Speech, and Hearing Services in Schools, 30*, 228–230.

Apel, K., & Swank, L. (1999). Second chances: Improving decoding skills in the older student. *Language, Speech, and Hearing Services in Schools, 30*, 231–242.

Balason, D., & Dollaghan, C. (2002). Grammatical morpheme production in 4-year-old children. *Journal of Speech, Language, and Hearing Research, 45*, 961–969.

Catts, H. (1997). The early identification of language-based reading disabilities. *Language, Speech, and Hearing Services in Schools, 28*, 86–89.

Catts, H., Fey, M., Zhang, X., & Tomblin, B. (2001). Estimating the risk of future reading difficulties in kindergarten children: A research-based model and its clinical implications. *Language, Speech, and Hearing Services in Schools, 32*, 38–50.

Catts, H., & Kamhi, A. (2005). *Language and reading disabilities*. Boston: Allyn & Bacon.

Chappell, G. (1985). Description and assessment of language disabilities of junior high school students. In C. Simon (Ed.), *Communication skills and classroom success: Assessment of language-learning disabled students*, San Diego, CA: College-Hill.

Fleming, J., & Forester, B. (1997). Infusing language enhancement into the reading curriculum for disadvantaged adolescents. *Language, Speech, and Hearing Services in Schools, 28*(2), 177–180.

Fujiki, M., Brinton, B., Isaacson, T., & Summers, C. (2001). Social behaviors of children with language impairment on the playground: A pilot study. *Language, Speech, and Hearing Services in Schools, 32*(2), 101–113.

Fujiki, M., Brinton, B., & Todd, C. (1996). Social skills of children with specific language impairment. *Language, Speech, and Hearing Services in Schools, 27*, 195–202.

Graham, S., & Harris, K. (1999). Assessment and intervention in overcoming writing difficulties: An illustration from the self-regulated strategy development model. *Language, Speech, and Hearing Services in Schools, 30*, 255–264.

Haynes, W., and Pindzola, R. (2004). *Diagnosis and evaluation in speech pathology*. Needham Heights, MA: Allyn and Bacon.

Johnson, C., Beitchman, J., Young, A., Escobar, M., Atkinson, L., Wilson, B., et al. (1999). Fourteen-year follow-up of children with and without speech/language impairments: Speech/language stability and outcomes. *Journal of Speech, Language, and Hearing Research, 42*, 744–768.

Kavale, K. (1980). Learning disability and cultural economic disadvantage: The case for a relationship. *Learning Disability Quarterly, 3*, 97–112.

Kestner, J., & Borkowski, J. (1979). Children's maintenance and generalization of an interrogative learning strategy. *Child Development, 50*, 485–494.

Kratcoski, A. (1998). Guidelines for using portfolios in assessment and evaluation. *Language, Speech, and Hearing Services in Schools, 29*, 3–10.

Larson, V., & McKinley, N. (1995). *Language disorders in older students*. Eau Claire, WI: Thinking.

Larson, V., McKinley, N., & Boley, D. (1993). Service delivery models for adolescents with language disorders. *Language, Speech, and Hearing Services in Schools, 24*, 36–42.

Lasky, E. (1985). Comprehending and processing of information in clinic and classroom. In C. Simon (Ed.), *Communication skills and classroom success: Therapy methodologies for language learning disabled students*. San Diego, CA: College-Hill.

Lasky, E., & Tobin, H. (1973). Linguistic and nonlinguistic competing message efforts. *Journal of Learning Disabilities, 6*, 243–250.

Masterson, J., & Crede, L. (1999). Learning to spell: Implications for assessment and intervention. *Language, Speech, and Hearing Services in Schools, 30*, 243–254.

McKinley, N., & Larson, V. (1985). Neglected language-disordered adolescent: A delivery model. *Language, Speech, and Hearing Services in Schools, 16*, 2–15.

Miller, G. (1947). The masking of speech. *Psychological Bulletin, 44*, 105–129.

Miller, L. (1989). Classroom-based intervention. *Language, Speech, and Hearing Services in Schools, 20*(2), 153–169.

Naus, M., & Halasz, F. (1979). Developmental perspectives on cognitive processing and semantic memory structure. In L. Cermak, & F. Craik (Eds.), *Levels of processing in human memory*. Hillsdale, NJ: Lawrence Erlbaum Associates.

Paul, R. (2001). *Language disorders from infancy through adolescence: Assessment and intervention* (2nd ed.). St. Louis, MO: Mosby.

Prendeville, J., & Ross-Allen, J. (2002). The transition process in the early years: Enhancing speech-language pathologist's perspectives. *Language, Speech, and Hearing Services in Schools, 33*, 130–136.

Rescorla, L. (2002). Language and reading outcomes to age 9 in late talking toddlers. *Journal of Speech, Language, and Hearing Research, 45*, 360–371.

Schwartz, L., & McKinley, N. (1984). *Daily communication*. Eau Claire, WI: Thinking.

Schworm, R., & Abelseth, J. (1981). Evaluating instructional interactions: Where do we begin teaching? *Learning Disabilities Quarterly, 4*, 101–111.

Simon, C. (1987). Out of the broom closet and into the classroom: The emerging SLP. *Journal of Childhood Communication Disorders, 11*, 41–66.

Wallach, G., & Butler, K. (1994). *Language learning disabilities in school-age children*. Baltimore: Williams and Wilkins.

TERMS TO KNOW

figurative language	pragmatics
metalinguistics	semantics
morphology	syntax
phonology	

TOPICS FOR DISCUSSION

1. How do the current methods you have learned for the teaching of reading incorporate metalinguistic skills?

2. What alterations could you make to these methods for a student with language disorder who had particular trouble with metalinguistics?

3. Obtain several textbooks used in reading instruction and evaluate the extent to which they really communicate ideas as opposed to facilitate phonetic drills. Then, find some books that focus on phonics.

4. Record yourself giving instructions to an imaginary class on how to do a specific assignment. Play back the tape and analyze the complexity, rate, and disfluency in your instructions. Note your use of figurative language. How would you change these instructions if you had a chance to do them again? How do you think a child with language-learning problems would understand the instructions?

5. Take a specific lesson plan that you have written for one of your education classes and use it for this exercise. Pretend that you have two children with language disorders in your class and indicate how you would teach the lesson differently because they are in the class. Describe any use of visual aids, handouts, explanations, questioning, and class discussion.

chapter seven

Dialectal Differences: African-American English as a Case Example

Student (excitedly): Miss Jones, you remember that show you tole us bout? Well, me and my momma 'nem—

Teacher (interrupting with a warm smile): Bernadette, start again, I'm sorry, but I can't understand you.

Student (confused): Well, it was that show, me and my momma—

Teacher (interrupting again, still with that warm smile): Sorry, I still can't understand you.

(Student, now silent, even more confused than ever, looks at floor, says nothing.)

Teacher: Now, Bernadette, first of all, it's Mrs. Jones, not Miz Jones. And you know it was an *exhibit,* not a *show.* Now, haven't I explained to the class over and over again that you always put yourself last when you are talking about a group of people and yourself doing something? So, therefore, you should say what?

Student: My momma and me—

Teacher (exasperated): No! My mother and I. Now, start again, this time right.

Student: Aw, that's okay, it wasn't nothin.

Geneva Smitherman (1977, p. 217) *Talkin and Testifyin*

■ 193 ■

The present chapter considers a highly controversial topic. On one hand there have been several popular sociopolitical movements advocating that all Americans should speak only English and that even the use of dialectal variations should not be encouraged or tolerated in educational and business environments. On the other hand, sociolinguists promote the view that multiculturalism and its associated language differences are not disorders and should be embraced because they are an inherent part of a person's culture. In fact, *everyone* speaks a **dialect**. This perspective is well supported by federal laws mandating bilingual education for students and guidelines regarding nondiscriminatory testing for non-English speaking persons. It is even controversial to talk about the type of language to which we compare a dialect. For instance, we have used the term **Standard American English (SAE)** for years when describing the contrastive features of dialects. We compare the grammatical, phonological, morphological, and pragmatic rules of a dialect with SAE to illustrate language differences. A problem, however, is that SAE does not exist in reality. Lippi-Green (1997, p. 64) describes SAE as a "bias toward an abstracted, idealized, homogeneous spoken language that is imposed and maintained by dominant bloc institutions." The institutions she refers to are the mass media and entertainment industry, the educational system, and corporate America. Typically the "standard" language is the one used by people with power and money in a society, and it is the language best understood by the majority of people. Another commonly cited component of SAE is that it does not carry with it regional or ethnic variations. The most common area of the country identified as speaking SAE is the Midwest. These notions carry with them some significant problems. First, if SAE is the "prestigious" language spoken by those with institutional power and wealth, then other forms of language (i.e., dialects) are automatically devalued, along with the people who speak them. Just the name *standard English* implies that dialects may be substandard versions of English. A second problem is that if SAE is Midwestern, it is really just another regional dialect itself. In a recent PBS documentary entitled "Do You Speak American?" it was noted: "Ask a group of experts to define Standard American English, and you'll find, paradoxically, there's no standard answer." Some have suggested the use of *Mainstream American English (MAE)* or *General American English (GAE)*, but in reality, these are not much better than SAE because they have their own set of implications and problems. In this textbook we will continue to use SAE to refer to the mainstream language variety for several reasons. At the time of this writing (2005), a search of Web sites for the American Speech-Language-Hearing Association (www.

asha.org), The Center for Applied Linguistics (www.cal.org), and the Linguistic Society of America (www.lsadc.org) shows that all these professional organizations continue to use *SAE* as the most common term referring to mainstream language. At the present time, we can see no persuasive evidence that professional organizations or researchers are moving away from using the term *SAE*. In the recent PBS special previously referred to, the term *Mainstream (Standard) American English* was used, which in some ways is even more confusing. Finally, the current issues of professional journals in communication disorders all use the term SAE in research articles (Craig & Washington, 2004; Craig & Washington, 2002; Thompson, Craig, & Washington, 2004).

To address cultural issues, many school systems have incorporated a more multicultural approach to teaching academic content that includes examples and contributions from a variety of cultures. Although specific data on the issue are difficult to obtain, the present authors believe that most students in this country are being taught using SAE curriculum materials with some degree of sensitivity to cultural variations. We will discuss this in more detail in a later section.

Speaking a dialect can carry with it certain disadvantages when the educational "standard" is SAE. In special education, for example, we are aware that students who are bilingual or bidialectal may perform poorly on standardized tests because of linguistic interference or cultural factors (van Keulen, Weddington, & DeBose, 1998). Decades ago there were unfortunate examples of children who spoke another language being tested in SAE. Shockingly, if the tests were measuring intelligence, some normal children were "diagnosed" as being mentally retarded, not because of cognitive difficulties, but because the test was in English and did not take into account that the child was bilingual. Historically, there have been many more children of color than white children in special education programs receiving special education services. In the case of communication disorders, many of these "problems" were language based (van Keulen, et al., 1998). A significant percentage of these children no doubt had normal language skills within their dialect or language group, but performed poorly on tests that focused on Standard American English and were culturally biased. In the past 20 years, test developers have made a concerted effort to reduce linguistic and cultural bias on tests and to include a variety of cultural groups in normative samples. Today, most school systems have increased their vigilance to ensure that a disproportionate number of minority students are not enrolled in special education programs because of cultural or linguistic interference factors. In spite of these advances, we still hear tales of misdiagnosis and insensitivity to multi-cultural issues.

A major issue implied in the controversy just described is whether a person speaking a dialect of English has a *disorder* of language and whether that person should be enrolled in therapy to change his or her way of talking. While some people may not see this as a problem, the speech-language pathologist (SLP) certainly is faced with the issue on a daily basis. If he or she is required to work with students on changing their dialect, then he or she is ultimately faced with an overwhelming caseload of children who are essentially normal with regard to their language community. With a caseload of this size, there would be little time to serve those students with legitimate communication disorders in the areas of voice, fluency, language, and phonology. Thus, you will find that most SLPs have a clear position on what constitutes a disorder and what, if anything, to do with dialect speakers.

One goal of this chapter is to illustrate the significant impact of social dialects on communication and academic performance in educational settings. It is impossible to cover all regional, ethnic, and racial dialects of American English in a single chapter and include all their rules, conventions, and differences from Standard English. Therefore, we have elected to illustrate social dialects using **African-American English (AAE)** as a case example for several reasons. First, census figures from the year 2000 show that Hispanics and African-Americans are the largest minority population groups in the United States. This means that most teachers will encounter African-American students in their classrooms. A second reason for using AAE as an illustration is that even though we have known about the features of this dialect for decades, many people remain unaware of its rules and historical origins. Many still view AAE as an impoverished form of speaking and are not aware that the dialect has a legitimate connection to African languages (Rickford, Sweetland, & Rickford, 2004). While we use AAE as an example of social dialects in the present chapter, readers should bear in mind that the points we make could be applied to *any* dialect of English. If you are a teacher in a system that has a large Hispanic population, we would hope that you become familiar with information on local Hispanic dialectal variations and cultural mores. Similarly, if you teach Navajo children or Asian/Pacific Islanders you should familiarize yourself with important cultural mores and dialectal variations. This information should be at least as in-depth as that provided in the present chapter.

Most people from a variety of different cultures tend to be *ethnocentric* (Lynch & Hanson, 1992). That is, they view the world from a perspective of their own culture and place value judgments on the practices, mores, and languages of other cultural groups. Ethnocentricity may be a natural tendency, but it is one that can be overcome with exposure to other cultures and systematic study. People are said to have increased their *cultural literacy* when they have learned about and accepted the value of the differences among various cultural groups. Cultural literacy is not the province of *any* cultural group. For example, being a member of a minority group does not guarantee a high level of cultural literacy. The only road to cultural literacy is the study and experience of other cultures and keeping an open mind. Historically, school systems in the United States have been driven by a largely white, European, middle-class value system, although this has changed significantly in the last quarter century. Failure to consider other cultures and their contributions is an example of ethnocentricity and gives a relatively narrow view of the world to students. Interestingly, if we look at the broader picture we find that almost 85% of the world's population is made up of people of color. Recent population projections in the United States suggest that by the year 2050, one-half of America's population will probably be nonwhite. In some states at the present time, whites are in the minority or approaching this status (e.g., California, Texas, New Mexico). This gives a whole new meaning to the notion of *minority group* for many readers. Whether or not one is considered a minority is largely a matter of context. An African-American in Utah may be a minority, but in Washington, D.C., he or she is a majority group member. Many people today reject the term *minority*, considering it meaningless because it changes with context. Also the term *minority* suggests that the group is less important as compared to a *majority*. There is also ethnocentricity with regard to languages. Most people feel that their own language is the "best." It is interesting that in the United States some feel that we should only learn and speak English. Yet, bilingualism, not monolingualism, is the norm throughout the world. There are over 3000 different languages and dialects in the world and over 150 in the United States. Most people in the world speak several languages.

As mentioned above, school systems have made significant changes in recent decades, including more sensitivity to cultural variations. This practice allows us to pull away from an ethnocentric view that white, European, middle-class expectations and practices have value for all students regardless of cultural group. It also prepares teachers and SLPs for the steady increase of different cultural groups in schools. There are many different cultural groups represented, and we must develop strategies for accommodating all children regardless of their background.

Most people are aware that there are a number of different ways to speak in the United States. For instance, it is not uncommon to hear reports that African-Americans or Hispanics speak differently from whites. People of Italian, Polish, or German descents often speak with an accent. Further, it is often said that people from lower socioeconomic levels speak differently than middle- or upper-class persons. Regional differences abound in this country, with people in the South speaking differently than those in the Midwest or on the East Coast. Despite these manifold racial, ethnic, social, and regional differences in speech and language, Americans seem to be able to communicate with each other. Although it may take some careful listening for an Anglo to understand a heavy Hispanic dialect, ideas *can* be passed from one person to another. The fact that communication can take place between these diverse groups attests to the fact that they are all basically speaking English, and that there are many more similarities than differences among the various versions of English.

A dialect is a "variety of a national language" (Taylor, 1986, p. 386) that is shared by a particular **speech community** for purposes of frequent interaction. A speech community may reflect any of the groups mentioned such as racial, ethnic, social, or regional. According to Taylor (1986, p. 395) these variations in language may be the product of any of the following:

(a) the languages brought to the country by various cultural groups. That is, speakers of English, Polish, Chinese, Wolof, and such; (b) the indigenous Native American languages spoken in the country; (c) the mix of the various communities and regions where the cultural groups settled; (d) the political and economic power wielded by the various cultures settling in the regions; (e) the migration patterns of the cultural groups within the country; (f) geographic isolation caused by rivers, mountains, and other features, as in the dialects of the Ozark and Appalachian mountains; and g) self-imposed social isolation or legal segregation.

In the sections that follow, we will describe and give some examples of how a variety of factors affect the way people speak English. None of these versions of English are defective and thus, none require speech or language therapy.

THE DIFFERENCE–DEFICIT ISSUE

Historically, there was a time when various authorities regarded dialectal variations as representing a *deficit* in language ability. Dialects, then, were viewed by some as impoverished forms of English, spoken by people who were attempting to use Standard American English, but were falling short of their goal. Some deficit theorists even implicated the intellectual abilities of certain groups. Their reasoning was that since language is used in the service of thought and if these speakers have imperfect language, then they also must have impoverished thinking abilities. Certain groups, especially African-Americans, were singled out as examples of the deficit model. People were quite generous with some dialects in attributing them to the mixing of two different languages. For instance, most people viewed a German or French accent as charming and attributed the language changes in these dialects to the influence of a person's native language. These generous views were often not extended to African-American English. Many thought it was neither charming nor legitimate because it had no obvious linguistic roots to another language and because of underlying racism.

As linguists began to investigate African-American English, however, it was determined that it did, in fact, have its roots on the western coast of Africa (Dillard, 1972). There was a well-developed historical path that could be traced from African-American English to African languages, and this connection gave African-American English the same legitimacy accorded to other dialects. African languages have features that are similar to those used in African-American English. This historical validation shows that African-American English is not simply an impoverished version of SAE, but a dialect that has its roots in other languages. AAE, like other dialects, is rule governed, which further demonstrates its status as a language system, not a deficiency.

Today, linguists prefer to talk about dialects as being *language differences*, as opposed to **language deficits**. This term means that dialects are simply different ways of speaking English, and no implication is made regarding levels of acceptability, capabilities of speakers, or the superiority of one dialect over another.

ETHNICITY, RACE, AND FIRST LANGUAGE COMMUNITY

Every culture has its customs, social conventions, and linguistic differences. These unique characteristics are interwoven in a very complex manner, and it is difficult to define a culture without delineating its peculiar differences. Language is an integral part of a person's ethnicity or racial definition; it cannot be removed without irreversibly altering the nature of the ethnic or racial group. For instance, a speaker of Yiddish may use unique vocabulary (*nebbish, schlemiel, putz*) with distinct stress and intonation patterns when talking to members of his or her ethnic group. Rosten (1971, p. 72) provides an example from Yiddish that illustrates: "*Two* tickets for her concert I should buy?" Littell (1971, p. 85–86) gives examples of syntax differences in Pennsylvania Dutch, such as "Don't eat yourself so full already—there's cake back yet—and Sally you chew your mouth empty before you say." African-American speakers may also use vocabulary (crib = residence; kicks = shoes; homey = friend; tight = pleasing to the eye, etc.) not typically spoken by people who are not members of this culture. Every racial or ethnic group has its own unique vocabulary items, sentence structures, ways of changing the sounds of English, and different social uses of language. These linguistic changes are part of the complex of behaviors that actually define the culture. When people make fun of the way ethnic or racial minorities talk, they are really making fun of an important determinant of a person's culture. Further, if a speech-language pathologist or educator suggests that a person must change the way he or she talks, this really amounts to altering a significant aspect of a person's culture and should not be done lightly. Essentially, if one says that a person's dialect is unacceptable, it is really being said that the culture is also unacceptable.

In the United States, the two largest racial/ethnic groups are African-Americans and Hispanics. These groups have distinct dialects, which will be described in more detail later. Other groups are immigrants or refugees from East Asia, Southeast Asia, and the Pacific Islands. The Asian/Pacific Island people in America speak the following major languages: Mandarin, Cantonese, Taiwanese, Hakka, Tagalog, Ilocano, Japanese, Korean, Vietnamese, Khmer, Lao, Hmong, Mien, Chamorro, Samoan, and Hindi (Cheng, 1989). Most white Americans have not even heard of these languages, but as these speakers are incorporated into the mosaic of our culture, dialects, and **language differences** will emerge. Most Americans are familiar with the language differences in first-generation immigrants from Europe (Germany, Poland, Italy, Ireland, France, Czech Republic, and Russia). These dialects have been portrayed in many popular films, and in large cities one can still hear the various ethnic language variations being perpetuated by second- and third-generation Americans. Finally, teachers in some areas of the country encounter other major dialectal variations when dealing with Native American, Eskimo, and Hawaiian children. Each of these cultural groups has its own variety of English.

REGIONAL VARIATIONS

Most Americans are aware that people in various parts of the country speak a dialect of English that is peculiar to their geographic region. There are many more regional dialects in the eastern portion of the United States, and regional differences become far less dense in the western states. For example, dialects in Boston, New York City, and Pennsylvania are quite different within a relatively small geographic area. Yet, it is sometimes difficult to hear differences in dialects in individual states west of the Mississippi River. Some dialects are composed of many variations from the SAE pattern, and others have only a few features that distinguish them from other regions. It should be noted that each region might have its own unique alterations in speech sounds, syntax, vocabulary, and social language rituals. For instance, carbonated beverages are known in the Midwest as *pop*, on the East Coast as *soda*, and in the South as *co-cola* (even if the person is referring to root beer). People in the Midwest say *hi* or *hello* when greeting someone, while people in the South say *hey*. People in Chicago use a *shopping cart* and Southern shoppers use a *buggy*. As Owens (1988) says, "The Italian sandwich changes to submarine, torpedo, hero, wedge, and hoagie as it moves about the United States" (p. 366). He could also have added *grinder*, common in Rhode Island, to the sandwich list. These are just examples of semantic differences around the country.

There are also differences in the phonetic elements used in the various regions. Most people are aware that speakers in Massachusetts and Maine pronounce the r̲ sound differently than speakers in the Midwest. In Maine a person might say, "paak youh caa" for "park your car." Actually, this grossly resembles the Southern pronunciation of the same sentence because in Southern dialect the r̲ sound also is affected. Even syntax is influenced by regional dialect variation. In the South, for instance, an acceptable sentence may involve two modals such as, "He might could do that." In the Midwest, *might* and *could* would not be placed together in the same utterance. In the South, people are always "fixing to go" somewhere. People on the East Coast, however, do not "fix to go" anywhere; they just go. Thus, there are many regional alterations to language, and the SLP and teacher must be aware that these variations are part of a particular culture and acceptable to use in that region.

SOCIAL CLASS VARIATIONS

Every culture has a number of social classes. You might recall the film *My Fair Lady* in which a speech expert named Henry Higgins stood outside a theater after a performance and was fervently scribbling phonetic transcriptions of speech he overheard from the patrons. When a flower girl named Eliza Doolittle spoke, Higgins exactly knew not only where she was from geographically, but also to which social class she belonged. Similarly, in some lower socioeconomic areas in New England, people might say things like *youse guys* and *dere* for *there*. These are examples of social class variations in language. Many people from lower socioeconomic classes use *ain't*. Studies of the language used by lower social classes have revealed that they speak a vernacular of English that has a system all its own. The term *vernacular* refers to an informal way of expressing ideas within a speech community. These investigations also show that most versions of a language spoken by lower social classes are more restricted than the elaborated standard language. By restricted, they mean that many words are omitted or shortened by the speakers of a vernacular of a language than in the standard language. Thus, "I am not going" is longer than "I ain't goin."

PEER GROUP IDENTIFICATION

When a teenager or adult becomes a member of a definable peer group, a language variation often occurs. Parents complain that their teenage sons and daughters do not speak English, or they are sloppy in the way they talk. While not a dialect per se, peer groups do serve to perpetuate unique ways of talking, and these linguistic varieties include all areas of language (e.g., syntax, semantics, pragmatics, etc.). Instead of a dialectal variation, many would consider peer group language as *slang*, which serves a very important social solidarity function for group members. Contemporary teenagers may show their respect for someone by saying, "You're the bomb!" This, of course, has nothing to do with explosives. They may also acknowledge a mistake by saying, "My bad." Specific groups such as street gangs, military personnel, musicians, and such have many distinct language variations when compared to Standard American English.

COMMUNICATIVE CONTEXT

Throughout the day, every speaker in a culture experiences a variety of **communicative contexts**. By communicative context we mean the situation in which the communication is taking place. The situation is not simply the physical place of communication but also includes the identity and characteristics of the listener. For instance, an adult SAE speaker might speak differently to a group of African-American teenagers because of a variety of factors (age, cultural differences, and social class differences). We all change the way we talk depending upon the circumstances of communication. You probably would talk quite differently to your roommate than you would to the president of the university. You would talk differently to a person with a hearing loss than you would to a person with normal hearing. You would talk to a 4-year-old differently than you would to a teenager. You would talk differently in a neighborhood bar than you would at a formal dinner. The many changes that a person makes in language as a response to communicative context is called *style shifting* or *code switching*. Style shifting has been studied in the African-American culture. It has been reported that many speakers of AAE change their style of communication when addressing members of mainstream culture (Hecht, Collier, & Ribeau, 1993; Seymour & Seymour, 1979). Cazden (1970) examined African-American children and found that they used a **street register**, which is a relaxed manner of talking to their peers at school and on the street. They also used a **school register** when addressing authority figures in the school environment. Interestingly, speakers of the school register used shorter sentences, were less syntactically complex, were more disfluent, and had quite different content as compared to speakers of the street register. Like any other dialect, communication style differences in AAE are affected by such variables as age, gender, and socioeconomic status. These examples illustrate the process of switching the way we talk to fit the communicative context. In reality, most speakers engage in style shifting. For instance, an African-American doctor might use some features of an African-American dialect when talking to patients of his or her own cultural group and switch to more of a Standard American English production when dealing with white patients.

DIALECTAL CONTINUA

When talking about the dialects spoken by various groups in the United States, it would be erroneous to give the impression that every member of a particular culture, region, or peer group speaks the same way. For example, the term *African-American English* is somewhat inaccurate because it gives the impression that everyone who is of African-American descent speaks this dialect. In reality, there are many African-Americans who speak SAE or some regional dialect that has no features of African-American English. There are many New Yorkers who are African-American and simply sound like they are from New York. We know of some white children in the rural south who attend a predominantly African-American school and come home incorporating many features of AAE into their language. There are many people from lower socioeconomic levels that speak more of a middle-class version of English. There are teenage girls from the San Fernando Valley area in Southern California who do not sound like Valley girls (e.g., "Totally, Fer Sure"). Thus, it is productive to think of every dialect and **vernacular** of English as existing on a continuum.

For example, say that AAE and SAE have about 29 features that they produce differently from one another (Williams & Wolfram, 1977). One African-American speaker may incorporate all 29 of the features and thus represent a maximal difference between African-American and SAE. Another African-American speaker, however, may only incorporate 10 of the possible 29 features and thus show more similarity to a SAE speaker. Finally, a third speaker may only use two or three of the features of AAE and represent a language use that is almost indistinguishable from Standard American English. These examples could have been from Hispanic English or regional dialects as well. A person in Maine may or may not have a heavy New England dialect for a variety of reasons (business, long-standing cultural ties, and frequent moves around the country). We should, therefore, not stereotype a person in terms of language just because he or she may represent a particular group or region of the country. There is a **dialectal continuum** upon which each person may incorporate many or few of the features of a dialect.

Another important notion is that dialects are in a constant state of flux. Whenever two dialects are put in close geographical proximity to one another a phenomenon takes place known as **dialect importation**. This means that each dialect borrows from the other, and there is a mutual influence on the dialects. For instance, in south Texas there is a way of speaking called *Tex-Mex*. It is a special dialect created because of the influence of the geographical relations between Mexico and Texas. In Europe, there are many small countries that are located right next to each other, and in the border areas distinct dialects have developed from the influences of two languages. Some linguists have indicated that Southern English may have been influenced by African-American English because historically many Southerners were raised by African-Americans employed on plantations to care for children. Some authorities indicate that the Southern dialect is becoming less pronounced (no pun intended) because of the large influx of northerners moving to warmer climates. Thus, dialects influence each other.

It has been said that America is a melting pot in which many cultures become homogenized into the population. This is partly true with dialects because the ways of talking influence each other and dialects gradually change. Others have said that a better analogy than melting pot to characterize America would be to use a salad. In a salad, the ingredients are together in a bowl, but to a large degree retain their identities. Although dialects change very gradually over time, they are a reflection of a person's culture, and there is much preservation of dialects as well as a result of efforts to perpetuate important cultural attributes. There are many reasons why dialects are preserved. For example, forced or voluntary segregation is one factor. Many large cities have areas where concentrations of ethnic and cultural groups live and work. Some cities have areas known by such names as *Chinatown* or *little Italy*. In some cities where there are large Latino populations, even the signs on businesses are written in Spanish. This kind of segregation helps to preserve dialects. Another example of preserving dialects is illustrated by different socioeconomic groups. If people from lower socioeconomic groups live in close proximity to each other, it helps to perpetuate their use of the vernacular of their dialect. Whatever variables account for affecting dialects, we know that forces exist to both perpetuate and change dialectal forms.

SPECIFIC DIFFERENCES BETWEEN AFRICAN-AMERICAN ENGLISH AND STANDARD ENGLISH

As mentioned previously, differences between SAE and AAE can be phonological, syntactic, semantic, and even pragmatic. Tables 7-1 and 7-2 outline only some of the more obvious phonological and syntactic features of African-American English. There are many descriptions of AAE linguistic features that consider this topic in great detail (Green, 2002; Rickford, 1999), but these are beyond the scope of the present chapter. Rickford and Rickford (2000) provide a readable summary for those without a background in linguistics. Clearly, if one considers all of the grammatical rules in SAE and the relatively few differences between AAE and SAE, there are far more similarities than differences between the dialects. We mention the few features of AAE in Tables 7-1 and 7-2 only to illustrate to teachers that a small number of linguistic differences can explain many of the variations they may encounter in the speech and writing of African-American students. Rickford and colleagues (2004) report that there is great variation in teacher-preparation programs in terms of including information on dialectal features. Many of the variations are accounted for by the consonant cluster reduction rule, which affects not only final consonant blends, but also the inclusion of past tense, possessive, and third person -s markers. The other major rule that affects many types of utterances is the use of the verb *to be* and its variants.

Table 7-1 Phonological Features of African-American English

Consonant cluster reduction: If a consonant cluster (blend) is located in the final position of a word (e.g., test, build) one member of the cluster may be deleted or reduced in African-American English. There is a very specific rule that operates here so only certain cluster types experience deletion. For instance, if both members of the cluster are the same with regard to voicing (both voiced sounds or both voiceless sounds), the final member will be reduced. Some examples of words that end in clusters that are both voiceless are as follows: test, mask, gasp, gift, wished (wisht). These words would be pronounced tes, mas, gas, gif, and wish. The same rule applies if both members are voiced sounds: build, hand, warmed. These words would be pronounced buil, han, and warm. When the two members are different in their voicing (i.e., one voiced and one voiceless), the cluster is typically not reduced. For instance, in the words jump, count, rent, belt, and gulp, the two sounds in the cluster differ in terms of voicing—one is voiced and the other is voiceless. These words are pronounced with both members of the cluster present. Thus, the cluster reduction rule in African-American English is lawful in nature. Clusters at the beginning and middle of words are not reduced.

The th phonemes: The voiced and voiceless th sounds in Standard American English are changed in a lawful way in African-American English. The specific changes made depend on the position of the th in the word. In the initial position, the voiceless th can be changed to a t sound (tink for think). The voiced th sound can be changed to a d sound (dem for them). When the voiceless th sounds are in the medial or final word position the f sound is substituted for them. For example, a child may say bafroom for bathroom. A similar rule applies for the voiced th sound in the medial position (bruvah for brother). At the end of a word the same rule applies with the substitution of f and v for the voiceless and voiced th sound (baf for bath: bave for bathe).

The r and l phonemes: A very similar rule applies in African-American English and in Southern English regarding the r and l sounds. In both dialects, the l or r often become uh as in sistuh for sister. Also, the r and l are sometimes absent in both dialects (hep for help; doe for door; foe for four; show for sure).

Final b, d, and g devoicing: At the end of a syllable, voiced plosives (b, d, g) may be replaced by their voiceless counterparts (p, t, k). Thus, an African-American speaker may say pik for pig, or but for bud.

Final omission of nasal sounds: At the end of words the nasal phonemes (m, n and ng) are often omitted and the preceding vowel is nasalized (e.g., pa for pan, ma for man). This is often noted as one of the economical features of African-American English because the nasal feature of the word is superimposed on the vowel, thus making the nasal consonant at the end of the word redundant.

STR blends: The str blends in African-American English are often changed to skr (string and street are changed to skring and skreet).

Table 7-2 Syntactic Features of African-American English

Past tense -ed: In African-American English, the bound morpheme *-ed* is omitted. This is because of the consonant cluster reduction rule referred to in Table 7-1. When a SAE speaker puts the *-ed* ending on a word, it is sometimes pronounced as one phoneme, either a t or a d. Thus, making the word *walk* past tense involves adding a t to the end of the word as in *walkt*. Since both members of the cluster kt are voiceless, the consonant cluster reduction rule eliminates the t sound in pronunciation. So, the following words are pronounced without the *-ed* ending: *cashed, cracked, named, slammed*.

Third-person singular present tense -s: In Standard American English, when a third-person form is used (*he, she, the boy*) it is required that an *-s* be attached to the verb (*he runs, she cooks, the boy eats*). In African-American English, the *-s* is omitted (*he run, she cook, the boy eat*).

Absent forms of the verb to be: In Standard American English, sentences must either have a verb or a form of the *be* verb such as *is, am,* or *are*. In African-American English, these forms of *be* can be omitted in many sentences. The forms are not totally absent in African-American English as certain sentence types do include them, such as tag questions (She not going, is she?) or exposed clauses (I know where he is).

Invariant *be*: The *be* verb in SAE changes its form depending on the type of sentence spoken. For example, *be* changes among *is, am, are, was,* and *were* with the effect of tense, plurality, and person. In African-American English, *be* does not change its form and may even be used as *be* (*He be workin*).

Double negatives: Like many other dialects and languages, African-American English use double negatives (*Couldn't nobody do it?*).

Possessives: In African-American English, the possessive morpheme *'s* can be omitted (*the girl car*). Possession is indicated by the order and proximity of words rather than adding the *'s*.

Plurals: In Standard American English the *-s* morpheme is placed at the end of words to mark plurality (*cars, cats, dogs*). African-American English speakers omit the plural morpheme largely because of the consonant cluster reduction rule and also because of the nonobligatory nature of the plural morpheme when talking about nouns of measure (money, time, and such). This leads to utterances such as two dollar, three year, and two cat.

From a semantic standpoint, we have already mentioned that there are a host of words and phrases in African-American English that are unique to this dialect (Major, 1994; Smitherman, 2000). Many of these terms become popular in the general American culture (e.g., chillin = relaxing; hood = neighborhood; the man = police; sup = what's up?) and then are often gradually relinquished by the speakers of African-American English (Andrews & Owens, 1976).

The syntactic changes listed in Table 7-2 are certainly not all-inclusive. There are some other subtle differences between Standard American and African-American English that are beyond the scope of the present chapter. The above differences, however, represent some major points of dialectal variation of syntax in African-American English.

In terms of language use, it is important to note that speakers of AAE prize the ability to communicate effectively. One's ability to "rap" or use language in social rituals of one-upmanship is valued in African-American culture.

THE EFFECTS OF DIALECTAL VARIATION ON THE STUDENT

There are two major implications of speaking a dialect in our school systems. First, most school systems are largely geared to SAE speaking, reading, and writing. Early surveys of parents of African-American children overwhelmingly supported the idea of using SAE in the schools (Taylor, 1971). In fact, early attempts at teaching literacy through the use of reading books written in AAE have not had a history of acceptance. van Keulen and colleagues (1998, p. 198) indicate that "The failure of a pilot series of dialect readers to gain widespread acceptance is often attributed to black parents' rejection of the concept." Perhaps the most popular approach to dealing with dialectal variation in schools is **bidialectalism** (Rickford et al., 2004). According to them (2004, p. 234), bidialectalism refers to:

> The perspective that vernacular speakers can and should command the standard variety as well as their native vernacular. It is an additive, rather than an eradicative, perspective, in that it seeks to expand speakers' linguistic repertoires instead of replacing one linguistic competence with another, more prestigious competence.

Thus, AAE speakers are entering a system that uses and reinforces language that is different in some respects from the language that they speak, and this can create some potential problems in learning (Gemake, 1981; Harber & Bryen, 1978; Laffey & Shuy, 1973). Imagine for instance, that the dialect you speak has some phonological and syntactic differences from the language you are being taught to read and write. Some sentences will have extra words in them, as in the case of *is* or *was* for an African-American English speaker. Some words will have extra sounds or letters in them, as in the case of plurals, possessives, and consonant clusters for the AAE speaker. Hispanic speakers may have the same difficulties of being faced with a code to learn that differs from the one they typically use. Reading and writing are difficult enough to learn for young SAE speakers, but AAE speakers are at an even greater disadvantage. Thus, one effect of speaking a dialect is that you may have a bit more difficulty learning to read, write, and speak Standard American English. This difficulty may result in lower grades, lower self-esteem, and less success in school.

The second implication is that a dialect speaker may be at a disadvantage when taking tests that are designed for SAE speakers. Fagundes, Haynes, Haak, & Moran (1998, p. 148) discuss some of the types of bias associated with standardized testing:

> The typical types of bias on standardized tests that can have a negative effect on culturally diverse children are *situational bias* (examination format is threatening to child), *directions bias* (directions for test can be misinterpreted by child), *value bias* (asking child to give moral/ethical judgments that may differ culturally from the examiners'), *linguistic bias* (presumption that the child is a standard English speaker), *format bias* (test procedures are inconsistent with child's cognitive style), *cultural misinterpretation* (negative interpretation of client behavior when it is culturally appropriate), and *stimulus bias* (test is highly object/picture oriented when child is socially oriented).

Although standardized language testing has a long history of not considering multicultural variables in test development, more recently developed examinations have been designed to remedy this important problem. For example, most newer tests depict people from a variety of cultures and norms and have been developed using standardization samples that include groups and numbers of children consistent with recent census information. In fact, Seymour, Roeper, and deVilliers (2003) have developed a criterion-referenced test that is specifically designed to take dialectal variation into account. Other nonstandardized testing approaches have also made significant contributions to reducing cultural bias in language testing. For example, some researchers have developed a minimal competency core that includes types of language that any child, regardless of dialect, should be able to produce because the items are not specific to a particular culture (Schraeder, Quinn, Stockman, & Miller, 1999; Stockman, 1996). Another approach involves the use of *contrastive analysis,* in which spontaneous language samples are gathered and analyzed to determine if variations produced by the child are accounted for by a dialect or if the variations are not dialectal but possibly evidence of a language disorder (McGregor, Williams, Hearst, & Johnson, 1997; Seymour, Bland-Stewart, & Green, 1998). Finally, some researchers have found that children with language impairment have difficulty repeating sequences of nonsense words, and since the stimulus items are not part of any culture, these processing tasks could be used to discriminate children with disorders from those that are speaking dialects (Bishop, North, & Donlan, 1996; Campbell, Dollaghan, Needleman, & Jamosky, 1997; Dollaghan & Campbell, 1998; Ellis-Weismer et al., 2000; Rodekohr & Haynes, 2001).

The SLP must constantly be aware of the possible negative effects of dialectal variation on formal tests and carefully examine errors to see if they are possibly the result of a student's dialect or culture. Taylor (1986, p. 405) indicates:

> The use of culturally and linguistically discriminatory assessment instruments is specifically prohibited by such federal mandates as the Education for All (Handicapped) Children Act of 1975 (PL 94-142) and its updated version (PL 98-199); the Bilingual Education Act of 1976 (PL 95-561); and Title VII of the Elementary and Secondary Education Act of 1965. In addition, several court decisions have declared illegal the use of culturally and linguistically discriminatory assessment procedures for determining the presence of handicapping conditions.

The two implications of speaking a dialect just discussed cannot be overemphasized. Classroom teachers must deal with the first problem of teaching their students to read and write. This requires that teachers be more aware of the characteristics of dialects spoken by their students so that they might be more able to effectively teach these children differences between SAE and their dialect. It is especially important for the teacher to be able to understand that a student may be confused about certain reading or writing fundamentals because of interference from his or her dialect (van Keulen et al., 1998). We will discuss this issue in greater detail in a later section. The second problem of test construction currently is being addressed by major test developers through the careful selection of more normative samples than were previously used. The American Speech-Language-Hearing Association (ASHA) has instructed SLPs to familiarize themselves with the characteristics of various social dialects and methods of culturally unbiased testing (Battle et al., 1983).

HOW CAN THE CLASSROOM TEACHER DEAL WITH THE DIALECT ISSUE?

Like any controversial issue, dealing with dialectal variations in the school curriculum has been approached from a variety of directions (Rickford et al., 2004). As mentioned earlier, bidialectal approaches emphasize the learning of SAE while still respecting a student's dialect. Some classroom materials have been developed specifically for a bidialectal approach (Anderson, 1990; Love, 1991; Parker & Crist, 1995). Some of the earlier bidialectal approaches emphasized drill work that was not as engaging for students, but some of the more recent programs have incorporated literature, the media, and writing in exercises that are more interesting (LeMoine, 2001; Maddahian & Sandamela, 2000; Rickford, 2002). Some successful programs have even enlisted students in the gathering and analysis of various linguistic samples to emphasize dialectal differences (Wolfram, Adger, & Christian, 1999).

One of the primary aspects of any bidialectal approach is that the teacher communicate respect for all varieties of English during interactions, classroom assignments, and discussions (Alexander, 1985; Birch, 2001). The following suggestions are taken from Alexander (1985, p. 24) and are ways the teacher can work more effectively with students who speak dialects. The examples concern African-American English, but they can be easily altered to apply to any dialect:

1. Develop an understanding of language and how it develops and changes.
2. Become familiar with the dialect of students.
3. Develop a respect for African-American dialect as a language system that reflects its culture.
4. Transmit this respect to all students.
5. Recognize that African-American dialect is a low-prestige dialect and that some students are very aware of this.
6. Demonstrate to students your belief that they are capable of handling two or more dialects.
7. Introduce them to other English dialects, such as those to which we are exposed when we travel in the United States.
8. Help students to understand the role of lingua franca. At one time French was the international language. Today, English is a language which is spoken all over the world. Advise students that they may have no idea now of

what paths they will take when they are older and that it is wise to be prepared and to learn this standard language now.

Alexander (1985, p. 27) also provides some interesting suggestions for classroom activities. Here are only a few of them:

1. Have the students read some of the poems of African-American writers that offer opportunities for a performance and a response. Consider the poetry of Gwendolyn Brooks and Langston Hughes. Rap music also provides many examples of the use of dialect in a musical art form that can be analyzed and discussed along with other types of poetry or lyrics.
2. Use student-developed stories (experience charts) that reflect their shared experiences. Allow students to read them orally.
3. Discuss the major dialect areas in the United States.
4. Discuss reasons for the different dialects and why dialectal differences should be respected.
5. Read aloud or play recorded passages in other English dialects to help students to appreciate the variability of English and the legitimacy of their own dialect.
6. Discuss and role-play different situations in which vernacular African-American English dialect and Standard American English dialect would be used.
7. Teach the grammatical constructions of the SAE dialect. Provide time for practice of these grammatical constructions.
8. Use pattern practice drills to help students develop an understanding of both African-American English dialect and Standard American English dialect. For example:
   a. I talked to Mary Ellen every day. I been talkin to Mary Ellen.
   b. I talked to Mary Ellen a long time ago. I been done talked to Mary Ellen.
9. Have the students conduct a television survey or evaluate current motion pictures and note which programs use noticeable dialects.

Some additional suggestions are made by Edwards regarding African-American speakers in the inner cities (1985, p. 79):

1. Learn the linguistic rules of African-American English.
2. Use the linguistic information to predict where speakers will have pronunciation, prosodic, and grammatical difficulties in speaking and writing SAE.

3. Prepare teaching materials that address the specific difficulties that you anticipate your students will have or which they already have.
4. Integrate these tactics with your regular methods and programs for teaching written and spoken Standard American English.
5. Above all, do not approach the teaching of English to African-American English speakers in a manner that can cause them to feel that their natural speech habits are deficient.

There are many examples available of effective teaching that takes these issues into account (Bohn, 2003; Foster, 2001; Irvine, 2002). Some of the points mentioned here are overlapping; however, these suggestions basically support the notion that teachers and other education professionals *should* emphasize SAE in the school environment. It is unrealistic for teachers to be expected to instruct students in a variety of dialects or have differing criteria for correctness in grading papers based on dialectal variation. A teacher with several different types of minority students in a class would have difficulty with such an approach.

Smitherman (1977, p. 219) indicates that it is wise to allow children to use their dialect when appropriate in the educational setting, especially when the main objective is for a child to express a point of view:

> At the many educational workshops and teaching seminars I have conducted, teachers often ask: "Are you saying we should teach the kids African-American dialect?" To answer a question with a question, why teach them something they already know? Rather, the real concern, and question, should be: How can I use what the kids *already* know to move them to what they *need* to know? This question presumes that you genuinely accept as viable the language and culture the child has acquired by the time he or she comes to school. This being the case, it follows that you allow the child to use that language to express himself or herself, not only to interact with their peers in the classroom, but with you, the teachers, as well.

From reading a broad base of sociolinguistic literature the present authors believe that the majority of authorities advocate the teaching of SAE in the educational system together with sensitivity to dialectal variation in instructional methods. Further support comes from sources suggesting that over 90% of African-American parents surveyed feel their children should be taught in Standard American English (Taylor, 1971). Covington (1976, p. 261) reported conducting parent seminars on the educational implications of African-American English at the University of Pittsburgh. She asked parents to make recommendations about the educational implications of African-American English after taking a 10-week seminar and hearing many expert guest speakers:

> They were totally against language intervention programs, textbooks written in African-American English, teaching Standard American English as a second language, and anything that would suggest that their children were disadvantaged. They recommended (1) that teachers speak Standard American English in instruction; (2) that their children use the same textbooks as white children and that the textbooks be revised to be more representative of a pluralistic culture; (3) that their child not be reprimanded for speaking African-American English in school; and (4) that standards in written work be the same for all children.

The suggestions also strongly support the practice of teaching SAE not as a substitute for an impoverished language system, but as a socially, educationally, and possibly economically advantageous linguistic code in the larger society. Many children style shift between SAE and AAE as appropriate and when dictated by various social contexts. We are not in the business of eradicating dialectal variations, only increasing the students' linguistic facility to switch between SAE and AAE when it is appropriate. The student must not be made to feel that his or her dialect is wrong. Many of these suggestions also emphasize that *all* students should be made aware of the many dialects in the United States, and an attitude of acceptance of these varied ways of talking should be fostered. This practice will broaden the views of SAE-speaking students as well as the other dialect speakers, and perhaps increase tolerance among all students and teachers. In using such an orientation, however, it is important that teachers are very clear about their criteria for grading in terms of language use. If departures from SAE in written work are to be penalized in grading, this should be clearly stated at the outset. It may not be a realistic expectation for teachers to assume dialect speakers can speak Standard American English in oral reports. It may not be in the student's best interests to penalize them for dialect usage. While students may attempt to style shift into their best approximation of Standard American English, there may always be some features of their dialect that remain. Teachers should be realistic about expectations and grading such oral performances.

DIALECTS, TEACHERS, AND THE SPEECH-LANGUAGE PATHOLOGIST

In the day-to-day interactions of teachers and SLPs, scenes such as these often unfold:

> Mrs. Steele, the second-grade teacher, has asked the speech-language pathologist to listen to little Maurice, an African-American child in her class. She says that Maurice leaves certain words out of sentences, omits sounds, and is generally hard for her to understand. When the SLP observes Maurice in the classroom setting, she notes that he omits <u>is</u>, plurals, possessives, and reduces consonant blends at the end of words. The SLP tells Mrs. Steele that Maurice is not exhibiting a communication disorder and is simply speaking African-American English. As a result, the SLP recommends that the teacher not initiate a referral for a speech–language evaluation. Mrs. Steele very politely nods her head, glaring at the SLP with her mouth drawn back in a tense red line.
>
> Hernando Sanchez was having a lot of trouble in school. His grades were low and his parents were worried. Mrs. Sanchez came in to talk to the teacher and was told that Hernando was having trouble because he was not learning English well enough to read or speak effectively. The teacher went on to say that since Hernando was speaking a Hispanic dialect, this was probably the cause of his academic difficulties. She indicated she would not refer him for an evaluation to determine if he needed any special services. The parent wisely requested that the speech-language pathologist and learning disabilities teacher examine Hernando. It was later found that the child had a significant language problem that was unrelated to his Hispanic dialect and was also learning disabled.

It is exactly these kinds of interactions that result in miscommunication among professionals and parents. If the SLP had been performing in-service training with teachers regarding dialectal variations, these situations may never have occurred. The two most common problems that teachers have are referring *all* dialect cases to the SLP due to lack of knowledge about social dialects, and not referring *any* minority students because the teacher assumes that all of their language differences are because of dialectal influence. Make *no* mistake: Children who are dialect speakers can also have coexisting communication disorders such as language problems, articulation problems, fluency disorders, voice disorders, and other difficulties mentioned in the present text. If the teacher even suspects that a child is experiencing a legitimate communication disorder, it is best to have that child screened by the SLP.

SLPs typically will resist working with dialect cases in the absence of a communication disorder for a number of important reasons:

The ASHA Position

The American Speech-Language-Hearing Association (Battle et al., 1983) has indicated that the SLP has a primary responsibility to those children with significant communication problems (stuttering, voice, language delay, articulation problems, cerebral palsy, cleft palate, hearing impairment, and such). If the caseload of the SLP were filled with children who were *normal* and speaking dialects, children with communication disorders could not be adequately served. The ASHA position is clear in that it states the SLP should give preference to individuals with a disorder. The ASHA position also indicates that the SLP must become familiar with features of various dialects so that discrimination in testing or enrollment will not occur.

No Problem Exists

To enroll a child in therapy implies that he or she has a disorder. If a child is enrolled for dialectal variations and is a dialect speaker, by definition, no problem exists. Thus, children and their parents may object to placement in speech therapy. In fact, this issue was taken to court, as explained by Taylor (1986, p. 408):

> In 1977, a group of parents in Ann Arbor, Michigan, filed suit in federal court on behalf of 15 African-American preschool and elementary children, charging that teachers in a local school had failed to adequately take into account the children's home dialects in the teaching of the language arts. Among their charges, the parents claimed that the teachers were not sufficiently knowledgeable about these dialects and, as a result, did not fully appreciate their intrinsic worth and usefulness in the educational environment. In several cases, children of the plaintiffs had been inappropriately enrolled in speech programs to "correct" their home dialects. The judge in the case concurred with the parents and ordered the Ann Arbor School Board to develop an educational plan which, among other things, would educate the teachers in the students' dialects and in how

knowledge and value of the dialects can be used constructively in the language arts curriculum.

The SLP may be the person most knowledgeable in your school system regarding dialectal variation. Information about social dialects is incorporated into every ASHA accredited training program, and SLPs are encouraged to provide in-service training to interested teachers about dialects and to communicate their important role in dealing with dialectal variation.

So, how *does* the SLP deal with dialect in the educational setting? First, the SLP will provide in-service training to classroom teachers and assist in providing resources for teachers as they try to incorporate dialectal variations into their instruction. A most important point is for teachers to become familiar with the various dialects in their classroom so that they will be aware of how to help individual students in learning Standard American English. The SLP will be an invaluable resource in this effort. For example, an African-American child may want to receive some specific instruction in SAE because of a particular vocational or higher education target which may be more attainable by learning SAE. The SLP may act as a consultant in helping the classroom teacher to design a cooperative program to increase SAE proficiency. Koenig and Biel (1989) report an innovative program in an Ohio school system that teaches English as a Second Language (ESL) to bilingual students and English as a Second Dialect (ESD) to students who speak dialects of English. The ESD program is available for students K–12 and provides instruction to facilitate speaking, reading, and writing skills in Standard American English. Students can enter the program through teacher, parent, or self-referral. The goal is to develop effective cross-cultural communication skills that can generalize to academic areas. The program is conducted by language aides working with students individually and in groups several times per week. The aides are under the supervision of the SLP and undergo intensive training sessions prior to working with students. Underlying the whole program is the philosophy that students "are taught with respect for the integrity of the native language, home dialects, and cultures" (p. 347). Such a program allows the SLP to offer services to dialect speakers through the judicious use of aides and still not expend significant time away from his or her caseload of children with clinically significant communication disorders.

Several other important points need to be made here. There are resources in some school systems having high concentrations of bilingual students. Some of these systems have ESL teachers (English as a Second

Language) that can help to teach Standard American English. Parents and older students also may avail themselves of night classes offered in many communities that teach English. Teachers, however, are a critical influence in allowing minority children to learn Standard American English, and it is their *attitude* that is a crucial variable. Covington (1976, p. 260) states:

> I cannot stress too much my feelings that positive attitudes and acceptance are crucial in the educational process. It would seem to me that if a teacher really felt strongly about young African-American children learning to speak "Standard English," the ideal way to bring it about would be to show that child respect, love, and acceptance and to use the speech pattern you would like the child to learn. We all know that young children are very imitative beings and they are quick to emulate people they admire. They will imitate the way the teacher walks, talks, acts, etc. If they like the teacher, they want to be like the teacher.

CONCLUSION

The issue of how to deal with social dialects in an educational setting is a touchy one. No one yet has the definitive answer as to how to incorporate minority language into a Standard American English curriculum without offending someone. All we can say at the present time is that dialects are *not* disorders, dialects *are* important parts of cultures and should *not* be derogated, and that greater understanding of social dialects will benefit all the people involved in this thorny issue. The classroom teacher is at the forefront of this complex situation and is faced daily with minority students. We would only encourage you as a teacher to:

- Provide good models of Standard American English.
- Be consistent and up front about your language expectations for grading purposes.
- Allow each student the courtesy of expressing ideas in his or her own dialect in appropriate situations.
- Try to be sensitive to the possible influence of dialect on errors you find in your students' work and compensate for these in your teaching.
- Attempt to incorporate examples of a variety of social dialects into teaching language arts, social studies, history, drama, and other relevant topics.
- Do not regard dialects as pathological and something to be referred to the SLP for correction.

It will be an exciting opportunity to teach in the next few decades as our society becomes even *more* multicultural. The school systems, parents, and students must rise to this challenge. This chapter began with an example about a little African-American girl being hassled by her teacher about her language while she was trying to relate an experience relevant to class. Geneva Smitherman (1977, p. 219) refers to this particular example in the following quote:

> If the masses of African-American kids are ever going to catch up with their white counterparts, such negative attitudes and behavior must be replaced by a genuine kind of teacher warmth. One that sincerely accepts the inherent legitimacy of the many varieties of English. One that honestly respects the power of both written and oral communicative styles. One that recognizes the connection between language and oppression and thus motivates the teacher to work to sever that connection. Ultimately, *both* African-American and white students must be prepared for life in a multilinguistic, transnational world. This requires teachers able to cultivate in students a sense of respect for, perhaps even celebration of, linguistic cultural differences—balanced by the recognition that, on the universal, "deep structure" level, the world is but one community.

REFERENCES

Abrahams, R., & Gay, G. (1975). Talking African American in the classroom. In P. Stoller, (Ed.), *African American English.* New York: Delta.

Alexander, C. (1985). African American English dialect and the classroom teacher. In C. Brooks et al., (Eds.), *Tapping potential: English and language arts for the African American learner.* Urbana, IL: National Council of Teachers of English.

Anderson, E. (1990). Teaching users of diverse dialects: Practical approaches. *Teaching English in the Two-Year College, 17*(3), 172–177.

Andrews, M., & Owens, P. (1976). *African American language.* Berkeley, CA: Seymour-Smith.

Battle, D., Aldes, M., Grantham, R. Halfond, M., Harris, G., Morgenstern-Lopez, N., et al. (1983). Position paper on social dialects. *Journal of the American Speech-Language-Hearing Association, 25,* 23–24.

Birch, B. (2001). Grammar standards: It's all in your attitude. *Language Arts, 78*(6), 535–543.

Bishop, D., North, T., & Donlan, C. (1996). Nonword repetition as a behavioral marker for inherited language impairment: Evidence from a twin study. *Journal of Child Psychology and Psychiatry, 36,* 1–13.

Campbell, T., Dollaghan, C., Needleman, H., & Janosky, J. (1997). Reducing bias in language assessment: Processing dependent measures. *Journal of Speech, Language, and Hearing Research, 40,* 519–525.

Cazden, C. (1970). The neglected situation of child language research and education. In F. Williams (Ed.), *Language, and poverty: Perspectives on a theme.* Chicago: Rand-McNally.

Cheng, L. (1989). Service delivery to Asian/Pacific LEP children: A cross-cultural framework. *Topics in Language Disorders, 9*(3), 1–11.

Covington, A. (1976). African American people and African American English: Attitudes and deeducation in a biased macroculture. In D. Harrison & T. 'Irabasso (Eds.), *African American English: A seminar.* Hillsdale, NJ: Lawrence Erlbaum.

Craig, H., & Washington, J. (2002). Oral language expectations for African American preschoolers and kindergartners. *American Journal of Speech-Language Pathology, 11*(1), 59–70.

Craig, H., & Washington, J. (2004). Grade-related changes in the production of African American English. *Journal of Speech, Language and Hearing Research, 47*(2), 450–463.

Dillard, J. (1972). *African American English.* New York: Random House.

Dollaghan, C., & Campbell, T. (1998). Nonword repetition and child language impairment. *Journal of Speech, Language and Hearing Research, 41*, 1136–1146.

Edwards, W. (1985). Inner city English. In C. Brooks et al. (Eds.), *Tapping potential: English and language arts for the African American learner.* Urbana, IL: National Council of Teachers of English.

Ellis-Weismer, S., Tomblin, J., Zhang, X., Buckwalter, P., Chynoweth, J., & Jones, M. (2000). Nonword repetition performance in school age children with and without language impairment. *Journal of Speech, Language and Hearing Research. 43*, 865–878.

Fagundes, D., Haynes, W., Haak, N., & Moran, M. (1998). Task variability effects on the language test performance of southern lower socioeconomic class African American and Caucasian five-year-olds. *Language, Speech and Hearing Services in Schools, 29*(3), 148–157.

Foster, M. (2001). Pay Leon, Pay Leon, Pay Leon Paleontologist: Using call and response to facilitate language acquisition among African American students. In S. Lanehart (Ed.), *Sociocultural and historical contexts of African American English* (pp. 281–298). Philadelphia: John Benjamins.

Gemake, J. (1981). Interference of certain dialect elements with reading comprehension for third graders. *Reading Improvement, 18*(2), 183–189.

Green, L. (2002). *African American English: A linguistic introduction.* Cambridge, UK: Cambridge University Press.

Harber, J., & Bryen, D. (1978). Black English and the task of reading. *Review of Educational Research, 46*, 387–405.

Hecht, M., Collier, M., & Ribeau, S. (1993). *African American communication.* Newbury Park, CA: Sage.

Irvine, J. (2002). *In search of wholeness: African American teachers and their culturally specific classroom practices.* New York: Palgrave.

Koenig, L., & Biel, C. (1989). A delivery system of comprehensive language services to a school district. *Language, Speech and Hearing Services in Schools. 20*(4), 338–365.

Laffey, J., & Shuy, R. (1973). *Language differences: Do they interfere?* Newark, DE: International Reading Association.

LeMoine, N. (2001). Language variation and literacy acquisition in African American students. In J. Harris, A. Kamhi, & K. Pollock (Eds.), *Literacy in African American communities* (pp. 169–194). Mahwah, NJ: Lawrence Erlbaum.

Lippi-Green, R. (1997). *English with an accent.* New York: Routledge.

Littell, J. (1971). *The language of man* (Vol. 5), Evanston, IL: McDougal, Littell.

Love, T. (1991). *A guide for teaching Standard English to black dialect speakers.* Education Resources Information Center (ERIC Document Reproduction Service No. ED340248).

Lynch, E., & Hanson, M. (1992). *Developing cross-cultural competence.* Baltimore: Brookes.

Maddahian, E., & Sandamela, A. (2000). *Linguistic affirmation program evaluation report.* Los Angeles: Los Angeles Unified School District, Program Evaluation and Research Branch.

Major, C. (1994). *Juba to jive: A dictionary of African American slang.* New York: Penguin.

McGregor, K., Williams, D., Hearst, S., & Johnson, A. (1997). The use of contrastive analysis in distinguishing difference from disorder: A tutorial. *American Journal of Speech-Language Pathology, 6*, 45–56.

Owens, R. (1988). *Language development: An introduction.* Columbus, OH: Merrill.

Parker, H., & Crist, M. (1995). *Teaching minorities to play the corporate language game.* Columbia, OH: University of South Carolina, National Resource Center for the Freshman Year Experience and Students in Transition.

Rickford, J. (1999). *African American vernacular English: Features, evolution, educational implications.* Oxford, UK: Blackwell.

Rickford, J. (2002). Linguistics, education and the Ebonics firestorm. In J. Alatis, H. Hamilton, & A. Tan (Eds.), *Round table on language and linguistics, 2000: Linguistics, language and the professions* (pp. 25–45). Washington, DC: Georgetown University Press.

Rickford, J., & Rickford, R. (2000). *Spoken soul: The story of Black English.* New York: John Wiley.

Rickford, J., Sweetland, J., & Rickford, A. (2004). African American English and other vernaculars in education. *Journal of English Linguistics, 32*(3), 230–320.

Rodekohr, R., & Haynes, W. (2001). Differentiating dialect from disorder: A comparison of two processing tasks and a standardized language test. *Journal of Communication Disorders. 34*, 255–272.

Rosten, L. (1971). The joys of Yiddish. In J. Littell (Ed.), *The language of man,* Evanston, IL: McDougal, Littell.

Schraeder, T., Quinn, M., Stockman, I., & Miller, J. (1999). Authentic assessment as an approach to preschool speech-language screening. *American Journal of Speech-Language Pathology, 8*, 195–200.

Seymour, H., Bland-Stewart, L., & Green, L. (1998). Differences versus deficit in child African American English. *Language, Speech and Hearing Services in Schools, 29*, 96–108.

Seymour, H., Roeper, T., & deVilliers, J. (2003). *Diagnostic evaluation of language variation (DELV) criterion-referenced.* San Antonio, TX: The Psychological Corporation.

Seymour, H., & Seymour, C. (1979). The symbolism of Ebonics: I'd rather switch than fight. *Journal of Black Studies, 9*, 397–410.

Smitherman, G. (1977). *Talkin and Testifyin.* Boston: Houghton Mifflin.

Smitherman, G. (2000). *Black talk: Words and phrases from the hood to the Amen Corner.* Boston: Houghton Mifflin.

Stockman, I. (1996). The promises and pitfalls of language sample analysis as an assessment tool for linguistic minority children. *Language, Speech, and Hearing Services in Schools, 27*, 355–366.

Taylor, O. (1971). Some sociolinguistic concepts of African American Language. *Today's Speech, Spring*, 19–26.

Taylor, O. (1986). Language differences. In G. Shames, & E. Wiig (Eds.), *Human communication disorders: An introduction.* Columbus, OH: Merrill.

Thompson, C., Craig, H., & Washington, J. (2004). African American and Caucasian preschoolers' use of decontextualized language: Literate language features in oral narratives. *Language, Speech and Hearing Services in Schools, 35*(3), 240–253.

van Keulen, J., Weddington, G., & DeBose, C. (1998). *Speech, Language, Learning and the African American Child.* Needham Heights, MA: Allyn & Bacon.

Williams, R., and Wolfram, W. (1977). *Social differences vs. disorders.* Washington, DC: American Speech and Hearing Association.

Wolfram, W., Adger, C., & Christian, D. (1999). *Dialects in schools and communities.* Mahwah, NJ: Lawrence Erlbaum.

TERMS TO KNOW

African-American English (AAE)
bidialectalism
communicative context
dialect
dialect importation
dialectal continuum
language deficit

language difference
Standard American English (SAE)
school register
speech community
street register
vernacular

TOPICS FOR DISCUSSION

1. What potential problems are faced by dialect speakers in an educational environment that emphasizes and rewards SAE? Focus on social, academic, and psychological aspects.

2. What do you feel would be the prevailing attitude of teachers and laypeople in your geographical area toward the notion of dialect in minority speakers? What are the possible reasons for these attitudes being negative or positive?

3. What are five specific ways a teacher can address the dialect issue in language arts classes?

4. Learning SAE can have several potential advantages to dialect speakers. Discuss the advantages of learning SAE.

5. Discuss ways in which parents, teachers, SLPs, and students can cooperate in dealing with the dialect issue in the public school system.

chapter eight

Fluency Disorders

INTRODUCTION

The word fluency means flowing along (Starkweather, 1981). Speech is **fluent** when words are produced easily, effortlessly, smoothly, quickly, and in a forward flow. Speech is **disfluent** when one word does not flow smoothly and quickly into the next.

Speakers occasionally exhibit disfluencies, such as pausing, interjecting "uhm," backing up and revising the wording of an utterance, or repeating part of the utterance over again. These are normal errors in speech fluency, as judged by society, and we all commit them from time to time. Table 8-1 lists and describes types of normal disfluency. Some fluency failures are not judged so kindly by society. Persons that utter too many disfluencies or say types that are conspicuously unusual are considered to have a **fluency disorder**. Disorders of fluency include developmental stuttering (often just called stuttering or stammering), cluttering, and acquired stuttering, either neurotic or neurogenic in nature. Each of these fluency disorders will be discussed, with emphasis on stuttering, as it is the fluency disorder most often encountered in the classroom.

Table 8-1 Speech Errors Typical of Normal Disfluency Versus Stuttered Speech

I. Typical Nonstuttering Categories
  A. Hesitation pauses (must be without undue tension and of brief duration)
    1. Silent pauses (also called *unfilled hesitations*) are brief periods of silence between words or sentences.
    2. Interjections (also called *filled pauses* or the *ah* phenomenon) include interjected sounds, syllables, and words, such as: *ah, er, uhm, well uhm.*
  B. Non-*ah* phenomena
    1. Sentence changes
      a. Revisions or false starts alter the original wording, as in "I think . . . I know you're right."
      b. Corrections or parenthetical remarks also change the original wording, but with an overt correction indicated, for example "Turn on the stove . . . I mean the heater switch."
    2. Repetitions of whole-words, particularly multisyllabic words
    3. Repetitions of phrases, such as "It's on the, on the top shelf."
    4. Omissions of sentence parts, such as "I (do) not like it" or "The client finished his hierar(chy)."
    5. Sentence incompletions and incomplete phrases, as the abandoned statement, "She never has . . . (liked me)."
    6. Slips of the tongue (also called spoonerisms and malapropisms) are of numerous types.
      a. Anticipations, such as "bake my bike" for "take my bike."
      b. Perseverations, such as "pulled a pantrum" for "the child pulled a tantrum."
      c. Reversals, such as "with this wing I thee red" intending to say "with this ring I thee wed."
      d. Blends, as in merging two words being thought of simultaneously, such as grizzly and ghastly but saying "grastly."
      e. Hapologies, as in merging two consecutive words, such as Post Toasties, into one, "Posties."
      f. Misderivations involve the use of a wrong prefix or suffix, such as in saying "an intervenient node" when meaning to say "an intervening node."
      g. Word substitutions often involve saying a word opposite in meaning or related in meaning to the intended word, such as saying "before the place closes" but intending to say "before the place opens."
    7. Intruding and incoherent sounds disrupt the forward flow of speech as in "She went . . . (Throat clearing) . . . to school" (assumes sound not used as avoidance tactic).
II. Typical Stuttering Categories
  A. Sound repetitions
  B. Syllable repetitions
  C. Word repetitions, particularly single-syllable words
  D. Sound prolongations
  E. Blocks

Source: Ambrose & Yairie, 1999; Campbell & Hill, 1993; Clark & Clark, 1977; Fromkin, 1973; Goldman-Eisler, 1968.

Stuttering is a disorder affecting the rhythm of speech. The individual knows precisely what he or she wishes to say, but at the time is unable to say it because of an involuntary repetition, prolongation, or cessation of a sound. Clearly, the loss of fluency conveyed in this definition is involuntary in nature and is due to a temporary loss of speech production ability rather than a problem with language formulation.

Authorities have struggled for years in trying to agree on the best definition of stuttering. The classic definition provided by Wingate (1966) probably best differentiates normal disfluencies from pathological stuttering.

> The term *stuttering* means . . . disruption in the fluency of verbal expression, which is characterized by involuntary, audible or silent, repetitions or prolongations in the utterance of short speech elements, namely: sounds, syllables, and words of one syllable. These disruptions usually occur frequently or are marked in character and are not readily controllable. Sometimes the disruptions are accompanied by accessory activities involving the speech apparatus, related or unrelated body structures, or stereotyped speech utterances. These activities give the appearance of being speech-related struggle. Also, there are not infrequently indications or reports of the presence of an emotional state, ranging from a general condition of "excitement" or "tension" to more specific emotions of a negative nature such as fear, embarrassment, irritation, or the like. The immediate source of stuttering is some incoordination expressed in the peripheral speech mechanism . . . (p. 488).

In clinical practice, many speech-language pathologists use simplified, operational definitions for identifying and counting stuttered moments. Some count syllables stuttered as a function of syllables spoken (Lincoln & Harrison, 1999) while others advocate counting stuttered words per minute of talking (Ryan, 1974; Ryan & Ryan, 1999). Regardless of the frequency method used, it is common practice to assess types of stuttering in terms of whole-word repetitions ("My my ball went under the car"), part-word repetitions ("B-but you said I could"), prolongations ("Mmmmmy dog had puppies"), and instances of struggle behavior (e.g., squinting of the eyes while trying to get a word out). Indeed, these are the types of disfluencies that teachers are apt to notice in students, and they suggest a true fluency disorder.

The World Health Organization scheme known as the International Classification of Impairment, Disabilities, and Handicaps (ICIDH-2) focuses attention on the *consequences* of stuttering, not the underlying causes (Yaruss, 1998; Yaruss & Quesal, 2004). Thus, the impairment of stuttering (the interrupted forward flow of speech) is both disabling and handicapping: stuttering and its affective, behavioral, and cognitive reactions limit a student's ability to communicate with others or to engage in social or school-related activities.

THE INCIDENCE AND PREVALENCE OF STUTTERING

You may wonder: "How many people stutter?" There are two ways to answer this question. The prevalence of stuttering is somewhat less than 1%. The **prevalence** of a disorder indicates how many people are afflicted by it at any given point in time. Hull, Mielke, Willeford, and Timmons (1976) assessed the speech of 38,802 public school students in the first through twelfth grades and found 0.8% of them to stutter. Furthermore, the study confirmed a well-established observation that males who stutter outnumber females who stutter 3 to 1. Young (1975), in reviewing the literature on prevalence of stuttering, suggests that a reasonable figure for both school-age and young adult stutterers is 0.7% of the population. With the population of the United States being approximately 281 million (*Encyclopaedia Britannica Almanac 2003*, 2002), these data suggest that more than 1.9 million Americans stutter.

A second way to address the question of how many people stutter is to measure its incidence. The **incidence** of a disorder can be measured over time to include those who presently stutter, as well as those who used to stutter but do so no longer. The incidence of stuttering among the general population is approximately 4–5% (Bloodstein, 1995; Conture, 2001), suggesting that, indeed, many recover from stuttering. Estimates are that some 50–85% of the children who stutter spontaneously recover (Andrews & Harris, 1964; Martin & Lindamood, 1986; Yairi & Ambrose, 1992; Yairi, Ambrose, & Niermann, 1993). Most children outgrow their highly disfluent speech by age 9 years; others still manage to recover by puberty. Recovery ranges however are so great that it makes clinical use of the information difficult. Yet this is an important aspect of stuttering that merits further study. No doubt teachers and SLPs will be asked many questions about recovery.

Parents will want to know the probability of *their* child outgrowing stuttering. There is no easy answer, but the speech-language pathologist may be the person most equipped with knowledge of the disorder, and knowledge of the child, to formulate the best response. Research shows that a child's chances of outgrowing stuttering worsen with age, the severity of characteristics exhibited, and the length of time stuttering has existed. A generalization is that a child who has stuttered for more than one to two years and/or who is past age nine years, probably will not recover without help. Parents and teachers may wonder, then, whether it might be best to postpone fluency treatment in hopes the child will outgrow stuttering. The prevailing clinical opinion, however, is not to wait. Early intervention is important. Stuttering is a simpler problem to treat in a young child. With Public Law 99-457, schools are responsible for handicapped children ages 3 through 5 years, facilitating such early intervention. Prevention and early intervention of stuttering are extremely important. It should be emphasized, though, that treatment is appropriate at any age. There are a variety of approaches for children, adolescents, and adults for which successful outcomes are reported.

There are many other interesting aspects of stuttering. Below is a list of some of these facts:

- Stuttering is universal. The disorder has existed throughout recorded history and is found among all peoples of the world.
- Stuttering almost always begins in childhood, usually before age 6 years. Ages 2 to 4 years are particularly common periods for the onset of stuttering.
- Stuttering occurs more often among males than females. Reports of sex ratio vary from 3:1 to as high as 6:1.
- Stuttering tends to run in families. Family studies have shown that the risk of stuttering in relatives of a person who stutters is increased over that for the general population. Furthermore, the pattern of transmission in families is consistent with predictions derived from genetic models (Cox, 1988), yet genetic components of stuttering have not been proved.
- The amount of stuttering varies widely with situations. Persons who stutter often report excessive speech difficulties when they are excited or feel under pressure. Saying their name, talking on the telephone, ordering in a restaurant, talking to a person in authority (e.g., a teacher), and talking in front of a group (as in a classroom) also are situations which elicit much stuttering. Additionally, speakers have good days and bad days, meaning that the frequency and severity of their stuttering fluctuates.
- Stuttering is reduced or eliminated in a variety of conditions as well. Most affected people report being able to sing, whisper, and talk to themselves or their pets fluently. By talking in a prolonged, slow fashion, most become stutter free. Choral or unison speaking and talking to a rhythmical beat also improve fluency.

- For those who do not outgrow it, stuttering tends to change—and worsen—as the person matures. What began as a speech problem evolves into not only a speech problem, but also a personal-social-psychological problem.
- Stuttering need not hold a person back from achieving full potential. Many famous, brilliant and talented people stuttered, such as: Winston Churchill, Moses, Marilyn Monroe, Sommerset Maugham, Isaac Newton, Mel Tillis, Bob Newhart, and James Earl Jones.

This list of interesting facts points to aspects of stuttering of which you, as a teacher, need to be aware. Many also have obvious implications for treatment.

CAUSATION AND DEVELOPMENT OF STUTTERING

Stuttering remains a mystery. The ultimate cause of this perplexing speech disorder is unknown, yet theories abound. Parts of the stuttering problem seem to be learned behaviors; still other evidence suggests that there are neurophysiological reasons for the loss of speech coordination. Psychological theories, once popular, seem to have suffered from a lack of verifiable causal evidence. It is beyond the scope of this chapter to critically examine all of the theories of etiology. However, our years of research reveal that no intellectual or emotional behaviors distinguish children who stutter from those who do not (Bloodstein, 1995; Zebrowski & Schum, 1993).

No matter what the cause of stuttering, the student begins trying too hard to speak and starts having more and more trouble. Although the onset of stuttering is usually gradual, danger signs emerge and, over time, the symptoms change and worsen. It is a vicious cycle unless the problem is caught in time. It is incumbent upon classroom teachers to refer students who show any signs of stuttering to the speech-language pathologist in an effort to prevent a more severe problem in the future. Furthermore, although parents most certainly did not cause their child to stutter, one can speculate that there are some behaviors that might contribute to its exacerbation and continued development. Clearly, then, there are environmental conditions that need to be addressed through intervention.

The Danger Signs

Parents and teachers of young children often worry that a particular child might be beginning to stutter. Speech-language pathologists are trained to recognize early danger signs of stuttering and to differentiate them from periods of normal disfluency. It is important for parents and teachers to know that all children periodically demonstrate disfluencies; however, these disfluencies are of particular types and do not occur too often. The following are some examples of normal speech errors in children that need not be of concern:

1. Whole-word and phrase repetitions:
   "My, my ball went under the car." "I want, I want some ice cream."
2. Sentence revisions:
   "It went—My ball went under the car."
3. Pauses filled with *um, ah, uh*:
   "I want some . . . um . . . ice cream."
4. Unfilled pauses or relaxed hesitations:
   "Daddy, I want (pause) some ice cream."
5. Infrequent, easy single part-word repetitions: "B-but you said I could."

Certain danger signs should alert parents, teachers, and speech-language pathologists that stuttering may be developing. Symptoms indicating risk include:

1. Frequent part-word repetitions, especially when part-word repetitions occur more often than whole-word or phrase repetitions: "B-but" more likely than "But-but"
2. Part of a word repeated more than two or three times: "Ba-ba-ba-ba-ball"
3. Repetitions having an irregular rhythm: "B-ba-ba-b-ball"
4. A sound held longer than normal (perhaps one second or more) "Mmm-mmmmmmmmmy ball"

Warning signs may be present in addition to the disfluencies themselves. Tension and fear often are seen in children with a developing stuttering problem. Excessive tension in the speech musculature may cause explosive enunciations of speech sounds, voice tremors, or rises in pitch when speaking. Muscles in the neck and face may distend as children struggle to talk. Children may even show fear when anticipating a difficult word and may, in fact, learn to substitute easier words. Avoidance behaviors become habituated shortly after the child becomes adept at anticipating difficulties. By this time, stuttering is beyond its beginning stages.

Danger signs make their appearance gradually in a child's speech. Stuttering rarely occurs overnight! This dissolution of fluent speech often follows a predictable pattern of development.

Developmental Phases

Developmental stuttering is so-called because it begins in early childhood, especially between ages 2 to 4 years, and its characteristics and symptoms worsen with time. No assumption is made about the original cause of the stuttering. The majority of stuttering cases begin and develop with a regular, predictable pattern. Bloodstein (1960), after a cross-sectional investigation of more than 400 stutterers, described four phases through which stuttering develops. These are shown in Table 8-2.

Van Riper (1982) also described the onset and developmental course of stuttering which, he said, can proceed in any of four different directions. These developmental scenarios were termed Tracks (Track I, II, III, IV). The onset and developmental course of the most typical form of stuttering constitutes Track I. Track I encompassed all of Bloodstein's (1960) phases with cardinal characteristics including: onset in the preschool years; normal speech and language development; previously fluent; easy and rhythmical repetitions predominate; episodic fluctuations in fluency; unawareness of speaking difficulties; and absence of avoidance behaviors. It is no wonder that these early characteristics were termed **primary stuttering**. With the passage of time, these symptoms worsen to include tension in the speech musculature, appearance of irregular part-word repetitions, followed by prolongations and struggle behaviors, the awareness and predictability of speaking difficulties, and the development of a stylized system of avoidance behaviors to reduce or conceal stuttering. The person, by this time in the development of the disorder, truly has the self-concept of being a stutterer. Although the development of this **secondary** form of stuttering requires conditioning through experience and the passage of time, it can occur at any age. Young children, indeed, can be confirmed stutterers.

The Track I developmental scenario accounted for 54% of the more than 300 cases studied by Van Riper (1982), including 44 clients followed longitudinally. An additional 14% of the cases fit a different pattern of onset and development, what he called Track II. (Tracks III and IV occur rarely.)

Data reported by Daly (1981) agree well with the commonness of these so-called typical Track I stutterers. He reported that 54% of 138 persons who stutter (treated at the Shady Trails Summer Speech Camp) indeed fit the Track I description. Accounting for 24% of the 138 stutterers at the camp, Track II stutterers were found to be more common than as reported by Van Riper.

In Track II, fluency problems were evident from the time the child began to talk. Not only is there no history of good fluency, these children often are

Table 8-2 The Classic Four Phases in the Development of Stuttering

Phase One:
1. The difficulty has a distinct tendency to be episodic, that is, to come and go in cycles.
2. The child stutters most when excited or upset, when seeming to have a great deal to say, or under other conditions of communicative pressure.
3. The dominant symptom is repetition.
4. There is a marked tendency for stutterings to occur at the beginning of the sentence, clause, or phrase.
5. In contrast to more advanced stuttering, the interruptions occur not only on content words, but also on the function words of speech (pronouns, conjunctions, articles, and prepositions).
6. Most of the time children in the first phase of stuttering show little evidence of concern about the interruptions in their speech.

Phase Two:
7. The disorder is essentially chronic.
8. The child has a self-concept as a stutterer.
9. The stutterings occur chiefly on the major parts of speech (nouns, verbs, adjectives, and adverbs).
10. Despite a self-concept as a stutterer, the child usually evinces little or no concern about the speech difficulty.
11. The stuttering is said to increase chiefly under conditions of excitement or when the child is speaking rapidly.

Phase Three:
12. The stuttering comes and goes largely in response to specific situations.
13. Certain words or sounds are regarded as more difficult than others.
14. In varying degrees, use is made of word substitutions and circumlocutions.
15. There is essentially no avoidance of speech situations and little or no evidence of fear or embarrassment.

Phase Four:
16. Vivid, fearful anticipations of stuttering.
17. Feared words, sounds, and situations.
18. Very frequent word substitutions and circumlocutions.
19. Avoidance of speech situations, and other evidence of fear and embarrassment.

Source: Bloodstein, 1960.

also delayed in the onset of talking, have articulation problems, and possess poor language skills. The syllabic repetitions seem hurried and irregular; more silent gaps and hesitations are evident at an earlier stage than in the Track I scenario. Yet, like the Track I, Track II stutterers show little awareness or frustration in the early stage of stuttering development. Fears, especially of speaking situations, develop later.

These children certainly are candidates for team intervention. The presence of weak language skills may impact all academic areas, particularly reading and spelling. The speech-language pathologist (SLP) also is likely to design a combination of treatment strategies to simultaneously address the fluency, phonology, and/or language disorders within the individual. Data and a research summary reported by Louko, Edwards, & Conture (1999) suggest that, indeed, 33% of persons who stutter have coexisting articulation or phonological problems. Less often, persons who stutter exhibit other concomitant disorders.

ASSESSMENT ISSUES

Although typical and atypical forms of stuttering exist, for those that do not outgrow it, evidence suggests that the problem becomes more complex with the passage of time. What starts as overt disfluency evolves into a complicated disorder affecting one's thoughts, emotions, words, deeds, and lifestyle. Early identification and early intervention are considered critical by many specialists in the area of stuttering (Onslow & Packman, 1999). By knowing the difference between normal disfluency and beginning stuttering, a classroom teacher can recognize the student exhibiting danger signs and make an appropriate referral to the speech-language pathologist. A teacher's intuition about and observation of a child's speech, along with parental concerns expressed to teachers, are principal avenues for identifying students in need of fluency management.

The classroom teacher refers the student to the speech-language pathologist, who attempts to answer two key questions in a diagnostic evaluation. First, is the person stuttering or not? Fluency may be viewed, quite simply, on a continuum, as shown in Figure 8-1. Some normal speakers are silver-tongued yet others are highly disfluent. The bulk of the population has average fluency containing speech errors including pauses, interjections, revisions, and the like (recall Table 8-1). Other speakers are viewed by society as abnormally disfluent. Where does society draw the line to separate normal from abnormal? There is no magic number that defines such a border, yet speech-language pathologists collect information and data to do just that. A trained, experienced speech-language pathologist gathers the necessary information to determine whether the person is stuttering or not; this is termed making a **differential diagnosis**. Often the diagnosis is more straightforward in the evaluation of an adult or adolescent than in a young child.

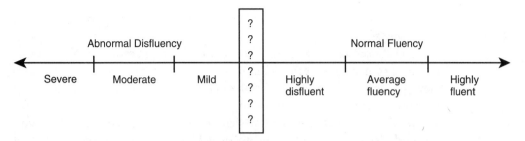

Figure 8-1 Fluency Depicted on a Continuum Illustrating the Process of Differential Diagnosis and Severity Determination

A second diagnostic question follows the first. If the person is stuttering, how bad is the problem? Here, the SLP is addressing the issue of **severity**; it, too, can be placed on the continuum, as shown in Figure 8-1. Information and data collected in the diagnostic evaluation help categorize the severity of the stuttering along the dimensions of mild, moderate, or severe.

Many assessment scales exist for the evaluation of a stuttering disorder and a thorough discussion may be obtained in the book by Haynes and Pindzola (2004). A classroom teacher also may encounter assessment information through a cooperative, working relationship with the speech-language pathologist. Certainly, information of this kind is contained in the student's speech-language file, is summarized on the student's individualized education program (IEP), and is discussed during the IEP meeting with the classroom teacher present. Two scales typical of stuttering assessment will be described—one useful in differential diagnosing and the other a well-known severity scale. Knowledge of their content is a good foundation for understanding the disorder itself.

Differential Diagnosis

Explicit identification procedures that can distinguish between persons who stutter and normally disfluent students are needed to make a differential diagnosis. Gordon and Luper (1992) reviewed six often-used protocols for identifying beginning stuttering, including *A Protocol for Differentiating the Incipient Stutterer* (Pindzola, 1988, 1999; Pindzola & White, 1986). This is an appraisal tool that synthesizes existing knowledge into a format that guides the speech-language pathologist through clinical observations, data collection, and interpretation. The protocol quantifies eight auditory behaviors perceived by the listener, assesses visual evidence of speaking difficulties, and examines subjective feelings as well as historical and psychological indicators of chronic stuttering.

The speech-language pathologist administers the protocol by obtaining a sample of natural speech. Often this is done by the SLP in a clinical interview. Listening to the student on the playground, in the cafeteria, or in the classroom also may provide the SLP with a natural sample of speech for analysis. The protocol uses a numerical scale for rating behaviors. The auditory and visual sections of the protocol yield a total score of between 14 and 42. Preliminary standardization studies (Pindzola, 1988) suggest that a total score of 14–21 is within normal limits, but a score greater than 21 may be indicative of incipient or confirmed stuttering. Some important information about stuttering from the protocol will be highlighted in the following sections.

The predominant type of disfluency that a speaker typically uses and the size of the speech unit affected by the disfluency influence the listener's judgments of speech normalcy. For example, repetitions of whole phrases are quite normal; whole-word repetitions are disfluencies typical of both stutterers and nonstutterers. Yet the predominance of part-word repetitions distinguishes stuttering from nonstuttering preschoolers (Yairi & Lewis, 1984). Hesitations or pauses before phrases or before words may, likewise, be less innocuous than such gaps within words (e.g., preceding syllables or sounds). The rule of thumb suggested by Perkins (1971) is that the smaller the speech unit affected, the more abnormal the disfluency. Recall again the types of speech errors listed in Table 8-1.

The frequency with which disfluent behaviors occur has long been recognized as important in the diagnosis of stuttering. There are various ways the SLP can determine frequency, and there are various data for interpreting normalcy. Suffice it to say that frequencies in excess of 2%, 5%, or 10% suggest a stuttering disorder, depending on the strictness of the criterion used by the SLP.

The duration of the disfluency may be expressed in two ways, either as number of times for repetitions or as length of time for prolongations. For example, in the sentence "My my my cat had kittens," the whole word *my* is produced twice before being uttered meaningfully. Likewise, silent or audible prolongations may be measured with a stopwatch, or simply estimated. If the typical duration of prolongations exceeds one second, or if repetitions involve numerous reiterations, these behaviors may be interpreted as a sign of stuttering.

Audible signs of effort while speaking generally are not noted among normal speakers and, therefore, are indicative of abnormality. A complete listing of these audible behaviors is not realistic, but typical behaviors include disrupted airflow, hard contacts (explosive, crisp articulation), and effort or tension heard in the voice.

Van Riper (1982) provides clinical reports that normal disfluencies and perhaps very early stutterings are characterized by repetitions that preserve the normal rhythm and rate of speech. Not until the tempo of the reiterations speeds up or their rhythm becomes irregular and choppy is there substantial reason for concern. The speech-language pathologist is asked to judge subjectively the student's rhythm, tempo, and the speed of disfluencies in using the protocol.

Behaviors that may be audible and learned are thought to develop as a means of minimizing stuttering. Concealment devices, such as word substitutions ("big fries" substituted for "large fries" to avoid the troublesome l sound) or circumlocutions (talking around *blue* by describing the color of the sky), may be used to avoid feared words. Postponement devices may consist of maneuvers (e.g., interjections) to delay attempts on a feared word and starting tricks (e.g., humming prefixed to the feared word) may be used to assist in initiating feared words. These and other mannerisms may help the SLP discriminate between stuttering and nonstuttering.

The second part of the protocol assesses visual evidence of a stuttering disorder. Visual signs of effort suggest to the listener that the act of speaking is unduly difficult. Such signs may reflect that a student is aware of the speaking difficulties, that he or she is trying to do something about the moments of difficulty, and that the disfluency has developed into a more severe problem. The SLP records the specific behaviors displayed by the student in the facial, head, and body regions. Frequently observed contortions are blinking, wrinkling of the forehead, distortions of the mouth, and overt tension in the jaw. Rhythmical head movements, head jerks, and the more subtle head turnings to divert eye contact also are observable in some persons who stutter.

The third section of the protocol assesses historical and psychological indicators of stuttering. The subjective evaluations made by a speaker while experiencing speech disfluencies, and in reaction to them, are diagnostically important. These covert reactions have been studied through the introspection of older persons who stutter but also may be present to some degree in younger children who stutter. The student's perception of the problem should be explored by the speech-language pathologist whenever possible;

additional information collected from parental reports and teachers is useful also. It is not uncommon for even young children to be aware and concerned about their disfluent speech as evidenced by parental reports of their child's being upset at peer teasing or crying over not being able to talk. Clearly, this early concern is testimony to the reality of a disfluency problem. Evidence exists that even preschool children are aware of stuttering (Ambrose & Yairi, 1994) and their degree of awareness may relate back to the developmental progression discussed earlier in the chapter (see Table 8-2).

These and other historical and psychological factors will be explored by the SLP by using Pindzola's *Protocol for Differentiating the Incipient Stutterer*. Clearly, much information should be collected on a student and used to shape clinical opinion. Only after weighing the evidence can a speech-language pathologist make an accurate diagnosis regarding stuttering.

Judging Severity

The individualized education plan adopted by most school districts requires a statement regarding the severity of the handicapping condition. The speech-language pathologist attempts to categorize the severity of the student's stuttering along the continuum of very mild to very severe. Many aspects of the stuttering condition contribute to such a severity determination, yet three parameters seem to be the most important. The frequency, duration, and physical concomitants of the stuttering should be quantified by the SLP. The *Stuttering Severity Instrument* (Riley, 1994), a severity scale in wide use, assesses these three parameters. The classroom teacher should be versed in the process of determining severity to appreciate what the modifiers mild, moderate, and severe represent and to contribute meaningfully to the discussions of a particular student held during the IEP meeting.

The *Stuttering Severity Instrument* (Riley, 1994) is useful with both children and adults and has provisions for testing those who can and cannot read. The number of syllables stuttered and the number of total syllables spoken are computed by the speech-language pathologist as the student reads or is engaged in conversation. Frequency, expressed as percentage of stuttering, is then computed (number of stuttered syllables divided by total syllables spoken $\times$ 100 = percentage) and converted to a corresponding task score. The SLP also monitors the amount of time a student is stuck during stuttered blocks, and averages the three longest. This measure is converted into a task score. Lastly, the speech-language pathologist watches and carefully listens to the student during reading and conversation samples, and rates the presence and conspicuousness of physical behaviors accompanying the speech attempts. A separate rating (on a 0 to 5 scale) is made for each anatomical area (facial, head, and extremity) and for distracting sounds; their sum constitutes the task score. Frequency, duration, and physical concomitant task scores are then combined for a total score. The severity of the student's stuttering can be ascertained by comparing the total score to the normative data provided by Riley. Stuttering severity may be described as very mild, mild, moderate, severe, or very severe in this manner.

Common Avoidance and Concealment Techniques

Sometimes a stuttering problem is not so obvious to a classroom teacher. Persons who stutter may become very adept at using **avoidance behaviors**, even at an early age. Avoidances are tricks and crutches. They are a complex series of behaviors that can be used by children and adults to cope with and perhaps hide stuttering. They are learned tactics. Persons who stutter begin to disguise behaviors by having someone talk for them, by refusing to talk at all, or by giving up and saying "I don't know." Fear grows and spreads; the student worries and may develop a low self-concept.

> Mario is moving through the school's cafeteria line. One of the day's selections is his favorite, spicy chicken tortilla soup. He wants to ask for some but has a feeling he will block on the word "soup." He says to the cafeteria worker, "I'd like some chicken, um so to speak, uh some chicken s-s-s-s—." The cafeteria worker hastily interrupts and says, "You want what?" Mario responds saying, "A cup of—you know—that stuff with chicken, onions, celery . . ." "You mean chicken salad?" snaps the cafeteria worker while trying to hand it to Mario and continuing, "You have to keep the line moving." Mario, in frustration, ekes out, "Well, just give me some fingers!" Mario continues down the line thinking to himself how sick he is of eating chicken fingers! In this scenario Mario is using a variety of avoidance tactics to **postpone** and/or **start** saying the feared word *soup*. By describing the ingredients, Mario is using the technique of **circumlocution** to talk around the feared word. Finally, in disgust, he gives up and **substitutes** an easier word, ordering fingers.

The presence of repetitions, prolongations, and struggle behaviors often is obvious. A teacher who hears and sees these behaviors in a child should refer the student to the speech-language pathologist. Avoidance behaviors, by their very nature, obscure recognition of a person who stutters. The covert tricks disguise speech difficulties; you may find it harder to recognize this type of stuttering in the classroom. The following is a list of commonly used avoidance techniques. Teachers should familiarize themselves with these techniques to be able to spot such cases.

- Remaining silent; giving the impression of being a quiet or shy person
- Avoiding situations that demand speech (e.g., not using the telephone, not participating in show-and-tell, not contributing to group discussions, refusing to give an oral report)
- Seldom interacting with the teacher and other persons in authority
- Agreeing easily; avoiding speaking by concurring with others rather than explaining reasons for disagreement
- Rehearsing speech and using preparatory techniques
- Using fillers excessively, such as *like*, *well*, *uhm*, and so on
- Avoiding certain words by substituting others
- Looking away while speaking; maintaining poor eye contact with a listener
- Pretending to think during pauses while really blocking
- Feigning a cough or yawn or shielding the mouth during a block
- Talking while moving a body part (e.g., foot tapping, arm swinging) or talking to a rhythm
- Altering breathing patterns during speech or before speech

Information the Teacher Can Provide

An open, working relationship between the classroom teacher and the speech-language pathologist is important. Teachers serve as a prime referral source of persons who stutter to the intervention program and can provide valuable information about the student's behaviors. The following list of teacher observations, compiled by Pindzola (1988), may be useful to the speech-language pathologist.

1. Describe as completely as possible what the child is doing that makes you suspect a stuttering problem exists.
2. Describe how often or with what frequency the stuttering occurs in your class.
3. How does the student react to the stuttering?
4. What struggle behaviors and facial contortions, if any, have you observed?

5. Are there particular situations or activities in school that seem to worsen the stuttering (e.g., during show-and-tell, oral book reports, on the playground)?
6. Are there situations or activities that the student tries to avoid because stuttering might occur?
7. Describe the student's peer relationships (e.g., well liked, shy, teased).
8. What is known about the home situation (pace of living, organization, discipline, sibling rivalry, divorce, emotional tension)?

In concert with a determination of fluency characteristics and disfluency severity, a thorough communication assessment is necessary, including appraisal of language and phonology skills. The SLP tries to determine the extent of the student's handicapping condition and this is discussed in the IEP meeting. Teachers and parents can be extremely valuable in helping the SLP make an accurate determination of the degree to which the student is handicapped by the stuttering problem (i.e., educationally, psychologically, and economically).

THERAPEUTIC PRINCIPLES

The speech-language pathologist should discuss a particular student's treatment approach with the classroom teacher and, whenever possible, enlist the teacher's aid and support. While it is beyond the scope of this chapter to discuss the myriad of treatment programs available, an overview of therapeutic principles is warranted. Before proceeding, we wish to alert teachers that children who display additional speech and language problems, or cognitive/intellectual deficits concomitant with stuttering, generally present a poorer prognosis in fluency treatment than those with "pure" stuttering (Louko, Edwards, & Conture, 1990).

Treatment Options for the Young Student

Different philosophies exist regarding the treatment of young persons between the ages of 3 and 9 years who stutter. Treatment options are shown schematically in Figure 8-2.

In the first option, environmental treatment, the speech-language pathologist determines that the most prudent course of action is to work through the significant others in the child's life—parents and teachers—to modify the daily environment. The goal is to structure the child's environment to make

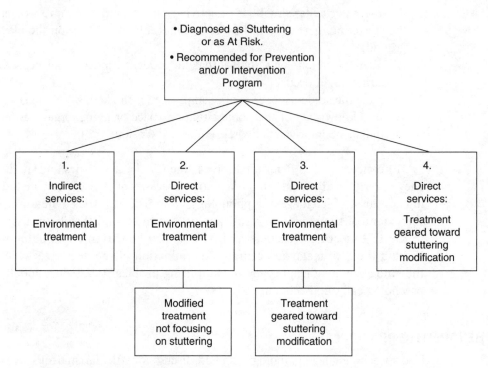

Figure 8-2 Treatment Options for the Young Child

it more conducive to fluency. The child is not seen for treatment; typically, parents and teachers meet regularly with the SLP to discuss environmental modifications and results. Opting for only environmental treatment is commonly done for the child at risk for developing stuttering or for the child beginning to stutter who displays early symptoms. Modifying parental and teacher reactions to disfluencies, altering the pace and organization of home and classroom, and generally educating significant others about fluency, disfluency, and the modeling of good speech habits are beneficial. Reduction in communicative pressures that the child is vulnerable to are a necessary and important aspect of treatment. Table 8-3 describes some common forms of communicative stress. Because these situations can occur at home and in school, it is vitally important that both the parents and teachers work with the SLP to reduce and, whenever possible, eliminate them. The payoff of environmental treatment for young children beginning to stutter or those at risk for this disorder generally is improved fluency in the child and the likelihood of recovery.

Table 8-3 Some Forms of Communicative Stress

1. Listener loss
2. Interruptions
3. Competition for the conversational floor (i.e., an uninterrupted turn to talk)
4. Cross-examination kind of questioning
5. Demands for display speech (e.g., "recite your poem for grandma")
6. Demands for confession
7. Having to talk under conditions of strong emotion (e.g., guilt, fear, anger), or when fatigued or distracted

Source: Van Riper, 1982.

A second treatment option (see Figure 8-2) is to combine the environmental treatment with direct but modified therapy for the child. Sessions may be individual but are often in groups. The treatment is considered modified as it does not focus on specific symptoms of stuttering. Rather, treatment may emphasize the concept of rhythm by having children sing, speak to a rhythm, practice rhymes, use choral speaking, and just generally experience much success in easy, fluent speech. Modified treatment often involves the strategies of language learning and discourse manipulation (Weiss, 2004a). The language skills of a young child who stutters may be somewhat delayed. The length and complexity of utterances affect the likelihood of even normal speakers having a disfluency. By shoring up weak language skills, and by systematically controlling the linguistic output of young clients (regarding sentence length and syntactic complexity), speech-language pathologists are able to reduce or eliminate stuttering (Weiss, 2004b; Weiss & Zebrowski, 1992). Additionally, some speech-language pathologists may include in the modified program mention of "smooth" and "bumpy" speech and train the children to identify samples of each. Altering the "bumpy" speech, however, is not done in this form of treatment.

A third option of treatment for the young person who stutters (see Figure 8-2) is to combine the environmental approach with direct intervention. The child attends individual or group treatment sessions (depending upon the severity of the problem) with the purpose of modifying specific stuttering symptoms. A variety of therapeutic emphases are possible. The student may be taught a new, fluent way of talking by learning patterns such as slow speech; breathy speech; stretchy speech; an easy speaking voice; slow, easy speech; and other similar strategies for fluency. Discussions of feelings and attitudes may be a component of the treatment program for children ready to address personal issues surrounding their speech difficulties.

The fourth option of direct stuttering modification alone (see Figure 8-2) expands the details involved in mastering strategies, techniques, or targets for fluency. The absence of simultaneously occurring environmental treatment may be a function of: (1) the setting in which services are provided (parents may not be available to participate fully in the intervention program); or (2) the possible progression of the student's stuttering symptoms beyond the level where environmental manipulations would be expected to have much effect. In such cases, efforts need to be focused on direct treatments using greater specificity.

Regardless of the option pursued, stuttering intervention with young children is both effective and efficient in clinical settings. An excellent overview of the leading approaches to childhood stuttering is in the book by Onslow and Packman (1999). Gregory (1990), however, cautions that for treatment to be effective, it should be fairly intensive in the early stages. He recommends at least three individual sessions of 30–50 minutes a week. Gregory goes on to say that one of the problems of effective stuttering treatment in the school setting has been the infrequency and short duration of the sessions. Innovative models of service delivery, such as the consultative/collaborative approaches discussed in this book, should be of great benefit to students who stutter.

Treatment for the Older Student

The treatment of stuttering among older children, adolescents, and adults of all ages is of the direct type. Obviously, programs differ in complexities and emphases for these disparate age groups. Since negative feelings and attitudes develop late in the evolution of stuttering, treatment for the older student may involve explorations into these psychological topics. The emotional crisis of stuttering escalates during the teenage years when social interactions become so critical. Physiological modifications of speech are often components in adolescent and adult fluency programs. Physiological targets may include breathing, voice onset, and rate, as well as a host of others. Computerized instrumentation may help in the training of these speech targets. Much practice is necessary to habituate new speaking patterns, and support from family, friends, and school personnel can be critical to success.

Some children who stutter, particularly older school-aged children and teenagers, do not want to participate in treatment. This desire to refrain from treatment may be related to such feelings or beliefs as fear of peer group judgments, fear of change, fear of failure to change, fear of disappointing oneself and one's family if progress in treatment is not made, lack of concern about stuttering, lack of sufficient motivation to work toward making changes in speech fluency, and the like.

Gregory (1987) describes why participating in class activities, interacting with fellow students and teachers, and receiving treatment as a school activity are topics that teenagers who stutter think about a great deal. Examples of school situations follow; as a future teacher, what might you do to alleviate these anxious times?

- Almost all who stutter have experienced the frustration of saying, "I don't know," when they did know, rather than take the chance of stuttering as they answered a question in class.
- Students who stutter refer to the anticipation of what they call "reading up and down the rows." They scan ahead in a reading passage to see if there are words on which they may stutter in the passage anticipated for their turn. Not only does the student fear being blocked, but also being laughed at.
- Giving reports is another commonly feared situation. (Some find that practicing a report many times alone makes it easier when giving the report in class.) Also, it is hard for the student to participate in class discussions when stuttering is anticipated. Avoiding these situations only increases tension and eventual stuttering.

Ways Teachers Can Assist in the Intervention Program

Once a treatment program has been established by the speech-language pathologist, significant others in the student's environment can—and should—contribute. The roles of the parents and teachers cannot be overemphasized. The student who stutters needs help and much practice to carry over, or generalize, the newly learned speaking patterns that may be part of the intervention program. Classroom teachers can assist both the student and the speech-language pathologist in this practice. The following list of suggestions may be useful (Pindzola, 1988):

1. Encourage the student to talk about the speech management sessions and to explain the fluency strategies that are being learned.

   Rationale:
   Explaining something newly learned helps cement one's understanding of it. Talking openly about one's problem is also very therapeutic. It is healthy

to admit a problem, and treating or overcoming it can be a source of pride. Furthermore, this discussion informs the classroom teacher of the fluency strategies being used (if any) so that the teacher may model them as well. By knowing the strategies, the teacher can monitor their application and reinforce their use or provide subtle reminders when they are needed.

2. Provide help with speech assignments. Work closely with the speech-language pathologist in adapting classroom activities to practice time, where fluency strategies may be applied in real situations. The speech-language pathologist will want to observe the student in real communication in the classroom, particularly in the later stages of treatment.

Rationale:
Newly acquired behaviors need much practice to become habituated. Also, mastery of a skill in the therapy room is meaningless until the skill can be applied in the real world.

3. Provide frequent verbal and social reinforcement for the student's use of fluency strategies. It is particularly important to reinforce fluent speaking in situations that have been difficult in the past.

Rationale:
Reinforcement increases the likelihood that the behavior will recur. Reinforcement of fluency and the use of strategies is done by the speech-language pathologist in the treatment session, but it is more important that such reinforcement be given outside in the real world.

4. Be a good speech model for the student to imitate. The following specific suggestions apply when speaking directly to the child who stutters; some, however, may be used routinely in addressing the entire class.

   a. Use short sentences.
   b. Use vocabulary appropriate for the child's age; do not pressure the child to be more advanced in language usage than other children of the same age.
   c. Speak slowly. An unhurried rate of talking is a good model for fluency.
   d. Pause before responding to a student's utterance. This models the concept of taking one's time and ignoring the pressures to speak quickly.
   e. Avoid interrupting the conversational speech of others. Through such modeling, students learn the importance of turn-taking, which is not only polite but is a pragmatic feature of language. Interrupting and being interrupted both tend to generate disfluent speech.
   f. Blend words together smoothly; speech should not sound choppy. Keeping the voice and air flowing between words in a sentence is a good fluency model.

g. Model speaking in a soft manner. A voice that is not loud and has less muscular effort driving it is less likely to tense or block (and result in stuttering).

A concise motto for teachers to remember in modeling good speech is simply to talk in a manner that is "soft, smooth, and slow."

When there is a student who stutters in the classroom, the teacher may find it helpful for all students to discuss openly and in a nonjudgmental manner the nature of stuttering. To promote adjustment and understanding, the teacher may wish to infuse literature that deals with stuttering into the language arts curricula. Bushey and Martin (1988) critiqued 20 works of children's fiction in which a character stutters. A sampling of this literature is shown in Table 8-4 and is listed according to reading age level.

Teacher Tips for Classroom Management

A classroom teacher has an opportunity to participate in the prevention and treatment of stuttering by properly structuring class activities. A teacher can structure the classroom environment to *facilitate* fluency or to *inhibit* it. Naturally, a good teacher will want to provide experiences that encourage fluency, but what is said, what is done, and how things are done make a difference. The disfluent student needs flexibility, not sympathy from the teacher. Good judgment is important. The following guidelines may help in the development of flexible classroom management skills (Pindzola, 1988):

- The student must not develop the attitude that normal responsibilities can be avoided because of stuttering. Classroom duties and responsibilities should be assigned as they are for other children. Perhaps modification or substitution of some activities is appropriate from time to time.
- Call on the person who stutters to answer questions in class but take care in phrasing the questions so that the answers may be very short. (Short sentences elicit less stuttering than long ones.) Call on the student who stutters only when you are confident he or she knows the answer. Avoid calling on the student on days when his or her speaking is unusually difficult.
- Oral recitation and reading aloud activities need not be abandoned just because a student who stutters is in the class. Excluding a person who stutters denies the chance for improvement and forces the acceptance of this defect. A chance to participate verbally helps establish self-confidence. Consider different methods of doing recitative and reading activities.

Table 8-4 Stuttering in Children's Literature

Emily Umily, by Kathy Corrigan. Toronto: Annick Press, 1984. Reading level: age 4–7 years. Emily begins kindergarten reluctantly. She tries to participate like all the other children, but is quite disfluent. The children laugh at her as she says "umm" every few words—hence the nickname *Umily*. Emily's emotional reactions worsen in the story until she experiences positive attitude changes.

Don't Worry Dear, by Joan Frassler. New York: Behavioral Publications, 1971. Reading level: age 4–8 years. This book is useful as a tool for counseling parents. The character, Jenny, sucks her thumb, wets her bed, and stutters on some words. Surrounded by warmth and acceptance, she is given an opportunity to overcome these habits.

The Legend of the Veery Bird, by Kathleen Hague. San Diego, CA: Harcourt Brace Jovanovich, 1985. Reading level: 4–10 years. This modern fairy tale is of a boy who stutters named Veery that lives at the edge of a forest. As a misunderstood child, he shuns the human world and embraces the world of the forest. The magical forest keeper helps him deal with his sorrows and grants him a lovely singing voice. The beautiful story is also emotionally satisfying and deals as well with the death of parents.

Glue Fingers, by Matt Christopher. Boston: Little, Brown, and Company, 1975. Reading level: age 5–9 years. In this sports story, Billy Joe is afraid of rejection, so he decides not to play football until he stops stuttering. Reluctantly, he joins the team late in the season and becomes the star. His teammates are impressed with his athletic prowess and accept his stuttering.

Seal Secret, by Aidan Chambers. New York: Harper and Row, 1980. Reading level: age 9–12 years. This is a wonderfully written adventure story in which stuttering is only a minor theme. Two very different boys are forced to become playmates at their vacation seaside home. One plans to keep a baby seal trapped in a cave to raise for meat and skins. The other boy is outraged and plans to rescue the seal. He is successful, but injures himself and nearly loses his life in the process.

The Skating Rink, by Mildred Lee. New York: Seabury Press, 1969. Reading level: age 13–18 years. Tuck is looking forward to his 16th birthday when he can drop out of school. He walks two miles to school every day to avoid his classmates' ridicule about his stuttering. Then he meets a husband and wife skating team who are building a rink. Tuck befriends them both only to discover his own hidden skating talents. The story is rich in details of stuttering experiences and explores many theories and superstitions about stuttering.

Source: Bushey & Martin, 1988.

Choral reading is especially good; rather than individual performances, have the students read or recite simultaneously with a partner.

- Reading aloud in a slow, easy manner with light articulation is a good method; this is an ideal time to practice fluency strategies learned in therapy. For severe cases, the student may practice reading for the teacher before reading to the class. It is characteristic of stuttering to adapt or become more fluent with successive readings of the same passage.

- It is best to call on students randomly. Activities such as alphabetical roll call or answering questions down rows of desks can create anticipatory anxiety. Anxiety interferes with the ability to coordinate speech muscles; stuttering often results.

- Make no great issue of speech and be patient. Give the student *time to speak* without pressure. Eye contact is important; show by your expression that you are interested in *what* the student has to say, not *how* it is said.

- Be a good listener; listen in a calm, relaxed manner. Allow the student to complete the sentence without being interrupted and without having the words supplied.

- Insist on conversational manners in the classroom. A person speaking should not be interrupted. No one should monopolize a conversation. Let the student who stutters have a chance to talk.

- Create an atmosphere of ease and relaxation in the classroom. Avoid an atmosphere of tension and pressure.

- Conduct the school day in a routine manner. Stick with a schedule so the student does not need to be hurried. Surprise and unexpected events seem to trigger more stuttering.

- Insist on discipline. Teachers and parents of children who stutter need to know that structure reduces anxiety. When children are not sure what is expected of them and/or what will happen next, uncertainty breeds anxiety and worry. Anxiety is an exacerbating component in children's stuttering problems (Zebrowski & Schum, 1993). In this context, then, both parents and teachers should be encouraged that positive discipline (i.e., setting firm and realistic limits in a positive manner) can reduce anxiety.

- Avoid competition among the students. Do not favor one student over the others. In particular, do not overprotect, pamper, or be extremely anxious about the student who stutters.

- Do not allow ridicule or sarcasm from class members. Discipline the guilty participant as you would under other circumstances. Educate the class to be tolerant of the differences among people. Just as some students have trouble with math or reading, others have trouble with talking.

- Think of the child who stutters as a normal student who presently has difficulty talking. The student is not learning disabled, retarded, nor emotionally disturbed. Do not let the stuttering bias your educational expectations.

- If the student mentions frustration about the inability to talk fluently, reassurance that everyone finds it difficult to talk at times may help.

Remind the student that the new way of talking (as learned in management sessions) would be appropriate and helpful in getting over the difficult moments.

- Talk openly about stuttering. It can be most helpful if parents and teachers engage children in objective, nonjudgmental discussions of stuttering. Indeed, when a child is experiencing a lengthy or struggled block, much support can be intimated by saying, "I can tell you're having a hard time," or by physical contact (touching the arm, shoulder, or back without verbalizing) (Zebrowski & Schum, 1993).
- Be frank with the student. If the student is called a stutterer or is teased and becomes embarrassed by the speech difference, it is wise to state that you recognize the hesitations and repetitions, but if he or she uses the new techniques learned in speech treatment it will be easier to talk.
- In the classroom, model *delayed responding* by taking a second before answering. The student who stutters should adopt this habit of "taking some thinking time" before responding and your assistance and understanding can be crucial.
- In the classroom, provide a model of smooth, unhurried talking. Speaking in a softer voice is also a good model for all students to emulate.

Table 8-5 provides additional information on booklets, videos, and Web sites that may be of interest to both teachers and students who stutter.

OTHER FLUENCY DISORDERS

A rare acquired fluency disorder is that of neurotic or hysterical stuttering, called Tracks III and IV by Van Riper (1982). **Neurotic stuttering** is characterized by a sudden onset of rather severe stuttering. The onset may occur at any age, including adulthood, yet usually happens in an older child. Some psychological trauma, emotional upheaval, or stress seems to precipitate the occurrence of stuttering (Deal, 1982; Mahr & Leith, 1992; Van Riper, 1982). The psychogenic stuttering pattern is severe from the beginning, with unvoiced prolongations, laryngeal blocks, tension, and/or lengthy repetitions typical. Although highly aware of these sudden and severe disfluencies, the person may or may not be frustrated by them. The level of concern and motivation to change are important elements for the speech-language pathologist to assess in determining a therapeutic outcome.

Stuttering also may be acquired following specific nervous system damage, such as from stroke, head trauma, infection, or tumor. Although similar-

Table 8-5 Selected Booklets, Videos, and Web Sites on Stuttering Useful for Classroom Teachers and Their Students Who Stutter

A homepage on stuttering is maintained by a faculty member at Minnesota State University-Mankato at www.mnsu.edu/dept/comdis/kuster/stutter.html. This excellent site also includes special pages, "Just for Kids" and "Just for Teens," as well as covering frequently asked questions and special topics, such as how to handle teasing or tips on making a presentation. A "kid-to-kid" chat room also exists at this Web site as does information on cluttering.

The American Speech-Language-Hearing Association maintains basic information on fluency disorders, risk factors, and communication tips for the general public at www.asha.org/public/speech/disorders/stuttering.

The National Stuttering Association is a self-help and support organization for people who stutter. The Web site www.nsastutter.org/ also provides information on local support groups, adult workshops, youth days, and the like.

Stuttering: Straight Talk for Teachers is a video and booklet set designed for every classroom teacher with a child who stutters; also useful for SLPs working with teachers individually or leading in-services. Covers teachers' frequently asked questions and has classroom suggestions. Available for $5 from The Stuttering Foundation at www.stutteringhelp.org.

Notes to the Teacher: The Child Who Stutters at School is a brochure with useful tips for teachers and parents, and is also available in Spanish. Available for 10 cents from The Stuttering Foundation at www.stutteringhelp.org.

Stuttering: For Kids By Kids—This videotape (or DVD) uses cartoon characters and real kids to talk about what stuttering is, what to do when teased about stuttering, what bugs a child who stutters, and what helps. Available for $10 from The Stuttering Foundation at www.stutteringhelp.org.

Sometimes I Just Stutter—Written for children who stutter, this 40-page booklet with activity pages provides helpful information on stuttering, why stuttering fluctuates, why teasing occurs, and what teachers and family members should know about stuttering. Available in English and in Spanish for $2 from The Stuttering Foundation at www.stutteringhelp.org.

The School-Age Child Who Stutters: Working Effectively with Attitudes and Emotions—This 192-page workbook for speech-language pathologists works with feelings and beliefs of school-age children; includes reproducible handouts and tasks to gather information from children, parents, and teachers. Available for $15 from The Stuttering Foundation at www.stutteringhelp.org.

ities exist, there are enough characteristic differences to insist that such a fluency disorder is not true (developmental) stuttering. The term **neurogenic stuttering**, then, establishes this as an acquired fluency disorder that results from neurological damage. Neurogenic stuttering may occur in conjunction with bilateral or unilateral brain damage, with focal or diffuse lesions, or with cortical or subcortical damage to the central nervous system (Van Borsel, Van Lierde, Van Cauwenberge, Guldemont, & Van Orshoven, 1998).

There are numerous reports of neurogenic stuttering in patients with aphasia, apraxia, cerebral palsy, neurological diseases (e.g., Parkinsonism), dementias (including dialysis dementia), and substance-abuse addicts. Although nervous system damage can occur at any age (even prenatally), most instances of neurogenic stuttering occur in adults.

Cluttering is a fluency disorder but not just a fluency disorder. Cluttering has varied symptomatology and occurs simultaneously with other speech, language, and behavioral disorders. According to Weiss (1964, 1968), cluttering symptoms may be categorized into obligatory, facultative, and associated types. The five obligatory symptoms of cluttering include: part- and whole-word repetitions, lack of awareness of the disorder, short attention span, perceptual weakness, and poorly organized thinking. Among facultative symptoms are: excessive speech rate (tachylalia), interjections, articulatory and motor disabilities, and grammatical difficulties. Some associated symptoms include: reading and writing disorders, lack of rhythm and musical ability, and restlessness and hyperactivity.

Similarly, Daly (1993) views cluttering as a fluency disorder syndrome. The many facets of the condition are noted in his definition:

> Cluttering is a disorder of both speech and language processing that frequently results in rapid, dysrhythmic, sporadic, unorganized, and often unintelligible speech. Accelerated speech (tachylalia) is not always present, but impairments in formulating language almost always are. . . . Those who clutter confuse their listeners with incomplete and awkward sentences, false starts, sound sequencing errors, and word-retrieval problems. Their garbled speech is confounded by a lack of clarity of inner language formulation. Equally frustrating for clinicians are the absence of self-awareness and the unconcerned attitude of many clients who clutter. Their self-monitoring skills for speech and social situations are deficient (p. 7).

In contrast, St. Louis and colleagues (1992, 2003, 2004) regard that rate problems are somehow central to cluttering, stating that persons who clutter talk too fast and fail to maintain normally expected sound, syllable, phrase, and pausing patterns. St. Louis and his colleagues do not include language difficulties in their definition of cluttering, noting that there are a few persons who clutter who do not evince language problems. Still, they cite other symptoms which are optional, if not frequent, in persons who clutter: lack of awareness of the problem; family history of fluency disorders; poor handwriting; confusing, disorganized language or conversational skills; temporary improvement when asked to slow down or pay attention to speech; misarticulations; poor intelligibility; social or vocational problems; distractibility; hyperactivity; auditory perceptual difficulties; learning disabilities; and apraxia.

With such a host of possible symptoms affecting all channels of communication and behavior in general, the teacher may have little difficulty in recognizing such an unusual child in the classroom, yet may not realize that speech-language problems are at the core. Referral to a speech-language pathologist is appropriate. As espoused by Preus (1996), cluttering is not only related to stuttering, but also to other disorders, notably psycholinguistic disorders, minimal brain dysfunction (MBD), language learning disorders (LLD), attention deficit disorders (ADD), and central auditory processing disorders (CAPD). The relationship between cluttering and a series of learning and related disorders necessitates interdisciplinary cooperation. After differential diagnosis of cluttering and all its components along the lines suggested by St. Louis et al. (2003), the speech-language pathologist will devise a treatment plan. Therapeutic efforts may be directed toward rate of speech, heightened monitoring, clear articulation, language formulation and organization, speech naturalness, attention and concentration skills, and remedial reading. A team of special education professionals should be involved in the total intervention program, with the classroom teacher as the central figure.

The fourth-grade teacher referred Adam to the school SLP, concerned that he might be stuttering because of his repeating and unclear speech. In the assessment Adam displayed a rapid rate of speech (as measured by overall syllables per minute but especially during articulatory rate when only fluent segments were measured). His speech sample was sprinkled with many syllable and word repetitions as well as numerous incomplete sentences. When answering specific questions it was necessary for the speech clinician to ask him to repeat many answers as it was difficult to understand what he had said. Intelligibility for spoken words and short phrases was excellent. No struggle behaviors were noted and Adam, upon questioning, was oblivious to any speech differences he might have. In follow-up with the classroom teacher, the SLP learned that Adam was a poor reader and that his handwriting was hard to read because it was both sloppy and contained many misspelled words. The school reading specialist was called in for assessment of possible dyslexia. At the IEP meeting the father, who was a physics professor at the nearby university, was observed to speak rapidly. The father also noted that growing up he too "had stuttered" but not as badly as an uncle who was plagued with it his whole life. The intervention decided upon was a team approach with classroom teacher, reading specialist, and speech-language pathologist working closely together. Among the initial strategies for speech were to increase Adam's awareness of his output and to train a slower, syllable-timed speech pattern.

CONCLUSION

Disfluent speech occurs among normal-speaking children and adults. But when certain types of speech errors predominate, or when the disfluencies occur too frequently, speakers often are judged to have a fluency disorder. Several kinds of fluency disorders exist but developmental stuttering, or simply stuttering, is the most common. The incidence of stuttering is approximately 4–5% but through spontaneous recovery the prevalence rate hovers around 0.7–1% of the population. When persistent, stuttering tends to worsen with time, developing more speech tension, struggle, and associated learned behaviors that affect the speaker's life. Certainly, stuttering and its affective, behavioral, and cognitive reactions limit a student's ability to communicate with others or to engage in social and school-related activities. There are many interesting aspects of stuttering that can be manipulated by teachers, parents, and speech-language pathologists. Positive classroom environments, speech production strategies, and emotional assistance can be provided to students who stutter by the classroom teacher, working in concert with the SLP.

REFERENCES

Ambrose, N., & Yairi, E. (1994). The development of awareness of stuttering in preschool children. *Journal of Fluency Disorders, 19*(4), 229–246.

Ambrose, N., & Yairi, E. (1999). Normal disfluency data for early childhood stuttering. *Journal of Speech, Language, and Hearing Research, 42*, 895–909.

Andrews, G., & Harris, M. (1964). *The syndrome of stuttering*. London: Heinemann Medteal Books.

Bloodstein, O. (1960). The development of stuttering: II. Developmental phases. *Journal of Speech and Hearing Disorders, 25*, 366–376.

Bloodstein, O. (1995). *A handbook on stuttering* (5th ed.). San Diego, CA: Singular.

Bushey, T., & Martin, R. (1988). Stuttering in children's literature. *Language, Speech, and Hearing Services in Schools, 19*(3), 235–250.

Campbell, J.H., & Hill, D. (1993). *Application of a weighted scoring system to systematic disfluency analysis.* Poster session presented at the annual meeting of the American Speech-Language-Hearing Association, Anaheim, CA.

Clark, H.H., & Clark, E.V. (1977). *Psychology and language: An introduction to psycholinguistics.* New York: Harcourt Brace Jovanovich.

Conture, E.G. (2001). *Stuttering: Its nature, diagnosis, and treatment.* Needham Heights, MA: Allyn & Bacon.

Cox, N.J. (1988). Molecular genetics: The key to the puzzle of stuttering? *Asha, 30,* 36–40.

Daly, D.A. (1981). Differentiation of stuttering subgroups with Van Riper's developmental tracks: A preliminary study. *Journal of NSSLHA, 9*(1), 89–101.

Daly, D.A. (1993). Cluttering: The orphan of speech-language pathology. *American Journal of Speech-Language Pathology, 4*(2), 6–8.

Deal, J. (1982). Sudden onset of stuttering: A case report. *Journal of Speech and Hearing Disorders, 47,* 301–304.

Encyclopaedia Britannica Almanac 2003. (2002). Chicago: Encyclopaedia Britannia.

Fromkin, V. (Ed.) (1973). *Speech errors as linguistic evidence.* The Hague, Netherlands: Mouton.

Goldman-Eisler, F. (1968). *Psycholinguistics: Experiments in spontaneous speech.* New York: Academic Press.

Gordon, P., & Luper, H. (1992). The early identification of beginning stuttering, I: Protocols. *American Journal of Speech-Language Pathology, 1,* 43–53.

Gregory, H. (1987). Coping with school. In J. Fraser, & W.H. Perkins (Eds.), *Do you stutter: A guide for teens.* Memphis, TN: Speech Foundation of America.

Gregory, H. (1990). Integration: Present status and prospects for the future. In J. Fraser (Ed.), *Stuttering therapy: Prevention and intervention with children.* Memphis, TN: Speech Foundation of America.

Haynes, W.O., & Pindzola, R.H. (2004). *Diagnosis and evaluation in speech pathology* (6th ed.). Boston: Pearson Education.

Hull, F.M., Mielke, P.W., Willeford, J.A., & Timmons, R.J. (1976). *National Speech and Hearing Survey* (Final Report, Project 50978). Washington, DC: Health, Education, and Welfare, Office of Education, Bureau of Education for the Handicapped.

Lincoln, M., & Harrison, E. (1999). The Lidcombe program. In M. Onslow & A. Packman (Eds.), *The handbook of early stuttering intervention.* San Diego, CA: Singular.

Louko, L.J., Edwards, M.L., & Conture, E.G. (1990). Phonological characteristics of young stutterers and their normally fluent peers: Preliminary observations. *Journal of Fluency Disorders, 15,* 191–210.

Louko, L.J., Edwards, M.L., & Conture, E.G. (1999). Treating children who exhibit co-occurring stuttering and disordered phonology. In R. Curlee (Ed.), *Stuttering and related disorders of fluency* (2nd ed.), New York: Thieme Medical.

Mahr, G., & Leith, W. (1992). Psychogenic stuttering of adult onset. *Journal of Speech and Hearing Research, 35,* 283–286.

Martin, R.R., & Lindamood, L.P. (1986). Stuttering and spontaneous recovery: Implications for the speech-language pathologist. *Language, Speech, and Hearing Services in Schools, 17,* 207–218.

Onslow, M., & Packman, A. (1999). *The handbook of early stuttering intervention.* San Diego, CA: Singular.

Perkins, W.H. (1971). *Speech pathology: An applied behavioral science.* Saint Louis, MO: C.V. Mosby.

Pindzola, R.H. (1988). *Stuttering intervention program: Age 3 to grade 3.* Austin, TX: PRO-ED.

Pindzola, R.H. (1999). The stuttering intervention program. In M. Oslow & A. Packman (Eds.), *The handbook of early stuttering intervention.* San Diego, CA: Singular.

Pindzola, R.H., & White, D.T. (1986). A protocol for differentiating the incipient stutterer. *Language, Speech, and Hearing Services in Schools, 17,* 2–15.

Preus, A. (1996). Cluttering upgraded. *Journal of Fluency Disorders, 21*(3–4), 348–358.

Riley, G.D. (1994). *Stuttering severity instrument for children and adults* (3rd ed.). Austin, TX: PRO-ED.

Ryan, B.P. (1974). *Programmed therapy for stuttering in children and adults.* Springfield, IL: Charles C. Thomas.

Ryan, B., & Ryan, B. (1999). The Monterey fluency program. In M. Oslow & A. Packman (Eds.), *The handbook of early stuttering intervention.* San Diego, CA: Singular.

St. Louis, K.O. (1992). On defining cluttering. In F.L. Myers & K.O. St. Louis (Eds.), *Cluttering: A clinical perspective* (pp. 37–53). San Diego, CA: Singular.

St. Louis, K.O., Myers, F.L., Faragasso, K., Townsend, P., & Gallaher, A.J. (2004). Perceptual aspects of cluttered speech. *Journal of Fluency Disorders, 29*(3), 213–235.

St. Louis, K.O., Raphael, L.J., Myers, F.L., & Bakker, K. (2003). Cluttering updated. *The ASHA Leader, 8*(21), 4–5, 20–22.

Starkweather, C.W. (1981). Speech fluency and its development in normal children. In N. Lass (Ed.), *Speech and language: Advances in basic research and practice,* Vol. 4. New York: Academy Press.

Van Borsel, J., Van Lierde, K., Van Cauwenberge, P., Guldemont, I., & Van Orshoven, M. (1998). Severe acquired stuttering following injury of the left supplementary motor region: A case report. *Journal of Fluency Disorders, 23*(1), 49–58.

Van Riper, C. (1982). *The nature of stuttering* (3rd ed.). Englewood Cliffs, NJ: Prentice-Hall.

Weiss, A.L. (2004a). What child language research may contribute to the understanding and treatment of stuttering. *Language, Speech, and Hearing Services in Schools, 35*(1), 30–33.

Weiss, A.L. (2004b). Why we should consider pragmatics when planning treatment for children who stutter. *Language, Speech, and Hearing Services in Schools, 35*(1), 34–45.

Weiss, A., & Zebrowski, P. (1992). Disfluencies in the conversations of young children who stutter: Some answers about questions. *Journal of Speech and Hearing Research, 35,* 1230–1238.

Weiss, D.A. (1964). *Cluttering.* Englewood Cliffs, NJ: Prentice-Hall.

Weiss, D.A. (1968). Cluttering: Central language imbalance. *Pediatric Clinics of North America, 15,* 705–720.

Wingate, M.E. (1966). A standard definition of stuttering. *Journal of Speech and Hearing Disorders, 29,* 484–489.

Yairi, E., & Ambrose, N. (1992). A longitudinal study of stuttering in children: A preliminary report. *Journal of Speech and Hearing Research, 35,* 755–760.

Yairi, E., Ambrose, N., & Niermann, B. (1993). The early months of stuttering: A developmental study. *Journal of Speech and Hearing Research, 36,* 521–528.

Yairi, E., & Lewis, B. (1984). Disfluencies at the onset of stuttering. *Journal of Speech and Hearing Research, 27,* 154–159.

Yaruss, J.S. (1998). Describing the consequences of disorders: Stuttering and the International Classification of Impairment, Disabilities, and Handicaps. *Journal of Speech, Language, and Hearing Research, 41*(2), 249–257.

Yaruss, J.S., & Quesal, R.W. (2004). Stuttering and the International Classification of Functioning, Disability, and Health (ICF): An update. *Journal of Communication Disorders, 37,* 35–52.

Young, M.A. (1975). Onset, prevalence, and recovery from stuttering. *Journal of Speech and Hearing Disorders, 40*(1), 49–58.

Zebrowski, P. M., & Schum, R.L. (1993). Counseling parents of children who stutter. *American Journal of Speech-Language Pathology, 2*(2), 65–73.

TERMS TO KNOW

avoidance behaviors
circumlocutions
cluttering
differential diagnosis
disfluent
fluency disorders
fluent
incidence
neurogenic stuttering

neurotic stuttering
postponement devices
prevalence
primary stuttering
secondary stuttering
severity
starter devices
stuttering (developmental stuttering)
substitutions

STUDY QUESTIONS

1. How can you distinguish between a child who is beginning to stutter from a child who is normally disfluent? Cite some of the danger signs for which you might look.

2. Describe, as if talking to a parent, the typical developmental sequence of stuttering.

3. Describe and give examples of stuttering behaviors, including repetitions, prolongations, and struggle behaviors.

4. Communicative stress is known to disrupt fluency. Cite common classroom examples of the stresses listed in Table 8-3. Be able to discuss these fluency disruptors without relying on the table.

5. Discuss as many things as you can think of that a teacher should do when a child who stutters is in the class.

6. List as many things as you can think of that a teacher should not do when a child who stutters is in the class.

7. What are some of the factors a speech-language pathologist might assess during an evaluation of a person suspected of stuttering? Include in your discussion, factors pertinent to making a differential diagnosis and in determining severity.

8. What are avoidance behaviors? Identify as many behaviors as you can that might suggest a person who stutters is in your class even though you have never heard him or her repeat or prolong sounds.

9. Differentiate between developmental and acquired types of fluency disorders.

chapter nine

Voice Disorders

INTRODUCTION

The voice carries a great deal of information about an individual. It is common to be able to identify a friend calling on the telephone when all the friend says is "Hi, how are you doing?" You know in an instant that the caller is Sarah, not Melissa, Kathy, or any of your other friends. It is also common to be able to identify from a voice sample a stranger's sex and approximate age without being able to see who is talking. The voice mirrors our emotions; we can tell from the tone of a friend's voice if anger, nervousness, or excitement is present. The voice also reflects our physical health, as in the statement, "You sound like you're coming down with a cold." Yes, the voice carries a great deal of information and has the responsibility of projecting us to the world.

A voice that is perceived as abnormal—too effeminate, too hoarse, too sing-songy, too soft, or too much of anything—may affect one's social acceptance, educational expectations, eventual type of employment, or cause one's personality to be inaccurately labeled (Jotz, Cervantes, Abrahao, Settanni, & Carrar de Angelis, 2002; Morton & Watson, 2001). These negative consequences underscore that a disordered voice may be a handicap. Recall that both PL 94-142 and the Individuals with Disabilities Education Act of 1997 incorporate the broad definition of a handicapping condition as including academic, social, and emotional impacts on the student. A voice disorder, therefore, may qualify as an educationally handicapping condition.

To underscore that contemporary health issues are concerned with the consequences of various disorders, the World Health Organization developed the International Classification of Impairment, Disabilities, and Handicaps (ICIDH). Updated, the ICIDH-2 emphasizes functioning as well as disability and health (WHO, 2001). Other attempts to quantify the impact and psychosocial consequences of voice disorders are still in the pioneering stages but include efforts toward a "voice handicap index" (Jacobson et al., 1997).

This chapter will review the anatomy and physiology of the larynx as was described more fully in Chapter 2, with an emphasis on normal versus abnormal vocal parameters. Vocal pathologies typically seen in the school-aged population will be discussed, and the roles of the classroom teacher and speech-language pathologist in the management of voice disorders will then be delineated. Later in this chapter, we will describe students who, for some medical reason, do not breathe through their larynx, and produce voice in an unusual way. Among other concerns, the environment of the classroom necessitates teacher monitoring for these special students.

It may be wise to state at the outset that voice disorders are typically divided into two types. **Phonatory disorders** are true disorders of the voice, as they stem from problems in the laryngeal mechanism. For example, the vocal folds may be inflamed, there may be a growth on or near the folds, or the folds may be paralyzed and unable to move. Voice disorders of this type will be the emphasis of this chapter. A second category of voice disorders is **disorders of resonance**. Structural or functional deviations in the vocal tract may affect the tone or resonance of the voice as it passes through the tract. The person may be judged as having a voice disorder because the quality of the voice sounds unusual. Examples include nasal obstruction causing hyponasality (which sounds like speaking with a head cold), velopharyngeal incompetence leading to hypernasality (which may be due to neuromuscular disorders, clefts of the palate, or tissue deficiencies), or the unusual haunting quality of cul-de-sac resonance, as often heard in the speech of persons with a severe hearing impairment. Disorders of resonance will be discussed only briefly in this chapter as they will be mentioned again in Chapters 10 and 11.

THE NATURE OF VOICE PRODUCTION AND VOICE DISORDERS

When we wish to talk, the respiratory musculature delivers exhaled lung air up through the bronchial passages and into the trachea. This air passes freely through the larynx when the vocal folds are opened, or **abducted**, merely to be compressed at some point in the upper vocal tract—perhaps by the tongue, teeth and/or lips, into sound. What is articulated, then, is a voiceless speech sound (such as the sounds associated with the letters p, t, s, f, and so on). Conversely the air released from the lungs may be momentarily blocked at the level of the larynx by vocal folds that are closed, or **adducted**. This blocked air accumulates and increases in pressure until it is strong enough to literally blow open the closed folds. The pressure beneath the vocal folds is termed **subglottic pressure**; not only does it blow the folds apart, but the rapid pressure changes and air velocities associated with this subglottic pressure explosion suck the folds together again. With continued air being supplied from the lungs, the folds are once again blown apart. This process of opening-closing-opening-closing continues at an incredibly rapid rate—about 120 times per second in an average adult male and about 200 times per second in an average adult female. Each opening-closing cycle of the vocal folds is termed a cycle of **vibration**, and the number of cycles per second is the **fundamental frequency** of vocal fold vibration. This vibratory pattern causes rapid, regular fluctuations of air pressure in the vocal tract and hence a crude sound is phonated. Simply put, voice is produced at the larynx, yet this sound wave must travel up the vocal tract to be shaped and articulated into recognizable (voiced) speech sounds (such as b̲, d̲, z̲, v̲, and all vowels).

It should be obvious from the foregoing discussion of voice production that problems may arise at many different levels. Voice disorders may be related to problems with the respiratory system and the generation of insufficient subglottic air pressures to drive the laryngeal mechanism; there may be laryngeal muscle weakness or paralysis affecting abduction and adduction abilities, or there may be growths, swellings, or sores on the glottal edges of the vocal folds which interfere with the regular and smooth vibrations so typical of healthy folds. These and myriad other problems may cause voice disorders.

To summarize then, the normal voice is supported by a healthy respiratory system, strong and coordinated laryngeal muscles, and even and smooth glottal edges that can vibrate regularly with changes in air pressures. Normal laryngeal conditions lead to normal parameters of the voice, meaning those attributes that compose our overall impression of a voice.

Voice disorders are prevalent in about 6% of the school-aged population (as reviewed by Wilson, 1987); this suggests an average of 2 students per class of 33 pupils has a voice disorder. However, it should be pointed out that the frequency of vocal deviations fluctuates as a function of age—higher in young children, and lower after adolescence. The prevalence of perceivable hoarseness in children attending first through fifth grades has been reported to be as high as 38% (Harden, 1986).

Elementary school-aged children, then, represent a significant group of persons with disordered voices. Why so? Statistics show that 45–80% of childhood voice deviations are the result of vocal abuse (Baynes, 1966; Herrington-Hall, Lee, Stemple, Niemi, and McHone, 1988). The vocal activities of children, especially boys, include frequent loud talking, yelling, and strained phonation.

Students in middle school through high school, while they may have a lower prevalence of voice disorders, nevertheless are at risk for developing problems. Students in these grades are likely to engage in extracurricular activities, such as cheerleading and competitive sports, in which vocal abuse frequently and insidiously becomes part of the activity.

CAUSATIONS OF COMMON VOCAL DISORDERS

Table 9-1 lists common etiologies or conditions that bring about voice problems, as typically seen in schools (Fox, 1985). The table also lists the most frequently occurring laryngeal conditions seen by **laryngologists**, or throat doctors, in a pediatric population ranging in age from 3 days to 18 years (Dobres, Lee, Stemple, Kummer, & Kretschmer, 1989). The implication is that, by the school years, some of the more serious medically related voice problems have been treated. Phonatory disorders, those due to laryngeal mass, or movement problems are much more commonly encountered than resonance problems of the vocal tract. Of this list, the conditions called *nodules* and *edema* are the most frequent causes of a voice disorder in the school years. The principal feature of both is hoarseness. Some of the conditions listed in the table will be discussed separately. And, although hundreds of Web pages that deal with voice disorders exist, Table 9-2 lists a few that might be of interest to teachers, especially those showing photographs of laryngeal disorders.

Nodules

Hoarseness is often due to the presence of **vocal nodules**. Nodules (or nodes) are calloused growths of tissue on the edge of one or both vocal folds. Whether unilateral or bilateral, nodules appear in the characteristic location shown in Figure 9-1, which is the place of greatest impact when the vocal

Table 9-1 Common Voice Disorders in Children and Youth

Phonatory Disorders Commonly Seen in Schools:

1. Nodules—Calloused growths on the vocal folds; see text
2. Edema—Swelling of the vocal folds; see text
3. Papilloma—Clusters of wartlike growths; see text
4. Paralysis—One or both vocal folds unable to move; if unable to open, the ability to breathe may be impaired; if unable to close the fold, voice may be weak and breathy; paralysis may be caused by trauma (such as nerve damage in an automobile wreck) or by a virus (with a good chance for spontaneous recovery)
5. Polyps—Fluid-filled growths on or around the vocal folds; often likened to blisters on the folds; usually caused by vocal abuse or misuse and linked to smoking as well; vocal symptoms are similar to nodules, particularly hoarseness and low pitch
6. Idiopathic—No visible pathology is present, yet the voice is judged to be abnormal sounding

Pediatric Laryngeal Pathologies Commonly Seen by Laryngologists (and Frequency of Occurrence):

1. Subglottic stenosis (31.2%)—A narrowing of the trachea; usually detected in infancy
2. Nodules (17.5%)—See above
3. Laryngomalacia (11.9%)—Usually seen in the newborn and often outgrown by age 2 years; a flabbiness of some laryngeal structures causing them to be indrawn during inhalation; stridor (noisy inhalation) and dyspnea (shortness of breath) usually result
4. Idiopathic (7.7%)—See above
5. Paralysis (6.2%)—See above
6. Papilloma (3.8%)—See above

Resonance Imbalances Commonly Seen in Schools:

1. Congenital palatal incompetence—Inability to close off the oral and nasal cavities; may be due to a variety of velar or pharyngeal problems
2. Structural deviations—Including palatal clefts, submucous clefts (hole in bony palate disguised by tissue coverage), nasal polyps, deviated septums (crooked interior nasal bone), and such
3. Neuromuscular disorders—Including velar paralysis, dysarthrias (motor speech disorders to be discussed in Chapter 12), cerebral palsies, and such
4. Functional—No structural cause of the resonance imbalance exists

Sources: Dobres, Lee, Stemple, Kummer, & Kretschmer, 1989; Fox, 1985.

folds adduct. Obviously, if adduction is done in a strained, forceful manner, the tissue here will become irritated and, over time, thickened. The young, still-forming nodule may be relatively small, soft, and compressible during vocal fold adduction, but with continued irritation, the nodule tends to enlarge, harden, and become less compressible. The size and callousness of

Table 9-2 Select Web Sites for Information on Voice Disorders

www.entusa.com/larynx_videos.html
This is an excellent site for seeing and hearing voice disorders. It is provided by an otolaryngologist, Kevin Kavanagh, MD. Color pictures of healthy and diseased vocal folds—including nodules, polyps, laryngitis, cancers, and paralyses—are shown along with audio samples of disordered voices and video clips.

www.hopkinsmedicine.org/voice/disorders.html
This site, provided by the Center for Laryngeal and Voice Disorders at The Johns Hopkins University School of Medicine provides concise descriptions of the symptoms, causes, and treatments of voice disorders. Some color photos are provided.

www.bcm.edu/oto/othersa5.html
This is the Baylor College of Medicine's guide to otolaryngology resources on the Internet. A large number of links exist for accessing information on laryngeal anatomy, vocal diseases, and a sundry of medical treatments.

www.asha.org/public/speech/disorders/voice-problems.html
The American Speech-Language-Hearing Association provides this site for the public. General information on the voice and its disorders is presented along with how to find treatment.

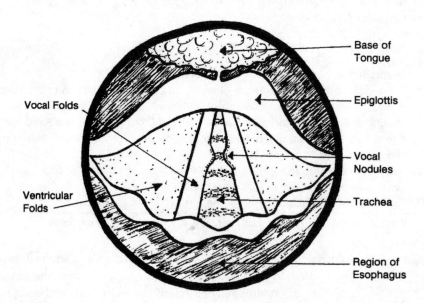

Figure 9-1 Schematic Drawing of the Larynx Showing Typical Location of Vocal Nodules

the nodules may, therefore, interfere with complete closure, leaving instead gaps (or chinks) where air can escape during adduction. The result will be a breathy quality to the voice and loss of overall vocal loudness. The nodular growth itself weights down the small vocal fold and causes the rate of vibration to slow. Consequently, the person's voice sounds lower pitched than it did when it was healthy. The mass also may interfere with the smoothness of these vocal fold vibrations, further adding a rough or harsh quality to the voice. In an attempt to produce a stronger, clearer voice with less breathiness and loss of loudness, the person may use extra tension or effort to close the vocal folds. This, however, begins a vicious cycle in that such strain merely increases the force of impact during adduction and aggravates the irritated nodule even more. Figure 9-2 schematizes these auditory symptoms of nodules.

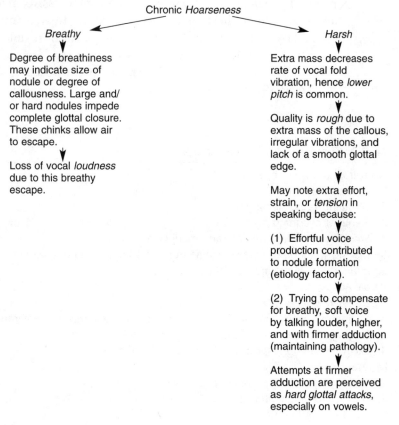

Chronic *Hoarseness*

Breathy

Degree of breathiness may indicate size of nodule or degree of callousness. Large and/ or hard nodules impede complete glottal closure. These chinks allow air to escape.

Loss of vocal *loudness* due to this breathy escape.

Harsh

Extra mass decreases rate of vocal fold vibration, hence *lower pitch* is common.

Quality is *rough* due to extra mass of the callous, irregular vibrations, and lack of a smooth glottal edge.

May note extra effort, strain, or *tension* in speaking because:

(1) Effortful voice production contributed to nodule formation (etiology factor).

(2) Trying to compensate for breathy, soft voice by talking louder, higher, and with firmer adduction (maintaining pathology).

Attempts at firmer adduction are perceived as *hard glottal attacks*, especially on vowels.

Figure 9-2 The Auditory Symptoms of Vocal Nodules

As we said, nodules are caused by chronic irritation and the force of impact when the vocal folds are slammed together. What causes some people to drive their laryngeal mechanism so forcefully? The answer is simply that they abuse and/or misuse their larynx too often. The implication for treatment is equally straightforward: identify the abuses and misuses of the voice, and help the person eliminate them. The nodule would, it is hoped, heal up and disappear. While the process really may not be this simple, and surgery may prove necessary, the identification of abuses and misuses is where the speech-language pathologist and laryngologist start. Some common situations of abuse and misuse are outlined in Table 9-3.

Nodules and the pattern of misuses and abuses that contribute to their formation tend to occur in certain types of people. Teachers, singers, and preachers are engaged in strenuous vocal activity as a function of their occupation. Table 9-4 provides a word of warning for classroom teachers. Middle- and high-school cheerleaders are vulnerable to frequent bouts of vocal strain, laryngitis, and the eventual development of nodules. Also children, particularly physically active boys with outgoing, aggressive, distractible, boisterous, talkative personalities, are predisposed to having nodules (Green, 1989).

Table 9-3 Common Misuses and Abuses in Students

I. Nonverbal (nonspeech) Abuses:
  1. Excessive crying
  2. Frequent throat clearing
  3. Frequent coughing
  4. Smoking (including tobacco and marijuana)
  5. Making strange noises (as machine gun, growling, siren noise during play, or grunting during football or karate practice)
II. Verbal Abuses:
  1. Excessive yelling, screaming, cheering
  2. Talking over noise (TV, radio/stereo, groups of friends, machine environments)
  3. Singing (especially out of natural range or in a forced manner)
  4. Excessive talking (especially if in a strained manner)
III. Misuses:
  1. Speaking at an inappropriate pitch level
  2. Using hard glottal attacks
  3. Speaking with tension
  4. Using excessively loud voice

Table 9-4 Information Classroom Teachers Should Heed About Their Own Voice

- Vocal nodules tend to occur in certain occupations, including the teaching profession.
- Over 11% of teachers, as compared to 6% of nonteachers, experience multiple voice symptoms.
- Vocal problems of teachers, especially elementary school teachers, include
  - Hoarseness
  - Voice/throat discomfort
  - Increased vocal effort
  - Tiring of the voice
  - Voice quality change after short use
  - Difficulty projecting the voice
  - Trouble speaking or singing softly
  - Loss of the singing range
- Teachers report that because of their vocal dysfunction they tend to reduce classroom activities and interactions with students, thus affecting the learning environment.
- Teachers feel they would benefit from a SLP's voice hygiene in-service directed at their personal vocal care as well as vocal strategies for handling classroom situations.

Sources: Roy, Merrill, Thibeault, Gray, & Smith, 2004; Yiu, 2002.

Referral to the speech-language pathologist is in order when a teacher notices a student with chronic vocal hoarseness. Consultation with a laryngologist may lead to one of three routes of intervention: medical, vocal hygiene, or voice treatment.

Based on the student's age and the maturity of the nodule, surgical removal may be recommended. Nodules often are removed by microsurgical stripping techniques or by laser surgery. Medical clearance for behavioral intervention also may be granted. In fact, Moran and Pentz (1987) found that 59% of laryngologists polled recommend behavioral intervention as the treatment of choice in children. Only 10% of these doctors opted for surgery as the treatment of choice. Once given medical clearance, the speech-language pathologist (SLP) has the choice of providing voice treatment or a vocal hygiene approach, as will be discussed later in the chapter.

Edema

Vocal **edema** refers to an inflamed swelling of the tissues on and around the vocal folds. To be sure, the abuses and misuses discussed earlier may lead to edema in the formative stages before the nodule appears. Edematous swelling also is commonly associated with respiratory tract infection (e.g., colds, flu) and allergies. Postnasal drip and sinus drainage, whether infected with bacteria or not, can irritate the mucous membrane linings of the larynx and cause fluid retention and edema. This fluidlike puffiness makes the vocal folds heavier. Consequently, they vibrate more slowly and perhaps unevenly. The auditory symptoms of hoarseness and lowering of the pitch are the result.

The teacher and speech-language pathologist need to gather information to help determine whether a student has vocal hoarseness because of edema associated with respiratory infection or allergy or because of some other more serious reason (such as nodules, tumors, cancers, and the like). Student and parent interviews can yield information regarding the student's health, whether the student claims to be experiencing a cold or allergy attack, whether the vocal hoarseness is worse in the mornings (indicating drainage while lying in bed is contributory), and whether the hoarseness is temporary. A student with hoarseness should be watched; colds and upper respiratory infections usually subside within 10 to 14 days. If the hoarseness persists longer than this period of time, a referral to the speech-language pathologist is in order.

Most schools have in place regulations which stipulate that the student must be seen by a laryngologist for differential diagnosis. Certainly, if the hoarseness is not due to edema but to a more serious, even life-threatening laryngeal condition, this should be discovered as soon as possible. If the hoarseness is attributable to edema, the student may benefit from decongestant or antihistamine medicines to relieve drainage. Care of the voice is important during these times of inflammation and vocal-fold edema. Care of the voice learned through vocal hygiene lessons may be taught by the teacher or the speech-language pathologist, as we shall soon discuss. Voice treatment by the SLP is generally not indicated for such cases.

Papilloma

A serious laryngeal condition is that of **papilloma** or, more accurately, juvenile laryngeal papillomatosis. Papilloma usually affects children, makes frequent recurrences throughout childhood, and gradually tapers off, becoming rare after puberty. Classroom teachers and special education personnel need to be cognizant of papilloma because of its life-threatening conditions.

Papilloma appear as clusters of wartlike growths and are thought to be viral related. These warty tumors often spread rapidly and interfere with the airway. Getting adequate air is more important than the hoarseness and breathiness that may co-occur with phonation. Students who are hoarse for more than 10 days should be referred to the SLP, who will in turn refer them to the laryngologist. Students with hoarseness also should be watched for daily changes in their ease of breathing. Once papilloma is diagnosed, it becomes a medical or surgical problem, especially if any obstruction of the airway is present.

Voice treatment per se by the speech-language pathologist generally is not indicated, as it will not resolve the papilloma, yet, vocal hygiene is important to impress on the student during the tumor flare-ups. Because papilloma tends to grow back quickly, repeated surgeries may be needed. Repeated surgeries scar the vocal mechanism and result in chronically abnormal vocal parameters, usually severe hoarseness, inadequate loudness, intermittent voice stoppages, and a lowered pitch. The SLP will offer voice treatment after surgery to help the student learn to use the scarred mechanism to its maximum potential.

VOCAL ASSESSMENT ISSUES AND PARAMETERS OF THE VOICE

Issues in the diagnosis and evaluation of vocal disorders are provided elsewhere, including the overview text by Haynes and Pindzola (2004). An overall judgment of a person's voice is insufficient for an evaluation; each parameter of the voice is best judged separately. *The Voice Assessment Protocol* (Pindzola, 1987) is a useful tool for appraising vocal characteristics. The speech-language pathologist may use this or a similar instrument as a guide in the decision-making process regarding normal versus abnormal voice-related features. The Voice Assessment Protocol appraises five parameters of the voice: pitch, loudness, quality, breath features, and rate/rhythm. The first three are by far the most salient of the vocal characteristics. As a teacher, your knowledge of these parameters will help in the classroom identification of students who may have voice disorders and thus may expedite their receiving assessment and intervention services.

Pitch

The student's pitch level during typical conversational speech is determined. This so-called **habitual pitch level** is the speaking fundamental frequency of vibration, and it is merely an overall average of the opening-closing cycles of the vocal folds. It is important for the SLP to determine by using normative data whether pitch level is appropriate for the student's age, sex, and body stature. For example, the fundamental frequency of a typical 6-year-old male or female first grader is about 320 Hz (or roughly E4 on the musical scale). By age 16, the fundamental frequency has dropped to an average of 150 Hz (D3 musically) for males and 215 Hz (A3) for females (Wilson, 1987).

The normal voice is characterized by variability in pitch known as intonation or inflection. The voice is abnormal when there is a lack of pitch variability, termed **monotone**, or when pitch fluctuations are excessive and sing-songy. Other pitch abnormalities the teacher and speech-language pathologist should listen for are diplophonia and pitch breaks. **Diplophonia** refers to the presence of two or more simultaneous pitches in the voice. These multiple tones are produced by separate or unequal vibratory sources and may indicate a serious problem with the vocal folds, or simply be an innocuous and temporary globule of saliva. **Pitch breaks** are intermittent and sudden changes in the pitch of the voice. The voice may jump upward, even into a squeak, or it may break downward. Frequent pitch breaks are associated with neurological problems and with growths on or around the vocal folds (and therefore may be serious), but also may be associated with puberty changes. Schoolteachers who interact with students at the age of puberty should be aware that rapid laryngeal growth during this developmental period, especially in males, causes random fluctuations of vocal-fold muscle length and tension. While upward and downward pitch breaks may be socially embarrassing to the student, they are of no consequence and generally subside within 6 months or so.

Loudness

Of interest during the assessment is whether **loudness** is appropriate for the speaking situation. If a voice is judged too loud or too soft, the speech-language pathologist should investigate possible reasons. The SLP should note if the typical loudness level can be maintained comfortably, without tension or strain. Loudness also should be maintained throughout the utterance and not trail off toward the end of the sentence. Furthermore, there should be no breaks or momentary skips of loudness.

It is of great importance for the speech-language pathologist to determine whether loudness abuse occurs. The teacher's daily observations and knowledge of the student's activities may prove extremely helpful here. Loudness abuses are often situation oriented rather than constant throughout the day. The student may use loud talking, strained phonation, or screaming only in certain situations, such as on the playground, in the cafeteria, or during physical education. A few abusive situations may be perpetuating a vocal disorder and, therefore, must become the focus of an intervention program, as we shall see later in this chapter.

Quality

The descriptive terminology used with disorders of vocal **quality** reflects the perceptual nature of the judgments. Words like breathy, harsh, hoarse, strident, rough, denasal, hypernasal, and husky are used commonly. Hoarseness, in fact, is the most common symptom of many vocal disorders. It is, therefore, desirable that all teachers be able to recognize a student with a hoarse voice. Simply stated, hoarseness is a combination of breathiness and harshness.

Breath Features

Breathing variables affect voice production and, as a result, should be assessed by the speech-language pathologist. The SLP will be interested in the adequacy of breath support, how many words (or syllables) are typically spoken per breath, how long the student can sustain a voiceless sound (such as s̲) and a voiced sound (such as z̲), and whether there are any distracting breathing noises, particularly during inhalation.

Rate/Rhythm

The rate at which a student talks can affect other variables of speech and the voice. In particular, rate may be related to poor breathing features and improper phrase grouping. The speech-language pathologist can best judge the impact of rate of speech; the teacher may lend an overall impression of a student's talking rate. The rhythm, smoothness, and coordination of speech reflect one's neurological integrity and, so, will be assessed by the SLP as well.

Instrumentation

Instrumental measures of vocal function have become increasingly available in most clinical sites, but less so in the public schools. Computer-based instrumentation holds much promise for enhancing the diagnostic process, treatment planning, and documentation of clinical effect (Behrman & Orlikoff, 1997). A discussion of sophisticated instrumentation and measures of specific vocal functions is beyond the scope of this book, yet comprehensive sources are available (Baken, 1987; Colton & Casper, 1996; Titze, 1994).

DIRECT AND INDIRECT INTERVENTION OPTIONS

From our discussions it should be obvious that the identification of students with voice disorders depends, to a large measure, on the ability of classroom teachers to recognize aberrant voices and make referrals. Comparing teacher referrals with actual voice evaluations, James and Cooper (1966) found that classroom teachers were able to identify voice disorders with only 10% accuracy. Fortunately, recognition of voice disorders has been shown to improve dramatically when teachers are trained to do so. DeGregorio and Polow (1985) presented a model for in-service workshops and planned interactions between teachers and speech-language pathologists. Classroom teachers can be effective listeners and facilitators of good speech and voice practice when taught the importance of their contribution.

Throughout this chapter we have alluded to two avenues of vocal intervention: the speech-language pathologist may enroll a student in a **vocal hygiene approach** or in **voice treatment**. These two avenues differ in their underlying philosophies and goals.

Vocal Hygiene Programs

Vocal hygiene programs are designed to be informative and are preventative; they can be offered to anyone and, as such, are the ultimate form of indirect intervention. Students with vocal disorders and even entire classrooms of students with normal voices can benefit from knowledge on the use and care of the human voice. Hygiene programs can be offered by the speech-language pathologist or by the classroom teacher, or the two professionals can work together in designing teaching units. Since no direct manipulation of vocal parameters is attempted, vocal hygiene programs do not require medical clearance, parental permission, or placement in the speech pathology program (hence no IEP is written).

Published vocal hygiene programs share common goals. First, the individual student or the entire class is educated in voice production. This typically entails a description of the normal larynx and how it functions, followed by discussions of what can go wrong. Nodules often are the principal example. This educational unit may be highlighted with pictures, movies, laryngeal models, and taped samples of healthy versus disordered voices. The Web pages cited in Table 9-2 may prove useful. A second goal is to identify abusive voice behaviors which can contribute to a voice disorder. Discussions may proceed from general abuses that anyone might do, to particular abuses that an individual student does. Depending on the maturity level of the students, this goal may be accomplished by brainstorming lists of abusive behaviors, cutting out magazine pictures of people engaged in abuses (e.g., screaming at a football game), coloring predrawn pictures symbolic of abuses (e.g., loud voice analogous to heavy walking boots and a soft voice like ballet slippers), and making scrapbooks or bulletin boards from these materials. A third goal of vocal hygiene programs, especially for students with disordered voices, is to help them reduce or eliminate their abusive behaviors. This may entail suggesting alternative behaviors for abusive ones where such alternatives exist, as in Table 9-5. Otherwise, overall reduction or complete elimination of abusive voice behaviors is necessary, particularly during situations with a high probability for abuse. Table 9-6 lists situations that may be troublesome for school-aged students.

The appendix summarizes sample hygiene programs for young children such as from Terrell and Morgan (1980) and Scott (1998) for preschool children, Nilson and Schneiderman (1983) for second and third graders, and from Cook, Palaski, and Hanson (1979) for third through sixth grade children. These synopses may provide ideas for use in classroom hygiene programs. Such units can be incorporated easily into health or science curricula. Additionally, some commercial vocal hygiene programs are available (Blonigen, 1980, 1991; Flynn, Andrews, & Cabot, 2004; Moran, & Zylla-Jones, 1998).

With regard to adolescents, and by way of example, the vocal activities of cheerleading include prolonged and strenuous use of the voice in the presence of tension and with inadequate breath support. It should not be surprising that cheerleading predisposes one to vocal troubles. Andrews and Shank (1983) found that 37% of high-school cheerleaders surveyed exhibited some degree of hoarseness or voice problem. Aaron and Madison (1991) designed a vocal hygiene program for high-school cheerleaders and for their advisors that explained voice production, identification of abusive vocal behaviors, and ways to self-monitor such abuses.

Table 9-5 List of Suggested Alternatives to Abusive Behaviors

Abuse	*Alternative*
1. Yelling to a friend	1. a. Walking closer to the person to talk b. Waving or whistling to get his or her attention
2. Cheering	2. a. Clapping hands b. Shaking a pom-pom at a sporting event
3. Singing	3. a. Mouthing the words to allow the voice rest
4. Coughing	4. a. Blow coughing (strong but silent exhalation of air) b. Sipping some water
5. Clearing throat	5. a. Using "sniff-and-swallow" technique b. Swallowing c. Sipping some water
6. Yelling for pet	6. a. Whistling b. Clicking the tongue

Table 9-6 Situations of High Probability for Abuse

1. Before school (at home in the morning)
2. On the way to school (especially noisy school-bus environment)
3. At recess
4. During lunch period
5. In physical education
6. In music class
7. On the way home from school
8. After school (playtime)
9. In the evening
10. During sports (football practice, cheerleading, pep rallies, competitive games, or activities)

Voice Treatment

Direct voice treatment is administered only to students demonstrating a voice disorder and having a reasonable prognosis for improvement. The National Center for Voice and Speech (1994) indicates that about seven genres of voice treatment are commonly used by speech-language pathologists. Pannbacker (1998) provides an excellent compendium of these voice treatment approaches and a critical review of their effectiveness. The type of voice treatment undertaken depends on the diagnosis, student characteristics, and the speech-language pathologist's preference.

Voice treatment programs for disorders stemming from abuse and misuse of the voice are strikingly similar to each other and, in the beginning, to vocal hygiene programs as well. Yet voice treatment goes further than vocal hygiene programs and seeks to actually alter vocal parameters. For this reason, voice treatment is always preceded by the SLP's comprehensive assessment, a laryngologist's consultation, and an IEP meeting in which the student's problem and the intervention plan are clearly explained to the parents and teachers. It is important that all of the teachers understand the need for specific recommendations (e.g., no singing for 3 months, return to laryngologist in 6 months, no loud talking or shouting, and the like). The involvement of teachers is therefore critical.

Not unlike vocal hygiene programs, voice treatment for disorders related to abuse and misuse usually begins with the same three goals. Goals four and five are unique to treatment programs:

1. Education in voice production
2. Identification of abuses and misuses of the voice
3. Reduction and/or elimination of these abuses and misuses

4. Identification of techniques that improve parameters of the voice
5. Modification and habituation of the improved voice

Treatment seeks to achieve a clear vocal tone and may use facilitating techniques to alter the student's pitch and loudness level; manner of vocal fold adduction; state of muscular tension in the larynx, throat, and mouth areas; depth and manner of respiration; and numerous other subgoals. A discussion of these techniques is beyond the scope of this text; suffice it to say that the speech-language pathologist has the responsibility of designing and executing the treatment program to facilitate the student's best possible voice. Teachers who actively support voice treatment programs provide immeasurable support to the student trying to master new vocal habits.

Before leaving this overview of treatment, we wish to acknowledge, like Andrews (1991), that although the middle- to high-school years are a vocally strenuous time for students, few adolescents perceive the need for voice treatment. Often those who are referred by teachers or parents prove to be apathetic or resistant to behavioral change. The intervention approach must first seek to change attitudes and promote motivation. Andrews and Summers (1991) describe an awareness phase of voice treatment that builds the attitudes, knowledge, and skills necessary for subsequent goals in adolescent vocal rehabilitation. In a similar vein, Beery (1991) presents an approach to voice treatment with adolescents that emphasizes the importance of psychosocial and family influences on vocal behaviors, while Haskell (1991) discusses the merits of adjusting adolescents' vocal self-perceptions.

SUGGESTIONS FOR TEACHERS

We agree with Kahane and Mayo (1989), who state that:

> A major component of the education process should be helping teachers recognize when to refer a dysphonic child to the speech-language pathologist. We need to educate teachers about what we do, the processes involved in remediation, and to encourage their participation in the treatment of the vocally abusive child. The classroom teacher serves as a model of good vocal usage and can facilitate therapy goals by monitoring and reinforcing appropriate targeted behaviors. His or her role in voice therapy should not be underestimated (p. 105).

It is the authors' hope that this book serves some of these noble purposes.

More specifically, a teacher can best contribute to the school's vocal hygiene campaign or to an individual student's voice treatment program by incorporating some of the following suggestions.

1. Participate in teacher in-service programs offered by speech-language pathologists. Your ability to identify and refer students with pitch, loudness, and quality aberrations may depend greatly on your training to listen with a critical ear. Degregorio and Polow (1985) and Deal, McClain, and Sudderth (1976) offer valuable procedures for the design of such in-services.
2. Liberally refer suspected voice cases to the speech-language pathologist. Voice abnormalities may indicate a medically serious problem, or they may not. It is always best to check them.
3. Volunteer to teach a vocal hygiene unit in your class or work closely with the speech-language pathologist's hygiene program. Remember that everyone can benefit from knowledge of the care and use of the human voice.
4. Attend the IEP meeting and discuss a student's voice disorder with the speech-language pathologist. The more you know, the better you will be able to help.
5. Assist the SLP in identifying daily abuses and misuses, and work with the SLP in developing effective methods of reducing abuse/misuse in the classroom.
6. Volunteer to assist in the treatment program. Make your classroom a situation of vocal practice and reinforce the work of the speech-language pathologist and the student.
7. Control the noise level in your classroom such that no one needs to speak loudly and forcefully. A quiet, controlled class is not only good for the student with a voice disorder but it is also preventative protection of the teacher's voice. A disciplined, quiet-speaking class also is conducive to student learning. To the extent possible, control excessive ambient noise from heaters and air conditioners. Also curtail everyone's talking when the loud grass mower is outside the window!
8. Model a soft speaking voice for your students. Not only is this excellent when a student with a voice disorder is in the class, it is good hygiene for everyone, including the teacher.
9. Avoid modeling whispered speech in class. Whispered speech is taxing to the laryngeal mechanism.
10. Allow a student with a voice disorder to drink water in the classroom. Frequent hydration can ease vocal distress and promote healing.

11. Allow a student with a voice disorder to suck on throat lozenges in class, if this is soothing and deemed appropriate by the SLP.
12. Follow and support any SLP recommendations for a particular student. This may involve, for example, altering assignments to involve less speaking, allowing a few days of voice rest, curtailing singing, or other temporary strategies.

BACKGROUND INFORMATION ON STUDENTS WITH ALTERED METHODS OF BREATHING

Not-so-subtle vocal changes or a complete absence of voice may occur in students who have undergone a rerouting of the airway. Following surgery or the management of certain medical conditions, students may be reintegrated into the schools with altered methods of breathing. Teachers, at first, may feel ill at ease at having a "neck breather" in the class. The teacher's understanding of the student's condition is necessary and important for structuring the optimal classroom environment.

Tracheostomized Students in the Classroom

For various medical reasons, some temporary and some permanent (including neuromuscular disease, head trauma, chronic obstructive pulmonary disease, upper airway obstruction, bilateral vocal cord paralysis, and sleep apnea), doctors may decide that to ensure reliable respiration, a person needs to have a **tracheostomy**. The tracheostomy is an opening made into the trachea just under the larynx. A tracheostomy tube is inserted to maintain the opening. During inhalation and exhalation, air passes through the tracheostomy tube in the neck rather than through the usual route through the larynx, throat, mouth and/or nose.

While the tracheostomy may help solve respiratory problems, it causes the loss of speech. Recall that exhaled lung air must pass through the larynx and blow the vocal folds into vibration to produce voice. With exhaled air routed out the hole in the neck, called a **stoma**, no vocal fold vibration occurs. There can be a simple solution. Most tracheostomized people (using a specific type of tracheal tube) simply put their thumb over the stoma to divert air back through the larynx when they wish to speak. As a classroom teacher, you should understand this method of speech and recognize the importance of the student maintaining clean hands. Always having to talk with one hand is not convenient, and it limits activities that can be accomplished simultaneously while speaking. Also some people, such as those with quadriplegia, cannot raise their hands to occlude the stoma and so are mute. Again, medical technology has provided a solution. A **speaking valve** can be connected to the tracheostomy tube at the stoma opening. The one-way valve opens upon inhalation and remains open during easy exhalation, allowing for neck breathing to occur. With a more forceful exhalation the valve closes the stoma opening and directs the air through the trachea, vocal cords, and up the rest of the vocal tract for articulation of speech. The valve, therefore, simply eliminates the need to talk with thumb occlusion. It is appropriate for use with infants, youths, and adults despite whether the tracheostomy is temporary or permanent. Classroom teachers should understand the basic operation of these valves and be tolerant of the appearance of the apparatus worn at the student's neck. Helpful Web sites are presented in Table 9-7.

> Tony M. has the inherited disease of Duchenne's muscular dystrophy. As a result of his progressive weakness, Tony became quadriplegic and was confined to a wheelchair but continued attending regular public school. His ability to breathe deteriorated and doctors decided it would be easier for Tony to breathe with a tracheostomy. Eventually, he was fitted with a speaking valve and operates his computer by voice control.

Table 9-7 Web Sites with Further Information on Altered Methods of Breathing and Speaking Valves

www.asha.org/public/speech/disorders/Tracheostomies+or+Ventilators.html
The American Speech-Language-Hearing Association provides a basic overview of speech issues found in patients with tracheostomies or ventilators. This is an excellent resource for the general public on this subject.

www.passy-muir.com
This commercial Web site describes tracheostomy and ventilator speaking valves used with children and adults. It contains excellent information and color pictures to aid understanding.

www.orl.nl/Voice_Rehabilitation/Blom-Singer/blom-singer.html
This site describes an indwelling low-pressure voice prosthesis typically used in a laryngectomy. Also, the site's "image atlas" has interesting pictures.

Students with Laryngectomy

Laryngectomy is surgical removal of the larynx. Often, this is done when cancer has invaded the larynx but, occasionally, removal is necessary in cases of burns (from acids, lyes), gunshot wounds, and other traumatic accidents. Laryngectomy, then, is often a procedure done on adults (especially those over age 60). There are, however, reported cases of laryngectomy in children, even infants as young as 10 days old (IAL News, 1981; Peterson, 1973). A student without a larynx obviously will not be able to produce voice and so will be trained by a speech-language pathologist to talk in an alternative fashion. Several options are available and these are beyond the scope of this book. In addition to loss of voice, laryngectomy also alters the breathing passageway. These students, like tracheostomized students, will breathe through the neck stoma.

Teacher Tips for Students with Altered Methods of Breathing

Students, especially young children, with tracheostomy tubes (with or without valves) represent a small yet challenging population to the speech-language pathologist and the school personnel. They have complex medical treatment needs, and their families often experience high amounts of stress. In large school districts, the SLP may wish to organize a support group for parents of these tracheostomized children, as done by Woodfin (1988).

Teachers also should realize that tracheostomized students are at high risk for many infections. Tracheitis, bronchitis, and pneumonia are frequent and may require ongoing antibiotics or occasional hospital stays. Teachers should assist in limiting exposure of other sick students (those with colds and respiratory infections) to the neck-breathing student. Teachers also should be understanding and helpful as the student works with a homebound teacher to make up missed schoolwork caused by frequent absenteeism.

Teachers also should try to maintain a clean classroom. Dusty environments are not good for neck-breathing students. Also, the temperature and humidity of the classroom air (or the outdoor air during special activities) are important. Breathing cold air or hot air that is dry can be quite painful to the mucous linings of the trachea, bronchi, and lungs. The student may wish to operate a humidifier in the classroom to help adjust the temperature and humidity of the air.

The school nurse needs to be aware that a student who breathes via the neck is in a particular class. It is prudent for the school nurse to review resuscitation techniques with a classroom teacher in case of an emergency. It should be obvious that mouth-to-mouth resuscitation is ineffective for anyone with a stoma—mouth-to-stoma techniques are needed.

Lastly, the teacher should assist the student in developing a sense of self-worth and of belonging to the class. Social relationships with classroom peers are not easy for the student that is different.

CONCLUSION

Voice disorders are more common among the school-aged population than would be predicted by SLP's caseloads. Several reasons may account for this paucity, including the teachers' reluctance to recognize and refer students with potential voice disorders. By working closely with SLPs, teachers can become attuned to differences and deviances in pitch, loudness, vocal quality, breath features, and rate/rhythm. Much can be done through vocal hygiene and voice treatment programs. By working together, teachers and SLPs can help students improve the voice, thereby ensuring that any academic, social, and emotional impacts are minimized, and that vocally related health issues, such as safe breathing in the classroom, are addressed.

REFERENCES

Aaron, V.L., & Madison, C.L. (1991). A vocal hygiene program for high-school cheerleaders. *Language, Speech, and Hearing Services in Schools, 22*(1), 287–290.

Andrews, M.L. (1991). The treatment of adolescents with voice disorders—some clinical perspectives: An introduction. *Language, Speech, and Hearing Services in Schools, 22*(3), 156–157.

Andrews, M.L., & Shank, K. (1983). Some observations concerning the cheering behavior of school-girl cheerleaders. *Language, Speech, and Hearing Services in Schools, 14,* 150–156.

Andrews, M.L., & Summers, A.C. (1991). The awareness phase of voice therapy: Providing a knowledge base for the adolescent. *Language, Speech, and Hearing Services in Schools, 22*(3), 158–162.

Baken, R.J. (1987). *Clinical measurement of speech and voice,* San Diego, CA: Singular.

Baynes, R.A. (1966). An incidence study of chronic hoarseness among children. *Journal of Speech and Hearing Disorders, 31,* 172–176.

Beery, G.C. (1991). Psychosocial aspects of adolescent dysphonia: An approach to treatment. *Language, Speech, and Hearing Services in Schools, 22*(3), 156–157.

Behrman, A., & Orlikoff, R.F. (1997). Instrumentation in voice assessment and treatment: What's the use? *American Journal of Speech-Language Pathology, 6*(4), 9–16.

Blonigen, J.A. (1980). *Remediation of vocal hoarseness.* Austin, TX: PRO-ED.

Blonigen, J.A. (1991). *Treatment of vocal hoarseness in children.* Austin, TX: PRO-ED.

Colton, R., & Casper, J.K. (1996). *Understanding voice problems: A physiological perspective for diagnosis and treatment,* Baltimore: Williams & Wilkins.

Cook, J.V., Palaski, D.J., & Hanson, W.R. (1979). A vocal hygiene program for school-age children. *Language, Speech, and Hearing Services in Schools, 10,* 21–26.

Deal, R.E., McClain, B., & Sudderth, J.F. (1976). Identification, evaluation, therapy, and follow-up for children with vocal nodules in a public school setting. *Journal of Speech and Hearing Disorders, 41,* 390–397.

DeGregorio, N., & Polow, N.G. (1985). Effect of teacher training sessions on the perception of voice disorders. *Language, Speech, and Hearing Services in Schools, 16*(1), 25–28.

Dobres, R., Lee, L., Stemple, J.C., Kummer, A.W., & Kretschmer, L.W. (1989). *Description of laryngeal pathologies in children evaluated by otolaryngologists.* Paper presented to the Annual Convention of the American Speech-Language-Hearing Association, St. Louis, MO.

Flynn, P., Andrews, M., & Cabot, B. (2004). *Using your voice wisely and well* (2nd ed.). Austin, TX: PRO-ED.

Fox, D. (1985). *Vocal screening and treatment techniques for public school population.* Paper presented to the Annual Convention of the Speech and Hearing Association of Alabama, Huntsville, AL.

Green, G. (1989). Psycho-behavioral characteristics of children with vocal nodules: WPBIC ratings. *Journal of Speech and Hearing Disorders, 54,* 306–312.

Harden, J. (1986). Voice disorders in children [Abstract]. *Asha, 28*(10), 164.

Haskell, J.A. (1991). Adjusting adolescents' vocal self-perception. *Language, Speech, and Hearing Services in Schools, 22*(3), 168–172.

Haynes, W.O., & Pindzola, R.H. (2004). *Diagnosis and evaluation in speech pathology* (6th ed.). Boston: Pearson Education.

Herrington-Hall, B.L., Lee, L., Stemple, J.C., Niemi, K.R., & McHone, M.M. (1988). Description of laryngeal pathologies by age, sex, and occupation in a treatment-seeking population. *Journal of Speech and Hearing Disorders, 53,* 57–64.

IAL News (1981, April). Baby born with cancer has larynx surgery at 10 days, now tries speech. *Newsletter of the International Association of Laryngectomees, 26,* 1.

Jacobson, B.H., Johnson, A., Grywalski, C., Silbergleit, A., Jacobson, G., Benninger, M.S., et al. (1997). The Voice Handicap Index (VHI): Development and validation. *American Journal of Speech-Language Pathology, 6*(3), 66–70.

James, H., & Cooper, E. (1966). Accuracy of teacher referrals of speech-handicapped children. *Exceptional Children, 33,* 29–33.

Jotz, G.P., Cervantes, O., Abrahao, M., Settanni, F.A., & Carrar de Angelis, E. (2002). Noise-to-harmonic ratio as an acoustic measure of voice disorders in boys. *Journal of Voice, 16*(1), 28–31.

Kahane, J.C., & Mayo, R. (1989). The need for aggressive pursuit of healthy childhood voices. *Language, Speech, and Hearing Services in Schools, 20*(1), 102–107.

Moran, M.J., & Pentz, A.L. (1987). Otolaryngologists' opinions of voice therapy for vocal nodules in children. *Language, Speech, and Hearing Services in Schools, 18,* 172–178.

Moran, M.J., & Zylla-Jones, E. (1998). *Learning about voice: Vocal hygiene activities for children, a resource manual.* San Diego, CA: Singular.

Morton, V., & Watson, D.R. (2001). The impact of impaired vocal quality on children's ability to process spoken language. *Logopedics, Phoniatrics, and Vocology, 26,* 17–25.

National Center for Voice and Speech. (1994). *Voice therapy and training.* Iowa City, IA: The University of Iowa.

Nilson, H., & Schneiderman, C.R. (1983). Classroom program for the prevention of vocal abuse and hoarseness in elementary school children. *Language, Speech, and Hearing Services in Schools, 14,* 121–127.

Pannbacker, M. (1998). Voice treatment techniques: A review and recommendations for outcome studies. *American Journal of Speech-Language Pathology, 7*(3), 49–64.

Peterson, H.A. (1973). A case report of speech and language training for a two-year-old laryngectomized child. *Journal of Speech and Hearing Disorders, 38,* 275–278.

Pindzola, R.H. (1987). *A voice assessment protocol for children and adults.* Austin, TX: PRO-ED.

Roy, N., Merrill, R., Thibeault, S., Gray, S., & Smith, E. (2004). Voice disorders in teachers and the general population: Effects on work performance, attendance, and future career choices. *Journal of Speech, Language, and Hearing Research, 47*(3), 542–551.

Scott, A. (1998). Vocal hygiene for preschoolers. *Advance for Speech-Language Pathologists & Audiologists,* July 13, 14.

Terrell, S.L., & Morgan, P.A. (1980). *The adventures of Mr. Gruff: A voice therapy program for pre-school children.* Paper presented to the Annual Convention of the American Speech-Language-Hearing Association, Detroit, MI.

Titze, I.R. (1994). *Principles of voice production.* Englewood Cliffs, NJ: Prentice-Hall.

Wilson, K.D. (1987). *Voice problems of children* (3rd ed.). Baltimore: Williams & Wilkins.

Woodfin, S.T. (1988). A support group for parents of tracheostomized children. *Texas Journal of Audiology and Speech Pathology,* 14(1), 7–9.

World Health Organization. (2001). *International Classification of Functioning, Disability, and Health (ICIDH-2).* Geneva, Switzerland: World Health Organization.

Yiu, E.M. (2002). Impact and prevention of voice problems in the teaching profession: Embracing the consumer's view. *Journal of Voice, 16,* 215–228.

TERMS TO KNOW

abducted

adducted

diplophonia

disorders of resonance

edema

fundamental frequency

habitual pitch level

laryngectomy

laryngologist

loudness

monotone

papilloma

phonatory disorders

pitch breaks

quality

stoma

speaking valve

subglottic pressure

tracheostomy

vibration

vocal hygiene approach

vocal nodules

voice treatment

STUDY QUESTIONS

1. List several behaviors that are considered abusive to the vocal mechanism.

2. Differentiate between disorders of phonation and resonance.

3. What are vocal nodules? Be able to discuss potential causal factors and general principles of intervention.

4. Discuss the major goals to be accomplished in a vocal hygiene program.

5. What are some things a teacher should do when a student with an altered method of breathing is in the class?

Appendix

HYGIENE PROGRAM BY TERRELL AND MORGAN (1980)

This program for reducing abusive vocal behaviors was designed for preschool children. It consists of an audiocassette recording of a conversation between two animal characters: a hoarse bear named Mr. Gruff, and a normal-voiced kitten named Mr. Gentle. The taped program is only 20 minutes in length but is segmented for use over a number of sessions. Additionally, time is spent each session reviewing portions of the tape through questions, further explanations, and demonstrations to ensure learning. Demonstrations include the use of a flannel board with pictures of Mr. Gruff and Mr. Gentle in various storylike situations.

In the pleasant conversation between the two characters, Mr. Gentle explains to Mr. Gruff the manner in which Mr. Gruff is abusing his voice and alterations that he can make to improve his voice quality. Mr. Gentle also offers a clear, precise explanation of the larynx, the normal vocal folds, vocal folds with nodules, and the ways that various types of vocal abuse can contribute to vocal nodules. Pictures for the flannel board accompany this explanation. At the end of the taped story, Mr. Gruff undergoes a dramatic change from a hoarse voice to a normal voice, much to the approval of Mr. Gentle.

In summary of Terrell and Morgan's program for preschool children, flannel board stories were used to demonstrate:

1. Types of vocal abuse
2. Situations of vocal abuse
3. Explanations of the larynx, including both normal folds and vocal folds with nodules
4. Alternatives for abusive vocal behaviors

HYGIENE PROGRAM BY SCOTT (1998)

A classroom of preschoolers was presented a hygiene program focusing on basic anatomy, using models, activities, and vocal habits, through coloring book activities. Coloring book pictures showed cartoon characters engaging in good and bad vocal behaviors. For example, a picture depicted a cartoon duck singing so loudly that his friend covered her ears. Kazoos were used to explain proper voice quality. By humming into the kazoo, the children focused on vocal quality rather than on meaning or articulation. The children felt their larynx while humming to also understand the source of their voice. Three 1-hour sessions were conducted with the children. One month later in a follow-up evaluation, the children "had retained much of the information about basic anatomy and identifying bad vocal habits in pictures."

HYGIENE PROGRAM BY NILSON AND SCHNEIDERMAN (1983)

Second- and third-grade children were enrolled in a preventative program for vocal hygiene. They did not need to demonstrate vocal abuse nor hoarseness to enter the program; the program was administered to entire classrooms with the teacher participating as well. Pretests were given to assess baseline knowledge. Each class received two half-hour sessions per week for 2 weeks. These four lessons are summarized.

Lesson 1: Basic laryngeal anatomy was explained. Quality terms (e.g., rough/smooth, hoarse) were discussed in general, and specific voices of the children were described in particular. Tape recordings of the children were made also.

Lesson 2: Adequate and inadequate voice qualities were discussed as were behaviors that were abusive to the voice. The children discussed alternatives to abusive behavior.

Lesson 3: Vocal qualities, vocal abuses, and abusive situations were discussed further. Lists were generated of abuses and high-probability situations for abuses. The students were read short stories containing characters that abuse and correctly use the voice. The children were encouraged to identify the vocal behaviors.

Lesson 4: All previous lessons were reviewed. Notebooks containing pictures of voice caricatures, the list of abusive and nonabusive voice behaviors, and an award for completing the program were presented to each child. A posttest was then given.

Five months later, the children were again given the posttest to see if the hygiene information had been retained. It had indeed.

HYGIENE PROGRAM BY COOK, PALASKI, AND HANSON (1979)

Third-, fourth-, fifth-, and sixth-grade children with hoarseness participated in a 6-lesson vocal hygiene program. The program consisted of two half-hour classes per week for 3 weeks. Instructional materials included tape recorded voice samples, handouts, and cartoon illustrations (such as Victor Voicebox).

The first lesson began with a 20-item pretest and was followed by an introduction to voice production. Each child's voice was recorded at this session. The second lesson taught concepts of vocal quality; taped examples (such as hoarseness) were played and discussed. Lesson Three discussed anatomy and voice production in more detail. Lesson Four discussed abusive vocal behaviors, using cartoon characters as illustrative material. Lesson Five gave the children an opportunity to determine their own vocal habits and identify possible sources of vocal abuse. A contractual agreement was made with each child to eliminate one form of vocal abuse. Each child received a booklet with pictures that summarized the program. Lesson Six was a summary of the program with emphasis on personal goals for eliminating vocal abuse. A posttest was given and an analysis of the results indicated that the children learned the vocal hygiene concepts. Through such educational awareness, the children should be able to prevent abuse and its damaging effects on the larynx.

chapter ten

Hearing Impairment

BACKGROUND INFORMATION

Nature of the Problem

Perhaps no communication disorder presents a greater challenge to students and teachers than the presence of a significant hearing impairment. Classroom teachers rarely have adequate training or experience to deal effectively with students who are hearing-impaired, and support services for the teacher and student may be inadequate or poorly coordinated. On the other hand, there is probably no greater reward for a teacher than to play a role in helping a student to overcome the barriers created by a hearing impairment and become a successful learner. Historically, children with severe or profound hearing impairments were educated in special schools. However, federal legislation such as the Individuals with Disabilities Education Act (IDEA) has resulted in the placement of many students with a wide range of hearing abilities in the "regular" classroom. The purpose of this chapter is to briefly describe the nature of hearing impairment, to discuss the possible effects of hearing loss on classroom performance, and to provide specific suggestions for the teacher who has a hearing-impaired student in a normal-hearing classroom.

The term **hearing-impaired** refers to a wide range of students, from those with a minimal reduction of hearing in one ear to those with no usable hearing in either ear. Some hearing-impaired students need only to be seated close to the teacher to compensate for their hearing loss; others require extensive support services, such as special teachers, sign language interpreters, electronic instruments, special classes, or special school placement.

The educational needs of the hearing-impaired child are determined by the interaction of several factors such as intelligence, parental involvement, early identification, and intervention. Two of the most critical factors determining the effects of a hearing loss are the extent of the hearing loss and the age at which the hearing loss occurred.

Extent of Loss

A hearing loss can be mild, similar to having "blocked" ears as the result of a severe head cold, or it may be so severe as to render hearing unusable for any purpose. It is apparent that the academic challenges facing the most severely hearing-impaired students are different from those facing students with milder losses. Traditionally, an effort has been made to distinguish the most severely hearing-impaired students from others by using the term **deaf** to describe students whose hearing loss is so great as to preclude the understanding of speech through the ear alone, and **hard-of-hearing** to describe students whose hearing loss makes difficult, but does not preclude, the understanding of speech through the ear alone (Moores, 1987). The dividing line between *deaf* and *hard-of-hearing* is not universally agreed upon, and these terms have been used with much imprecision. Even if the terms were more precisely defined, the hard-of-hearing category is still too broad to be helpful in planning educational intervention.

A more discriminating classification of hearing loss is one based on a measurement of **hearing threshold**. Threshold is the lowest intensity at which a person can hear a sound. The higher a person's threshold, the louder a sound must be to be heard. You will recall from Chapter 2 that intensity (which we perceive as loudness) is measured in decibels (dB). For children, an average threshold of 0 to 15 dB among the speech frequencies (500 to 2,000 Hz) is considered normal hearing. Thresholds above 15 dB indicate a hearing loss that can be categorized according to the following levels: slight (15–25 dB), mild (26–40 dB), moderate (41–55 dB), moderately severe (56–70 dB), severe (71–90 dB), and profound (above 90 dB). Table 10-1

Table 10-1 Effects of Various Degrees of Hearing Loss on Communication

Hearing Threshold	Effect on Communication	Possible Needs
0–15 dB **Normal hearing**	N/A	N/A
16–25 dB **Slight hearing impairment**	Difficulty hearing faint or distant speech in noise. Possible difficulty with tense and plural markers at the end of words.	Preferential seating. Possibly speech therapy. Possibly some form of amplification such as an auditory training unit.
26–40 dB **Mild hearing impairment**	Difficulty hearing faint or distant speech even in quiet setting. May miss up to 50% of class discussion. May be fatigued due to effort required to try to hear conversation.	Hearing aid. Assistive listening devices. Speech therapy.
41–55 dB **Moderate hearing impairment**	Hears normal speech completely only at close range. Possible limited vocabulary and delayed or defective syntax and speech.	Hearing aid. Assistive listening devices. Speech therapy. Possible assignment to special classes at least for some subject matter.
56–70 dB **Moderately severe hearing impairment**	Hears only loud conversational speech. May miss most or all of classroom discussion. Possible severe language delay, problems with speech intelligibility, and intonation patterns.	Same as above.
71–90 dB **Severe hearing impairment**	Cannot hear conversational speech. Spoken language may not develop without early intervention. Possible language delay and intelligibility problems.	Same as above. Likely assignment to special classes for some subjects.
>90 dB **Profound hearing impairment**	May hear or feel loud sounds. Hearing is not a primary communication channel. Possible language delay and intelligibility problems.	Same as above.

Sources: Flexer, 1994; Northern & Downs, 1991; and Stach, 1998.

describes the effect of these categories of hearing loss on communication. These thresholds represent the hearing level in the better ear. A student with a hearing loss in only one ear does not face the same challenges as the student whose loss is in both ears. It should also be noted that some hearing losses are progressive. Progressive losses become worse over time.

Although these categories are more precise than simply using the terms *deaf* and *hard-of-hearing*, it would be a serious mistake to judge the potential of a hearing-impaired student on threshold scores alone. Some students with severe or profound hearing losses have excellent speech and language skills and can function quite well in the classroom. Other children with less severe hearing losses may have unintelligible speech, poor language skills, and experience more difficulty in adjusting to a regular classroom. Although there are many factors that contribute to such individual differences, perhaps the most significant is the age at which the hearing loss occurred.

Age at Onset

Hearing loss can be **congenital**, that is, present at birth, or it can be acquired at any time during a person's life. For educators, the critical distinction is whether the hearing loss occurred before or after the development of speech and language. Hearing loss occurring prior to speech and language development is referred to as **prelingual,** and that occurring after speech and language develop is **postlingual**. Because children typically learn language skills through the auditory channel, prelingual hearing impairment can have a devastating effect on language development and, therefore, on academic performance.

Causation

There are three types of hearing loss: **conductive**, **sensorineural**, and **mixed**. The type of hearing loss is determined by the portion of the hearing mechanism that fails to function properly.

A conductive hearing loss results from disorders of the outer or middle ear. Recall from Chapter 2 that the outer ear consists of the pinna and the external canal. The outer ear has little function other than to direct the sound toward the eardrum. Therefore, hearing problems which originate in the outer ear most often result from blockage of the canal. Congenital malformations of the outer ear, known as **microtia** or **atresia**, narrow or occlude the ear canal and can result in a conductive loss. A buildup of excessive ear wax or **cerumen** also can impede the transmission of sound through the canal. Blockage of the external canal can also result from the tendency of children to place objects where they do not belong. This apparently powerful drive results in the placement of beans, peanuts, erasers, gum, and a variety of other objects into the ear canal. Fortunately, such obstructions can usually be removed quite easily by a physician.

Conductive hearing losses more often result from middle ear rather than outer ear disorders. Remember that the middle ear includes the eardrum, or tympanic membrane, and the three bones or ossicles known as the malleus, incus, and stapes. The most common middle ear disorder in children is **otitis media**. Otitis media means an inflammation of the middle ear. In most cases, this condition involves the presence of fluid in the middle ear cavity behind the eardrum. When fluid is present, the condition is known as otitis media with effusion (OME). The fluid interferes with the movement of both the eardrum and the ossicles, thereby reducing hearing sensitivity. In many cases the fluid is infectious and, left untreated, may perforate the eardrum, destroy the ossicles, and spread to other parts of the body. If there is no infection present, the existence of the fluid, and therefore the reduction in hearing acuity, may go unnoticed by the parents. Otitis media is extremely common among young children. Klein (1991) stated that "Otitis media is the most frequent diagnosis for illness when children visit medical facilities" (p. 140). Patrick (1987) indicated that in an average kindergarten class of 30 students, there could be between 5 and 11 cases of otitis media at any one time. Many children seem to be "otitis prone." According to Klein (1991), about one-third of all children experience recurrent instances of otitis media. Harrison and Belhorn (1991) identified situations and conditions which contribute to making a child otitis prone. These include:

- The presence of certain congenital anomalies such as cleft palate and Down syndrome
- A history of upper respiratory infections
- Early onset and frequent occurrences of otitis media
- Secondary or passive smoking (i.e., being around people who smoke)

There is significant disagreement as to whether the mild hearing loss associated with otitis media can delay speech-language development when the condition continues to recur. Several researchers report that speech or language may be delayed by the presence of otitis media during the period when a child is developing language (Friel-Patti & Finitzo, 1990; Northern &

Downs, 1991; Robb, Psak, & Pang-Ching, 1993; Teele, Klein, Chase, Menyuk, & Rosner, 1990). However, other studies (Grievink, Peters, van-Bon, & Schilder, 1993; Paul, Lynn, & Lohr-Flansers, 1993; Roberts, Rosenfeld, & Zeisel, 2004) have failed to find a relationship between the presence of otitis media and later language delays.

Otitis media is usually treated by the use of antibiotics over a period of about 2 weeks. However, in recent years a dramatic increase in antibiotic resistance has created great concern about the overuse of antibiotics for the treatment of otitis media. This has caused physicians to be more stringent in diagnosing the various types of otitis media and, in some cases withholding antibiotics (Harrison, 2004). When otitis media persists over a longer period, the condition may be treated by the surgical insertion of **ventilating tubes** (*pressure equalization* or *p.e.* tubes). These tiny tubes are inserted under general anesthesia through a tiny incision in the eardrum. The tubes ventilate the middle ear cavity, allowing the fluid to dissipate. The tubes come out on their own after several months.

The second type of hearing loss, sensorineural loss, occurs as a result of damage to the inner ear or the auditory nerve. There are many possible causes of sensorineural hearing loss. Among the most common are: genetic factors, maternal infection such as rubella, postnatal infection such as meningitis and encephalitis, drugs, and noise exposure. Unlike conductive losses, sensorineural losses are usually irreversible. Because different parts of the inner ear respond to different frequencies, sensorineural hearing losses often involve a specific range of frequencies. For example, a student might have normal hearing below 1,000 Hz, but sharply reduced hearing ability at higher frequencies. Since speech sounds occur over a wide range of frequencies, the child with a high frequency loss may hear enough of the speech signal to know someone is talking, but not enough to understand all of what is said. Teachers and parents sometimes mistakenly assume that hearing is an "all or none" ability. That is, if anything is heard, it is assumed that everything at that loudness level can be heard. Such is not the case in a sensorineural hearing loss.

To summarize, there are three important differences between a sensorineural and a conductive hearing loss:

1. Conductive losses are often reversible by medication or surgery. Sensorineural losses are generally irreversible.
2. Conductive losses tend to be the same at all frequencies. If speech is made loud enough, the student can understand. Sensorineural losses are

variable, with some frequencies worse than others. Even if speech is made louder, the student may not understand all words.

3. Conductive losses do not exceed 50 or 60 dB (moderate hearing loss) because after that level, the sound is transmitted directly to the inner ear by vibration of the bones of the skull. Sensorineural losses can be of any severity from mild to profound.

Some students have damaged inner ear structures and obstruction in the middle or outer ear. These children have hearing losses with both sensorineural and conductive components. Such losses are referred to as mixed losses.

Case Example

In addition to their academic burden, hearing-impaired students often must deal with insensitivity, misunderstanding, and prejudice. The following excerpt from a newspaper column chronicles the experiences of a student with a severe hearing loss who was mainstreamed in a public school system. This touching account points out many of the challenges that hearing-impaired children encounter in a school setting, particularly when the school personnel are not adequately trained to prevent such problems.

Marla frequently came home from school crying because other children made fun of her deafness. When Marla was in the first grade, there was one day when the children were to dress as if they were from the period on the TV series *Little House on the Prairie.* Marla did not hear the announcement. "You can imagine how she felt when she was the only one of six hundred students who did not show up dressed like that," said her mother.

One day when she was in the third grade, a teacher planned an April Fool's day joke on another teacher. Marla did not know that it was a joke because she did not hear the teacher tell the class. Somehow Marla gave the joke away, and the teacher who instigated the joke scolded Marla. "The teacher humiliated me in front of the class," said Marla. "I cried." Harassment from the other children increased after that. It was as if the teacher's action was a signal to the students that it was all right to ridicule the child with the hearing impairment.

There were endless incidents, such as children gathering around her at recess and moving their lips while pretending to talk to her. She would turn up her hearing aid and become frightened because suddenly there was no sound at all while the children would break into hysterics at her panic.

"It was the same old thing day after day," she said."I always wanted friends. There was really nobody. I was alone most of the time."

In the tenth grade she became so depressed over not having friends that she thought about killing herself. In the eleventh grade, a classmate named Pam began talking to her and persisted in showing Marla that she accepted her. Marla and Pam became close friends. "Some people even told me to stay away from her because she is deaf," said Pam. "I ignored them. She's just deaf. There's nothing wrong with Marla."

A few months ago, Marla started dating, and she has been accepted at a state university. She said her advice to other children with severe hearing impairments who are being mainstreamed is to be strong. "School is very important," she said. "No matter how bad it gets, just keep going."

Source: Lackeos, N. *Montgomery Advertiser-Alabama Journal,* May 25, 1986. Reprinted with permission.

ASSESSMENT ISSUES

Methods of Assessment

Severe or profound hearing losses are usually identified well before the student reaches school age. Children considered at risk for a hearing loss because of family history, events during pregnancy and delivery, or the presence of other medical conditions can be tested for possible hearing loss shortly after birth. In other cases, severe or profound hearing losses may be discovered as a result of delayed speech and language development. Such early identification is not always the case. Mild or moderate hearing loss may not be identified until after the student begins school and faces increased demands on auditory processing skills. In some instances, students may not acquire their hearing loss until after they begin school.

Because the presence of a hearing loss may not always be obvious, it is important that students have their hearing tested periodically. The instrument used to test hearing is an **audiometer**. There are several different kinds of audiometers, but the type used in most school settings is a portable **pure tone audiometer**. Pure tone audiometers present beeplike tones at various frequencies and loudness levels determined by the tester. The student is usually instructed to: "Raise your hand when you hear the beep." Many states require annual hearing screening tests for designated grade levels. A hearing **screening test** involves the presentation of tones at a predetermined loudness level at selected frequencies. If a student fails to respond appropriately to the hearing screening, additional tests are indicated. A speech-language pathologist may perform hearing screening tests; however, the additional hearing tests required to determine a student's hearing status are not within an SLP's scope of practice. These additional hearing tests must be performed by another professional with extensive training in the nature, assessment, and treatment of hearing problems known as an **audiologist**. The audiologist typically begins the hearing assessment by administering a **threshold test** to determine the student's precise level of hearing at each frequency. The threshold test also can indicate whether a hearing loss is conductive, sensorineural, or mixed by presenting the stimulus tone in two different ways. First, the tone is presented through earphones. This presentation, known as **air conduction**, requires the sound to pass through the outer, middle, and inner ear. If the student does not hear normally by air conduction, the examiner knows that a hearing problem exists but cannot determine whether it is conductive or sensorineural. To make this determination, sounds are next presented by placing a sound generator on one of the bones of the skull, most often the mastoid bone, directly behind the ear. In this type of presentation, known as **bone conduction**, the inner ear is stimulated directly by vibration of the bones, thus bypassing the outer and middle ear. The results of these tests are represented on a graphlike form known as an **audiogram**. Figures 10-1 through 10-4 show audiograms which reveal normal hearing, a conductive loss, a sensorineural loss, and a mixed loss respectively.

Because middle ear problems are so common among early elementary school children, some school districts use an additional instrument known as an **impedance bridge** or an **acoustic immittance bridge** as part of a routine hearing screening. By directly measuring the movement of the eardrum, the acoustic immittance bridge can reveal the presence of fluid in the middle ear cavity as well as expose a variety of other middle ear disorders. This is not a hearing test per se, but a very helpful assessment of the function of the middle ear.

How Teachers Can Help in Assessment

The formal procedures for identifying hearing-impaired students are not infallible. The classroom teacher may be the first person to detect behaviors that are associated with a hearing loss. Unfortunately, these behaviors are often attributed to a lack of attention, antisocial attitudes, or learning problems.

Normal

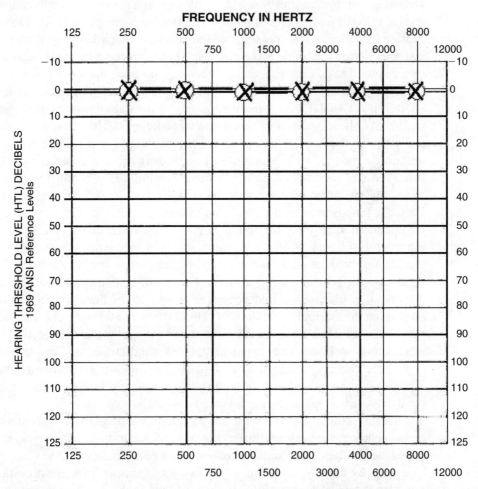

Figure 10-1 An Audiogram Showing Normal Hearing; 0 = Right Ear, X = Left Ear

The following behaviors, based on lists provided by Phillips (1975) and Flexer (1994), may indicate the presence of a hearing loss:

- Lack of attention during classroom discussions
- Noncompliant behavior
- Frequent requests for repetitions of what has been said
- Confusion and unusual errors in following directions

Conductive Loss

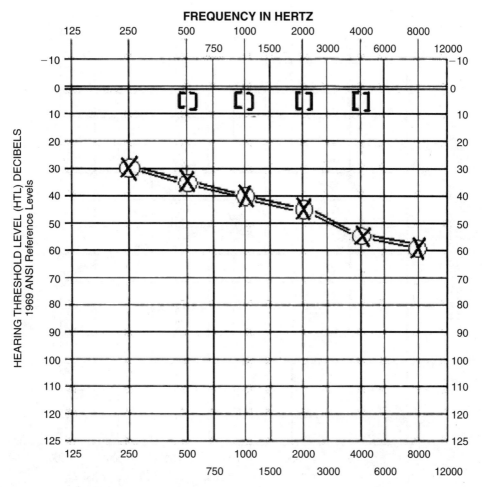

Figure 10-2 An Audiogram Showing a Conductive Hearing Loss; 0 = Right Ear by Air Conduction, X = Left Ear by Air Conduction, [= Right Ear by Bone Conduction,] = Left Ear by Bone Conduction. Notice Bone Conduction Thresholds are Better than Air Conduction Thresholds.

- Responding inconsistently or inappropriately to environmental sounds or spoken communication
- Turning the head to one side when listening to teachers or other students
- Paying close attention to the speaker's face
- Tendency to be withdrawn or isolated

Sensorineural Loss

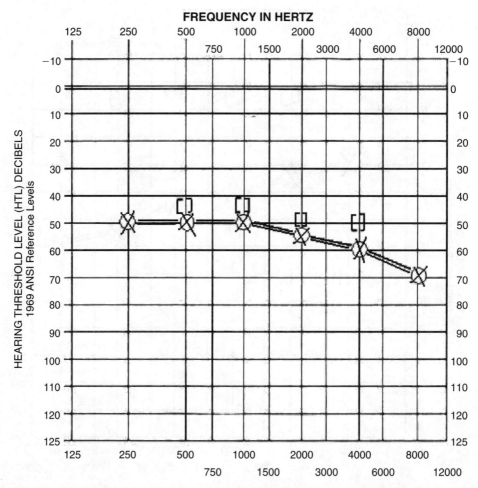

Figure 10-3 An Audiogram Showing a Sensorineural Hearing Loss. Notice that Both Air and Bone Conduction Thresholds are Below Normal

- Appearing uncomfortable or confused in noisy situations
- Earaches and pulling at the ears
- Dizziness
- Problems in speech, language, reading, and/or writing

Speech Problems

Most students with a significant hearing loss exhibit speech problems. The speech problems may be in articulation, voice, and/or resonance, and can

Mixed Loss

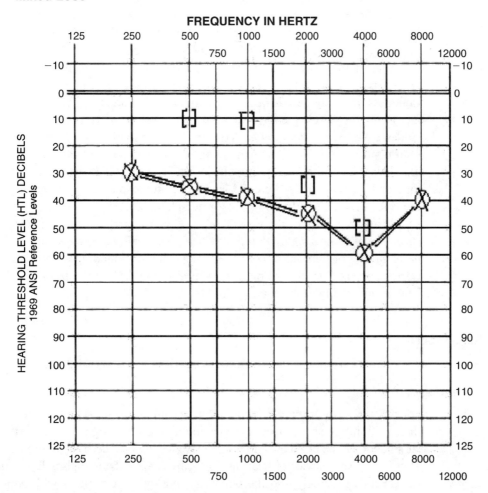

Figure 10-4 An Audiogram Showing a Mixed Loss. Notice that Bone Conduction Thresholds are Below Normal but Air Conduction Thresholds are Even Worse.

range from slight distortions of fricative sounds (such as s̲) to completely unintelligible speech or no speech at all. The nature and severity of the speech problem depend on several factors, including the extent of hearing loss, the type of loss, the age at onset, and the amount and type of early training. The speech problems of hearing-impaired students are caused by the inability to clearly hear the speech of others and the inability to monitor their own speech through the auditory channel. One can only imagine how difficult it must be for a child to learn to produce speech sounds without ever hearing those sounds. In addition to phoneme errors, hearing-impaired students may also exhibit problems with proper stress and accent patterns. Placing stress on the wrong syllable often makes it difficult for the listener to understand the word, especially in connected speech.

Hearing-impaired students frequently exhibit voice problems. Pitch may be unusually high, or the pitch may not vary, resulting in a monotone voice. Loudness also may be affected by hearing loss. An old stereotype associates all hearing-impaired speakers with an excessively loud voice. While many students with sensorineural losses do speak with a loud voice, many students with conductive losses may exhibit an excessively soft voice. The teacher may have to tell the hearing-impaired student when his or her voice is too loud or too soft to help the child learn to monitor loudness. The quality of the voice may be breathy and weak or harsh and strident.

Resonance is another aspect of speech affected by hearing loss. A speaker who is hearing impaired may be hypernasal (excessive sound in the nasal cavity) or denasal (a cold-in-the-nose quality sounding as if the nose were blocked). Speech also may be focused in the back of the throat, giving an unusual quality to the sound of the voice.

TREATMENT

Hearing Aids

For most hearing-impaired students, a hearing aid is a critical element in their habilitation and education. Selecting the best hearing aid for a particular student can be done only after extensive testing by a certified audiologist. There are several styles of hearing aids. Tiny **canal aids** or slightly larger **in-the-ear aids** fit snugly into the outer ear and are quite popular with adults because they are not as noticeable as other styles. Because children's ear canals grow and change dimensions along with the rest of their bodies, hearing aids that fit entirely into the ear are not used frequently for children. The two styles most commonly used with children are the **body aid** and the **behind-the-ear aid**. These aids are pictured in Figure 10-5. Several years ago, body aids were the most common type of hearing aid. These devices have the electronic parts in a small case which is worn in a pocket or special sling and is attached to an earpiece by a cord. More recently, the behind-the-ear aid has become the aid-of-choice for most children. This instrument is worn, as the name implies, behind the ear and is connected to the ear piece, or **earmold**, by a short section of tubing. Because body aids provide easier access

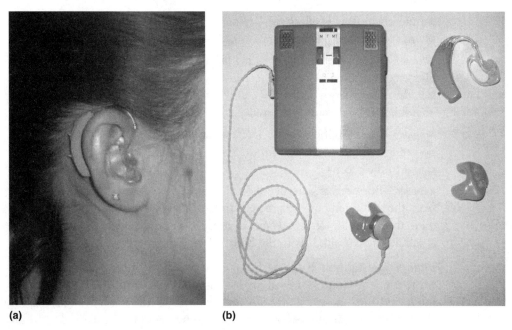

(a)   (b)

Figure 10-5 A Behind-the-Ear Hearing Aid (a), and a Body Style Aid (b).
Source: Hodgson, 1978. Reprinted with permission.

and manipulation of the controls, they are sometimes preferred for younger children or children with physical impairments.

Regardless of the style, all hearing aids have some features in common. Teachers should be aware of the following components of any hearing aid worn by a student:

Batteries Different hearing aids use different types of batteries. The teacher should know where the battery is located on the hearing aid and should request that the parents provide a replacement battery to be kept at school.

On-off switch As with most sophisticated electronic equipment, the first thing to do when the instrument is not working is to be sure that it is turned on. Many hearing aids combine the on and off function with the volume control. Others have a separate on-off switch. Labels and initials used to indicate functions on hearing aids vary with style and manufacturer, so the teacher should request that the student, a parent, or a speech and hearing professional demonstrate the functions of a hearing aid.

Volume control The volume control is usually set at a specified level. The teacher should know the level at which the student's aid is usually set and should check this level at the beginning of each day and when the student seems to be having difficulty with the aid.

Microphone Sound enters the hearing aid through the microphone. The microphone converts sound into an electrical signal. On a body aid, the microphone is in the portion worn on the body. On a behind-the-ear aid, it is at ear level. The microphone should not be covered or blocked by clothing or any other material.

Amplifier The amplifier, not visible on the outside of the aid, electronically boosts the signal received from the microphone and passes the strengthened signal to the receiver.

Receiver The receiver acts like a loudspeaker. It receives the boosted signal from the amplifier, converts the electrical signal back to sound, and passes it on to the earmold. On a body aid, the receiver is attached to the earmold. On a behind-the-ear aid, it is in the body of the aid.

Earmold The earmold is the part of the aid which fits into the ear. It seals the ear to prevent sound from leaking out into the surrounding air, and it directs the sound into the ear. Earmolds are made to fit the student's ear and are changed as the ear grows. On canal and in-the-ear aids, the earmold and the rest of the aid are a single unit. When the student's ear grows, the entire instrument must be replaced. On body aids and behind-the-ear aids, the earmold is separate from the rest of the aid.

Telephone switch Although this is not part of all hearing aids, many have an additional switch marked *T* and *M*. The *T* position is for use on the telephone, and the *M* or microphone position is for all other activity.

A properly functioning hearing aid is extremely important to the ability of the student with a hearing impairment to benefit from classroom instruction. Some students do not like their aids at first. They are not comfortable with them, or they feel that the hearing aid stigmatizes them. There are many stories of expensive hearing aids being thrown on the school roof or flushed down the toilet. The teacher should be certain that the student wears the hearing aid and that it is in working order. Some authorities suggest that on any given day over 50% of amplification devices might not be working (The Alexander Graham Bell Association, 2002). There are a few simple checks that a teacher can do to ensure that a student's hearing aid is working. Table 10-2 provides a simple check procedure that teachers may be able to incorporate into their daily routine with the hearing-impaired child. To complete the daily check, the teacher should have available two pieces of equipment, a battery voltage meter and a hearing aid stethoscope. The latter device is a

Table 10-2 Hearing Aid Check Procedure

Earmold (For body aids or behind-the-ear aids)	The hole at the end of the earmold that is directed toward the ear should be clear of cerumen. If cerumen is present it may be cleaned with a pipe cleaner or the mold should be washed in warm soapy water. If the earmold is washed, it must be thoroughly dried before replacing.
Hearing aid case, tubing and wire	Check for cracks or dents in the hearing aid case. With a behind-the-ear aid, be sure that the ear hook is not separated from the case and that the tubing leading to the earmold is not cracked. With a body aid be sure that the wire(s) leading to the ear piece(s) is fully insulated and not crimped or broken.
Microphone	Be sure that the microphone opening is clear and free from dirt. If dirty, it may be cleaned with a small brush.
Battery	The battery should be removed from the case and tested with a battery voltage meter. The battery contacts should be clear of corrosion. Be sure to replace the battery in the correct position.
Hearing aid controls	The hearing aid controls should be at the appropriate settings. The teacher should have a card with information provided by the audiologist or a parent to remind him or her of the appropriate settings for a specific aid and a specific child.
Listening check	If the teacher has a hearing aid stethoscope, it can be used to monitor the sound produced by the hearing aid. The sound should be clear and free from any distortion. Adjustments to the volume control should result in differences in the sound coming from the aid.

simple stethoscope designed to allow someone to hear the sound produced by a hearing aid without having to use the earmold. Table 10-3 provides some suggestions to help troubleshoot a malfunctioning hearing aid.

Teachers must keep in mind that the microphone of a hearing aid is at the student's ear, and the farther away from the teacher the student sits, the lower the intensity of the teacher's voice. Also, hearing aids amplify noise as well as speech. This means that if a child with a hearing aid is seated near a

Table 10-3 Troubleshooting the Hearing Aid

Problem	Possible Causes
No sound	• Aid turned off • Telephone switch in *T* position • Dead battery • Batteries placed incorrectly • Wrong batteries • Corrosion on battery contact • Earmold plugged with wax • Tubing blocked or twisted • Cord may be broken or disconnected (body aid)
Intermittent sound	• Broken cord or loose connection (body aid) • Faulty receiver • Faulty volume control
Weak sound	• Weak batteries • Earmold partially blocked • Kink in tubing • Wrong battery
Noisy unnatural sound	• Dirt buildup on on-off switch or volume control (move switch back and forth rapidly to clear these) • Corrosion on battery terminal • Weak battery • Incorrect tone control setting
Squealing	• Volume control set too high • Earmold loose • Tubing loose from earmold or ear hook • Tubing cracked

Sources: Davidson, 1995; Leavitt, 1984; and Smedley & Schow, 1998.

source of noise, and far from the teacher, the amplified noise may overwhelm the speech of the teacher. Tye-Murray (1998) identified three noise conditions that negatively affect the ability of students with hearing aids to hear classroom presentations. These conditions are:

Ambient noise: Tye-Murray (1998) defines **ambient noise** as noise that is present in a room when it is unoccupied. Such noise includes that emanating from heating and air conditioning systems, fluorescent lights, computers, and hallways.

Reverberation: The term **reverberation** refers to echoes caused by sound bouncing off walls, ceilings, and floors. Carpeting and heavy draperies tend to reduce reverberation, but not many classrooms are "sound treated" in that way. Therefore reverberation is a common problem in schools.

Background noise: Background noise is the noise made by other students in the room. Shuffling papers, talking, coughing, tapping a pencil on the desk, and so on.

Table 10-4 provides a checklist which may help teachers identify and reduce sources of noise and other factors which can interfere with communication between a teacher and a hearing-impaired student.

To overcome some of the problems with noise in the environment and distance between teacher and student, many schools use assistive listening devices as supplements to, or in place of, the student's hearing aid.

Assistive Listening Devices (ALDs)

The term *assistive listening device* refers to a broad range of devices that help people who are hearing impaired respond to auditory stimuli in the environment. Devices that cause a light to flash when a doorbell rings or a fire alarm sounds, or instruments that vibrate when a telephone rings, are assistive listening devices. However, we are concerned here with assistive listening devices used in educational settings. These devices, sometimes referred to as **auditory training units (ATUs)**, can be used instead of or with a hearing aid during class activity. An ATU serves the same purpose as a hearing aid, that is, to amplify sound. The major difference between a hearing aid and an ATU is that the microphone for an ATU is worn by the teacher. The advantages of the teacher wearing the microphone are that background noise in the immediate area of the student will not be amplified, and the teacher can move more freely around the room without concern about being too far from the hearing-impaired student. There are several types of ATUs. Most are wireless systems and use either FM signals or infrared signals to carry the message from the teacher's microphone to the student's receiver. Some classrooms are equipped with an induction loop system that involves installing a wire around the circumference of the room. Fortunately, it is not necessary to understand the electronics to use any of these instruments. After a brief orientation from a speech-language pathologist, audiologist, or company representative, most teachers can operate the equipment quite easily. All that is required is a genuine effort on the part of the teacher to use the instrument for the maximum benefit of the hearing-impaired student.

Table 10-4 Checklist for a Listener-Friendly Classroom

Concern	Yes	No	What Can Be Done to Improve the Situation?
Is there noise outside the classroom such as traffic, construction, playground?			
Is there noise inside the classroom from fans, lights, heating and/or cooling systems, etc.?			
Are there noisy student activities?			
Is there sufficient light in the room to aid students in speech reading?			
Are there bright lights, light from windows, or reflected light that makes speech reading difficult for the hearing-impaired students?			
Is the room arranged to maximize face-to-face contact between teacher and hearing-impaired students?			
Is the room arranged to maximize the use of visual aids (e.g., adequate chalk board space, electrical outlets for slides and transparencies, projection screen, etc.)?			
Is there carpeting and other reverberation-reducing features?			

Source: Some of the concerns above are based on those presented in "Teachers Guide to Hearing," a pamphlet produced by Oticon Corporation, Somerset, NJ.

Cochlear Implants

Many students with severe or profound hearing loss do not benefit from even the most powerful hearing aids or auditory trainers. The cochleas of these students are unable to generate neural impulses to be conducted along the auditory nerve (Stach, 1998). An exciting development in the treatment of such children has been the ability to directly stimulate the auditory nerve by the use of a surgically implanted device known as a **cochlear implant**. Cochlear implants have internal and external components. The external components resemble a conventional hearing aid. These components include a microphone, a processor, and a transmitter. The microphone, usually worn at ear level, receives the sound from the environment and converts it to an electrical signal. The processor, sometimes worn on the body (similar to a body type hearing aid) or at ear level, modifies the signal from the microphone into the type signal required by the specific instrument. The transmitter, which is attached to the head, transmits the processed signal to the internal components. The internal components, which have been surgically implanted into the skull and cochlea, consist of an internal receiver and an electrode array. The internal receiver picks up the signal from the outside transmitter, and the electrode array stimulates the auditory nerve.

It is extremely important that teachers understand that a cochlear implant does not provide normal hearing. The student with an implant is still hearing impaired. Tye-Murray (1998) indicates the performance of children who have received cochlear implants to this time leads us to expect that most children who have prelingual hearing loss achieve some sound awareness and some speech-reading enhancement when using their implants. Also, most children will show some improvement in their speech and language performance. However, Tye-Murray (1998) goes on to warn that in cautioning parents and teachers to have realistic expectations for children with cochlear implants, we should not lead them to expect too little either. Children with implants need to be challenged to maximally develop the hearing ability they do possess.

Human Resources

In addition to the devices listed above, the Alexander Graham Bell Society, in their pamphlet, *Mainstreaming the Student Who Is Deaf or Hard-of-Hearing* (2002), identifies the following human resources that might be employed to assist a hearing-impaired student in the classroom.

Sign language interpreter Students for whom auditory input is not sufficient may benefit from the presence of a sign language interpreter in the classroom. A sign language interpreter would use a manual communication system to convey the message of the teacher and other speakers in the classroom for the hearing-impaired student. In some cases, the student may respond in sign and the interpreter would then put the student's message into spoken language for the rest of the class. In classes where the student is expected to take notes, if a student is paying attention to a sign language interpreter, he or she may need another method to obtain those notes.

Transcriber or peer note taker Someone may be assigned to provide the student with a full set of notes to which the student may compare his or her own notes.

Peer note taker Another student who is a good note taker or who has had some training in taking notes may be employed to supplement the notes the hearing-impaired student is able to take.

The Gallaudet Research Institute survey for the 1999–2000 academic year indicated that for the more than 43,000 children with hearing impairments included in the survey, the most common support services were: speech training (63%), itinerant teacher (34%), sign interpreter (22.1%), counseling (8.3%), tutor (6%), and note taker (5.2%) (Gallaudet Research Institute, 2001).

SUGGESTIONS FOR TEACHERS OF HEARING-IMPAIRED STUDENTS

Classroom teachers are not expected to be experts on the habilitation of hearing-impaired students, nor should they be expected to provide one-to-one instruction for the hearing-impaired child at the cost of the other students. There are, however, several things that teachers can do to help meet the needs of the hearing-impaired student:

1. Provide favorable seating: The hearing-impaired child should be seated close to the teacher and away from background noise, such as the noise from a hallway or a street. Garwood (1987) suggests that movable desks and flexibility in arranging seating during various activities allows the hearing-impaired child an opportunity to observe and participate in classroom activities. Students with hearing aids should be seated to make maximum use of the aid. For example, they should not be seated with the aid against a wall (Kampfe,1984; Northcott, 1973). Also, children with hearing impairments should be seated with their back to windows and bright light sources, as many of these students depend on being able to see the face of the speaker clearly.
2. Remember that group activities may pose special problems for the child with a hearing impairment (Gildston, 1973). Some students with hearing impairments may not be aware that group members out of the line of vision are talking. Also, group activities can sometimes be associated with higher-than-normal levels of background noise.

3. Face the hearing-impaired student when speaking and be sure that the student is looking at you. Other children may be able to listen while looking at their work, taking notes, or while you are facing the board, but hearing-impaired students comprehend best when they can see the speaker (Reynolds & Birch, 1988). It is especially important for the teacher to remember not to talk while facing the chalkboard and not to cover his or her mouth with papers and/or books when giving information to the class.

4. Provide written instructions and summaries. Written information helps the hearing-impaired student keep in touch with lesson content. Simple lesson outlines, key vocabulary words, and homework assignments may be listed on the board (Harrington, 1976).

5. Speak clearly but naturally. Hearing-impaired children often depend on facial cues to aid understanding (Harrington,1976). To help remember critical factors in speaking to hearing-impaired students, Garwood (1987) suggested S-P-E-E-C-H as a mnemonic device.

   S State the topic to be discussed.

   P Pace conversation at a moderate speed, allowing occasional pauses to aid comprehension.

   E Enunciate clearly without exaggerated lip movements.

   E Enthusiastically communicate, using body language and natural gestures.

   CH Check comprehension before changing topics. Ask the hearing-impaired student questions to evaluate understanding. Do not simply ask, "Do you understand?" and rely on a nod or a yes. The student may not be willing to admit a problem understanding the material. Be alert to signs of confusion, such as a blank stare or unusual errors in following directions.

6. Rephrase and restate instructions and directions. This is especially important when it is apparent that the hearing-impaired student is having trouble understanding. Some words contain sounds which are not easily recognized by hearing-impaired students. Many hearing-impaired children have some delay in language development and may not be familiar with the vocabulary or grammatical structure used (Garwood, 1987).

7. Use a "preteach-teach-postteach" strategy (Reynolds & Birch, 1988). In this approach, the classroom teacher discusses upcoming lessons with other professionals who may be working with the hearing-impaired student, such as a teacher of the hearing-impaired or a speech-language pathologist. The special teacher or speech-language pathologist then ensures that the student understands key words and concepts to be used in the coming class presentation. The classroom teacher presents the

lesson and reports back to the other professionals any apparent difficulties the hearing-impaired student had with the lesson. The special teacher or speech-language pathologist then reviews the concepts with which the student experienced difficulty. This strategy is an excellent way to coordinate the efforts of several professionals, and a good example of a consultative model in action.

8. Establish positive attitudes toward the hearing-impaired child. Encourage participation in expressive activities such as reading, show-and-tell, and creative dramatics (Garwood, 1987). Have the speech-language pathologist or teacher of the hearing-impaired explain hearing loss (and hearing aids if appropriate) to the class (Brill, 1978; Harrington, 1976; Stassen, 1973). Teachers serve as models for the children in their classes. Recall from the story of Marla earlier in this chapter that it was a teacher's ridicule of a deaf student that seemed to trigger the same behavior by other students.

AUDITORY PROCESSING DISORDER (APD)

A problem which should be discussed here, although it is not a problem of hearing acuity, is the condition known as **auditory processing disorder (APD)**. Until recently this condition was frequently called central auditory processing disorder (CAPD). APD has many manifestations and therefore many definitions depending on the discipline of the person providing the definition. The situation is further complicated by the fact that APD is not universally recognized as a legitimate disorder category. Some feel that the symptoms suggesting APD are really symptoms of a broader language impairment or reflective of ADHD (Cacace & McFarland, 1998). Many definitions are highly technical and esoteric, but basically APD is a problem understanding the meaning of incoming sounds (Flexer, 1994) or as Lasky and Katz (1983) put it, a problem in what one does with what one hears. The ears work well and do their job in getting the signal to the brain, but the problem lies with the way the signal is decoded and interpreted in the central nervous system. Many children labeled as learning disabled may have APD. According to Baran and Musiek (1995) the symptoms of APD may include:

- Problems following complex auditory directions
- Problems hearing in noisy backgrounds
- Difficulty determining from where sounds originate (localizing sound)
- Trouble participating in long, quickly spoken conversations

- Distractibility
- More difficulty with verbally based subjects such as reading than with nonverbally based subjects such as mathematics
- Lack of musical appreciation
- Tinnitus (noise in the ear or head)
- Missing subtle acoustic cues
- Unusual difficulty learning foreign languages

It should be readily apparent that a child who exhibits various combinations of the above symptoms may experience difficulty in a typical classroom setting. These children may be perceived as less intelligent than they really are, inattentive, lazy, disruptive, and/or uncooperative. As with some language-impaired children, children with APD may experience greater difficulty in school as the demands for language processing increases, usually around third grade. Many of the suggestions provided earlier in this chapter for the hearing-impaired child would also be effective strategies for the child with APD. In addition to those suggestions, Johnson and Danhauer (1999) have provided the following additional suggestions for teachers of children with APD:

- Reduce distractions: Avoid extraneous noise and visual distractions, especially when providing new or important information.
- Be sure that you have the child's attention: Saying the child's name or gently touching his or her shoulder are easy ways to refocus attention. Words and phrases such as *listen, ready*, and *remember this* may be helpful in signaling an important message.
- Reduce those noises which cannot be eliminated: The use of sound attenuation earplugs or earmuffs may help the child to tune out those noises that cannot be eliminated from a school environment.
- Use visual aids: The use of overhead projectors, LCD projectors, and computers will likely enhance the learning experience for all children in the class but may be especially helpful to the child with APD.
- Avoid auditory exhaustion: Remember that children with APD must work hard at listening. This can lead to fatigue. The teacher may be able to schedule intensive listening activities early in the day or alternate auditory tasks with nonauditory tasks.
- Tape record important information. A tape may be made of critical information to provide the child with an opportunity to hear the information again at a later time when he or she is more receptive to this type of auditory input.

- Assign a "buddy": Another child who appears to be strong in auditory processing may be assigned to assist the student who is having difficulty. The nature of that assistance will differ with the specific individuals and class material involved.

One additional point should be made before ending the discussion of APD. As stated earlier, this condition is not recognized as a disorder that affects school-aged children (Cacace & McFarland, 1998). Therefore a diagnosis of APD does not qualify as an eligible condition for treatment in most school systems. Children showing the symptoms of APD are often treated under a diagnosis of receptive language disorder.

CONTROVERSIES

Most of the information and suggestions provided so far in this chapter are widely agreed upon in the field of communication disorders. Such agreement does not, however, characterize the entire area of education of the hearing impaired. Students classified as deaf, that is students with hearing losses of 70 dB or greater, often have different needs than students with less severe hearing impairment. How best to meet the additional educational needs of the student with a severe or profound hearing loss is a question that raises some of the most divisive and emotional controversies in the field. Two major controversies in which the classroom teacher might become involved include determining which type of educational placement constitutes the "least restrictive environment" for a deaf student, and whether oral speech is a desirable goal for all deaf children. In most cases, these issues will be decided by the evaluation team and specified in the individualized education plan (IEP).

Educational Placement

Moores (1987) described the various school placements for deaf children as follows:

Residential schools: These are schools designed exclusively for deaf students. The students reside at the school during the week and may live at home over the weekends.

Day schools: These are separate schools for the deaf that students attend during school hours then return home in the evening.

Day classes: These are special classes for students who are deaf in a regular public school. Instruction may be in completely self-contained classes, or students may spend part of their time in regular classes.

Resource rooms: In this plan, students who are deaf spend most of the day in regular classes but report to a special class for additional instruction. The additional instruction is usually in English or academic areas in which the student is experiencing some difficulty. The resource room usually provides individual or small-group instruction.

Itinerant programs: In an itinerant program, students attend regular classes on a full-time basis but receive support services from a special teacher who serves several schools. The support services vary from weekly to daily sessions according to the students' needs.

Tye-Murray (1998) reported that, in the years since the implementation of PL 94-142, there has been a dramatic decline in the number of students attending private residential schools and day classes for the deaf. Public schools have assumed more of the responsibility for the education of students with severe and profound hearing losses. This does not mean, however, that all students with hearing impairments are enrolled in regular public schools. The Gallaudet Research Institute survey for the 1999–2000 academic year indicated that of the more than 43,000 students with hearing impairment who were included in the survey, 28.7% were enrolled in special schools or centers, 30.4% in self-contained classrooms, 12.6% in resource room settings, and 44.8% were in a regular education setting (Gallaudet Research Institute, 2001). That same survey also reported the number of hour per week that students with hearing impairments were integrated with students with normal hearing. The survey indicated that 37.5% of students with hearing impairments had no integration with normal hearing students, 11% were integrated from 1 to 5 hours/week, 11.3% from 6 to 15 hours/week, 10.4% from 16 to 25 hours/week, and 29.8% with 26 or more hours/week.

Although there has been an increase in the number of students with profound hearing losses in regular classrooms for at least some academic subjects (Moores, Kluwin, & Mertens, 1985), there are those who feel that special schools for the deaf constitute a less restrictive environment than integrated settings. Proponents of special schools for the deaf say that the deaf child is isolated, socially stigmatized, and discriminated against in regular schools. Many regular schools and regular schoolteachers are not adequately prepared to deal with deaf children. In many cases, the major dissatisfaction with regular schools involves the method of communication the deaf child is taught to use. Regular public schools are based on oral communication. Many deaf children use communication systems that incorporate some form of manual signs.

Methods of Communication

There are several methods of communication used by deaf students. These can be categorized either as *oral* methods or *manual* methods. In oral methods, students use speech to express themselves, and depend on speech reading (lip-reading) and maximum use of amplified hearing to receive spoken language. In *manual systems*, students communicate through sign language and/or finger spelling. In sign language, a system of hand configurations and gestures are used to represent words. The most widely used system in this country is **American Sign Language** (ASL), also called **Ameslan**. In finger spelling, words are spelled letter by letter using a manual alphabet. Finger spelling is commonly used for proper names or words for which no sign exists.

Some methods combine oral and manual aspects. **Total communication** encourages the use of all available avenues of communication. Although it is primarily a manual system, total communication encourages students to use and to develop whatever speech, speech-reading and hearing ability they may have. *Cued speech* is primarily an oral method in which various hand configurations are used next to the mouth to cue the perception of less visible or easily confused spoken sounds.

Disagreements over oral versus manual communication have existed for centuries. At one time, oralism was the prevailing philosophy in the United States. Recently, a total communication philosophy with emphasis on sign language in addition to oral communication has grown in popularity. The proponents of total communication suggest that the manual signs facilitate language development in children. Opponents of a total approach point out that students who communicate through sign can communicate only to those who know sign. Another problem associated with the use of sign language is that the syntactic structure of ASL is not the same as that of spoken English. For example, the question: "Do you want to go to the movies?" in sign would have a syntactic structure more like, "Me you movies go." The ASL syntax can result in difficulties when the student is attempting to read and write in standard English; these are very much like the problems experienced by a dialectal speaker. In an effort to deal with this problem, sign language systems have been developed that use the syntax of spoken English. One of the most widely used of these systems is **Signing Exact English** (**SEE**). SEE emphasizes standard English word order, marks verb tense, and indicates irregular verb forms.

Until recently, deaf children who were mainstreamed were usually oral students with reasonably good speech and speech-reading skills. There has been little provision for the inclusion in the regular classroom of students who use total communication (Newton, 1987). Now, through the use of sign language interpreters, students using total communication are achieving success in the regular classroom setting. Finding a sign language interpreter is not always an easy task. There are local, state, and national registries of such interpreters. Also, local associations for the deaf, state agencies, and universities with training programs for teachers of the hearing impaired or for sign language interpreters might be helpful sources of information (Hayes, 1984).

Early Intervention

Calderon, Bargones, and Sidman (1998) state that early intervention with children who have severe and profound hearing losses has not been well researched. However, Marschark, Lang, and Albertini (2002), indicate that regardless of the type of school setting or the communication method used, early intervention can have a positive effect on the school performance of children with significant hearing impairment. Early intervention here refers to preschool programs and early parental involvement. Marschark and colleagues describe several types of preschool programs for children with significant hearing impairments. These include programs administered by public school systems, state health and human services departments, and residential schools. Some programs may take the form of home-based intervention involving periodic visits to the home and instruction provided to the parents. Marschark and colleagues indicate that preschool programs can help to prepare children for school by helping them to develop realistic and flexible social strategies and can promote language growth whether the communication system used is oral or total. Another benefit of preschool programs for children with hearing impairments is that they sensitize parents to the need to be involved in the education of their children. As most teachers would probably agree, parental involvement is often a key to any child's success in school. However, the parents of children with severe and profound hearing losses face unique problems. The presence of any child with a disability places unusual stress on the family (Luterman, 2001). In the case of a child with a severe or profound hearing loss whose parents have normal hearing, one source of stress may be how to communicate with the child. Because of this uncertainty about communication with the child, "active, hands-on involvement of the parents in deaf children's education is relatively infrequent" (Marschark et al., 2002, p. 150). Parents of children with severe and profound hearing losses may require some additional training and guidance to provide the type of involvement that will benefit the child. In fact, much of the benefit of early intervention for children with hearing impairments may be in helping parents understand and cope with the needs of their child. Calderon and colleagues (1998, p. 361) state:

> From a practical perspective, what early intervention programs seem to accomplish . . . is to help parents settle into their role of being a parent of a deaf or hard-of-hearing child, develop some level of awareness of the child's needs, fitting the child with hearing aids, and developing basic skills for communication with the child.

SUPPORT FOR THE CLASSROOM TEACHER

Often the difference between success and failure for the student with a hearing impairment in the regular classroom is the support services available to the classroom teacher. Chorost (1988) published the results of a survey of regular classroom teachers who had oral hearing-impaired children in their classrooms. After a full academic year, 40% of the teachers surveyed felt that the placement of the hearing-impaired child with whom they worked was not appropriate. These teachers most commonly cited two problems: (1) the child with whom they worked was so far behind normal hearing classmates that very little mainstreamed academic learning took place: and (2) too much of the teacher's time was taken from the other children. On the other hand, 60% of the teachers felt that the placement of the hearing-impaired child was appropriate and cited the support system available to them as being of help. This support system included:

- Visits to other programs with hearing-impaired students
- Annual conferences with hearing-impaired young adults and specialists in hearing impairment
- Circulation of texts and articles on hearing loss
- Strategies for modifying teaching techniques when working with hearing-impaired students (similar to the suggestions presented in this chapter)

- Instructions for using auditory training units
- Presentations to the class about hearing loss by the teacher of the hearing impaired

The above services may be of help to any teacher who has a hearing-impaired child in a regular classroom. In many cases, however, the teacher must request such services. To know what type of support system is available in a particular school system, the teacher must become familiar with the other professionals who work with hearing-impaired children.

The speech-language pathologist works to make the hearing-impaired student as effective a communicator as possible. This may involve work on speech and language development, speech-reading skills, a manual communication system, or all of the above. Regardless of the specific treatment goals, an open channel of communication between the SLP and the classroom teacher is essential to the success of the hearing-impaired student. The teacher is likely to encounter, or hear reference to, several other professionals involved in the education of the hearing-impaired student. A **teacher of the hearing impaired** (also called a teacher of the deaf, or educator of the acoustically handicapped) is a teacher who is trained specifically to work with hearing-impaired students. These teachers often hold professional certification by the Council on Education of the Deaf (CED). The teacher of the hearing impaired may work in a self-contained classroom, a resource room, or may serve schools on an itinerant basis. Because these teachers have training in both teaching and the special needs of hearing-impaired children, they are excellent sources of information for the regular classroom teacher.

An audiologist tests hearing, fits hearing aids, and provides suggestions for educational management. Audiologists hold at least a master's degree and should be certified by the American Speech, Language, and Hearing Association (ASHA). Audiologists should not be confused with hearing aid dealers who sell aids and have considerably less professional training. An **otolaryngologist** is a physician who treats disorders of the ear, nose, and throat. These physicians are sometimes referred to simply as ENTs or, if they limit their practice to disorders of the ear, **otologists**.

The hearing-impaired student will benefit far more from a coordinated effort on the part of these professionals than if each works in isolation. Depending on the individual situation, it may fall on the classroom teacher to take the lead in coordinating these efforts through meetings, phone calls, and letters. Although such efforts may take time and energy, they may often spell the difference between success and failure for the hearing-impaired student.

REFERENCES

Baran, J., & Musiek, F. (1995). Central auditory processing disorders in children and adults. In G.W. Lida (Ed.), *Hearing for the speech-language pathologist and health care professional.* Boston: Butterworth-Heinemann.

Brill, R.G. (1978). *Mainstreaming the prelingually deaf child.* Washington, DC: Gallaudet College Press.

Cacace, A.T., & McFarland, D.J. (1998). Central auditory processing disorder in school-aged children: A critical review. *Journal of Speech, Language, and Hearing Research, 41,* 355–373.

Calderone, R., Bargones, J., & Sidman, S. (1998). Characteristics of hearing families and their young deaf and hard of hearing children: Early intervention follow-up. *American Annals of the Deaf, 143,* 347–362.

Chorost, S. (1988). The hearing-impaired child in the mainstream: A survey of attitudes of regular classroom teachers. *The Volta Review, 90,* 7–12.

Davidson, S. (1995). Hearing aids. In G.W. Lida (Ed.), *Hearing for the speech-language pathologist and health care professional.* Boston: Butterworth-Heinemann.

Flexer, C. (1994). *Facilitating hearing and listening in young children.* San Diego, CA: Singular.

Friel-Patti, S., & Finitzo, T. (1990). Language learning in a prospective study of otitis media with effusion in the first two years of life. *Journal of Speech and Hearing Research, 33,* 188–194.

Gallaudet Research Institute. (2001). *Regional and national summary report of data from the 1999–2000 Annual Survey of Deaf and Hard of Hearing Children and Youth.* Washington, DC: Gallaudet University, GRI.

Garwood, V.P. (1987). Audiology in the public school setting. In F.N. Martin (Ed.), *Hearing disorders in children.* Austin, TX: PRO-ED.

Gildston, P. (1973). The hearing-impaired child in the classroom: A guide for the classroom teacher. In W.H. Northcott (Ed.), *The hearing-impaired child in the regular classroom: Preschool, elementary, and secondary years. A guide for the classroom teacher/administrator.* Washington, DC: Alexander Graham Bell Association for the Deaf.

Grievink, E., Peters, S., vanBon, W., & Schilder, A. (1993). The effects of early bilateral otitis media with effusion on language ability: A prospective cohort study. *Journal of Speech and Hearing Research, 36,* 1004–1012.

Harrington, J.D. (1976). The integration of deaf children and youth through educational strategies. Why? When? How? *Highlights, 53,* 8–18.

Harrison, C.J. (2004). How will the new guidelines for managing otitis media work in your practice? *Contemporary Pediatrics,* June 1. Retrieved February 17, 2005, from www.contemporarypediatrics.com/contpeds/articleDetails.jsp?id=108038.

Harrison, C.J., & Belhorn, T.H. (1991). Antibiotic treatment failures in acute otitis media. *Pediatric Annals, 12,* 600–610.

Hayes, J.L. (1984). Interpreting in the K–12 mainstream setting. In R.H. Hull, & K.L. Dilka (Eds.), *The hearing-impaired child in school.* Orlando, FL: Grune & Stratton.

Hodgson, W.R. (1978). Disorders of hearing. In P.H. Skinner, & R.L. Shelton (Eds.), *Speech, language, and hearing: Normal processes and disorders.* New York: John Wiley & Sons.

Johnson, C., & Danhauer, J. (1999). *Guidebook for support programs in aural rehabilitation.* San Diego, CA: Singular.

Kampfe, C.M. (1984). Mainstreaming: some practical suggestions for teachers and administrators. In R.H. Hull, & K.L. Dilka (Eds.), *The hearing-impaired child in school.* Orlando, FL: Grune & Stratton.

Klein, J.O. (1991). Prevention of acute otitis media. *Seminars in Hearing, 12,* 140–145.

Lasky, E.Z., & Katz, J. (1983). Perspectives on central auditory processing. In E.Z. Lasky, & J. Katz (Eds.), *Central auditory processing disorders: Problems of speech, language, and hearing disorders.* Baltimore: University Park Press.

Leavitt, R.J. (1984). Hearing aids and other amplifying devices for hearing-impaired children. In R.H. Hull, & K.L. Dilka (Eds.), *The hearing-impaired child in school*. Orlando, FL: Grune & Stratton.

Luterman, D.M. (2001). *Counseling persons with communication disorders and their families* (4th ed.). Austin, TX: PRO-ED.

Marschark, M., Lang, H.G., & Albertini, J.A. (2002). *Educating deaf students*. New York: Oxford University Press.

Moores, D.F. (1987). *Educating the deaf: Psychology, principles, and practices* (3rd ed.). Boston: HoughtonMifflin.

Moores, D.F., Kluwin, T., & Mertens, D. (1985). High school programs for the deaf in metropolitan areas. Washington, DC: Gallaudet College Research Monograph No. 3.

Newton, L. (1987). The educational management of hearing-impaired children. In F.N. Martin (Ed.), *Hearing disorders in children*. Austin, TX: PRO-ED.

Northcott, W.H. (1973). A speech clinician as multi-disciplinary team member. In W.H. Northcott (Ed.), *The hearing-impaired child in the regular classroom: Preschool, elementary, and secondary years. A guide for the classroom teacher/administrator*. Washington, DC: The Alexander Graham Bell Association for the Deaf.

Northern, J.L., & Downs, M.P. (1991). *Hearing in children* (4th ed.). Baltimore: Williams & Wilkins.

Patrick, P.E. (1987). Identification audiometry. In F.N. Martin (Ed.), *Hearing disorders in children*. Austin, TX: PRO-ED.

Paul, R., Lynn, T., & Lohr-Flansers, M. (1993). History of middle ear involvement and speech/language development in late talkers. *Journal of Speech and Hearing Research, 36,* 1055–1062.

Phillips, P.P. (1975). *Speech and hearing problems in the classroom*. Lincoln, NE: Cliffs Notes.

Reynolds, M.C., & Birch, J.W. (1988). *Adaptive mainstreaming: A primer for teachers and principals*. New York: Longman.

Robb, M., Psak, J., & Pang-Ching, G. (1993). Chronic otitis media and early speech development: A case study. *International Journal of Pediatric Otorhinolaryngology, 26,* 117–127.

Roberts, J.E., Rosenfeld, R.M., & Zeisel, S.A. (2004). Otitis media and speech and language: A meta analysis of prospective studies [Electronic version]. *Pediatrics, 113,*(3, Pt. 1):238–248.

Smedley, T.C., & Schow, R.L. (1998). Problem-solving and extending the life of your hearing aids. In R. Carmen (Ed.), *A consumer handbook on hearing loss and hearing aids: A bridge to healing*. Sedona, AZ: Auricle Ink.

Stach, B. (1998). *Clinical audiology: An introduction*. San Diego, CA: Singular.

Stassen, R.A. (1973). I have one in my class who's wearing hearing aids! In W.H. Northcott (Ed.), *The hearing-impaired child in a regular classroom: Preschool, elementary, and secondary years. A guide for the classroom teacher/administrator*. Washington, DC: The Alexander Graham Bell Association for the Deaf.

Teele, D., Klein, J., Chase, C., Menyuk, P., & Rosner, B. (1990). Otitis media in infancy and intellectual ability, school achievement, speech and language at age 7 years. *Journal of Infectious Diseases, 162,* 685–694.

The Alexander Graham Bell Association. (2002). *Mainstreaming the student who is deaf or hard-of-hearing: A guide for professionals, teachers and parents*. Washington, DC: Author.

Tye-Murray, N. (1998). *Foundations of aural rehabilitation*. San Diego, CA: Singular.

TERMS TO KNOW

acoustic immittance bridge	ambient noise
air conduction	American Sign Language

Ameslan
atresia
audiogram
auditory training unit (ATU)
audiologist
audiometer
auditory processing disorder (APD)
behind-the-ear aid
body aids
bone conduction
canal aids
cerumen
cochlear implant
conductive loss
congenital
deaf
earmold
hard-of-hearing
hearing-impaired

hearing threshold
impedance bridge
in-the-ear aids
microtia
mixed loss
otitis media
otolaryngologist
otologist
prelingual
postlingual
pure tone audiometer
reverberation
screening test
sensorineural loss
Signing Exact English (SEE)
teacher of the hearing impaired
threshold test
total communication
ventilating tubes

STUDY QUESTIONS

1. Identify the parts which all hearing aids have in common. Provide suggestions as to how a teacher can troubleshoot a faulty aid.

2. Provide specific classroom behaviors or teaching techniques that can be employed to enhance the learning of hearing-impaired students.

3. Why might a hearing-impaired student have difficulty with reading and writing?

4. Discuss the advantages and disadvantages of oral and manual communication methods for the deaf.

5. Identify other professionals who work with hearing-impaired students, and discuss how these other professionals could be of help to the classroom teacher.

chapter eleven

Cleft Lip/Palate and Related Craniofacial Syndromes

BACKGROUND INFORMATION

Nature of the Problem

Several birth defects are associated with malformations of the skull and/or the face. Such malformations are referred to as *craniofacial anomalies.* Because the craniofacial area includes the brain, cranial nerves, and the speech and hearing structures, children with craniofacial anomalies frequently exhibit speech, language, and/or hearing problems. Treatment of children with craniofacial anomalies is sometimes complicated by unwarranted beliefs and attitudes of parents and others. Conditions that include facial disfigurements seem to be associated with an unusual number of folk beliefs and old wives tales. Many of these folk beliefs vary from one culture to another. In some cultures, children with craniofacial anomalies are considered to be "witch-babies" and are left to die (Scheper-Hughes, 1990). In other cultures, such birth defects are blamed on some sin, indiscretion, or unkind attitudes of the parents during pregnancy (Meyerson, 1990; Toliver-Weddington, 1990). It is not uncommon to hear people express the belief that a cleft lip or palate is the result of the mother being frightened by a rabbit or other animal. Even relatively sophisticated people tend to assume that a facial disfigurement implies reduced intellectual capacity and, therefore, they underestimate the abilities of students with craniofacial anomalies. We believe that is important for teachers to understand the effects of craniofacial anomalies on a student's communication skills and academic performance, and to judge such students based on their performance rather than on any preconceived notions about such children.

Cleft Lip and Palate

Clefts of the lip and/or the palate are the most common craniofacial anomaly associated with communication disorders. A cleft is an opening or a separation. **Cleft palate** refers to an opening in the roof of the mouth, usually at the midline. The cleft may involve the soft palate only, or it may extend through both the soft and hard palate. In some cases, the membranous covering of the palate may be intact, but muscles underneath have failed to develop properly, resulting in a **submucous cleft**. Another condition frequently associated with cleft palate is cleft lip. This condition at one time was referred to as *hare lip*, but that term has not been used professionally for many years. **Cleft lip** involves a vertical separation of the upper lip on one or both sides. Occasionally, a cleft of the lip may occur at the midline. Cleft lip can exist alone, or it may involve the alveolar ridge as well. Frequently cleft lip and palate occur together, creating a cleft which extends through the soft and hard palate, the alveolar ridge, and the lip. Such an extensive malformation is referred to as a complete cleft. Figures 11-1 through 11-4 provide illustrations of various types of clefts.

Causation and Incidence

Both cleft lip and cleft palate result from a failure of the structures to grow together and fuse properly during embryonic development. This fusion occurs quite early, at about 6 to 8 weeks of gestation for the lip and about 10 to 12 weeks for the palate (Bzoch, 2004; Peterson-Falzone, Hardin-Jones, & Karnell, 2001). The causes of cleft lip and palate are not fully understood. It appears that most cases result from an interaction of genetic and environmental factors. Cleft lip and palate occurs in approximately one in every 750 live births. The incidence of cleft lip varies with race and is higher among Native Americans and Asians and lower among people of African descent.

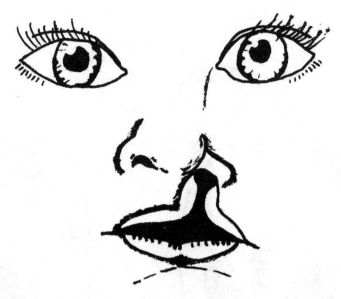

Figure 11-1 Unilateral Cleft of the Lip
Source: Illustration by Mark J. Moran.

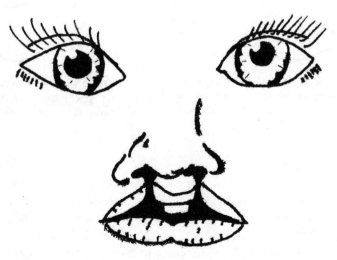

Figure 11-2 Bilateral Cleft of the Lip
Source: Illustration by Mark J. Moran.

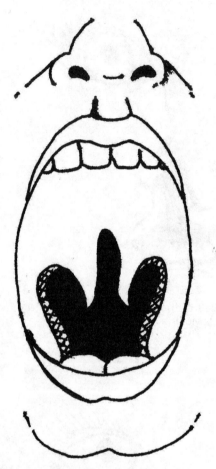

Figure 11-3 Cleft of the Soft Palate
Source: Illustration by Mark J. Moran.

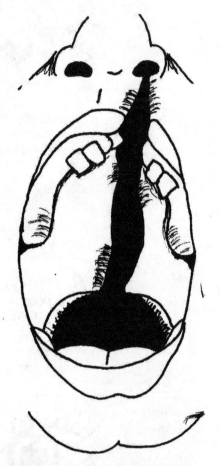

Figure 11-4 Complete Cleft Including Soft and Hard Palate, Alveolar Ridge, and Lip
Source: Illustration by Mark J. Moran.

Clefts of the palate do not show such a racial difference. Clefts of the lip occur more commonly in males, and isolated clefts of the palate are more common among females (Peterson-Falzone et al., 2001). There is some evidence that the incidence of clefts of the lip and palate is increasing because of factors such as increases in teenage pregnancies, pregnancies in older women, and consumption of drugs and alcohol during pregnancy (Slavkin, 1992).

Cleft lip and palate are most often repaired surgically. In the United States, surgery to repair a cleft lip is usually performed early in the first year of life, most typically at about 2 or 3 months of age (Seagle, 2004). The timing of surgery to repair the palate is somewhat more controversial and depends on factors such as the extent of the cleft, the general health of the child, and the philosophy of the surgeon. Surgery to close a cleft is most commonly performed by 12 to 18 months of age (LaRossa, 2000). While some surgeons prefer to wait until the craniofacial area is more fully developed (around age 5 years), clefts of the palate are typically closed by the time children begin school. Teachers must be aware, however, that surgical closure of the cleft may not eliminate all of the speech, language, and hearing problems associated with this condition. Even after surgery, cleft palate students may exhibit any or all of the communication disorders discussed here.

Speech Problems

A cleft palate affects speech primarily because it prevents the complete separation of the nasal cavity from the oral cavity. Although surgery can usually close the cleft, the soft palate (velum) may be too short or too immobile following surgery to adequately close off the nasal cavity. This condition is called **velopharyngeal insufficiency (VPI)**. Many cleft palate students require follow-up surgical procedures during the elementary school years to reduce or eliminate VPI. If surgery fails to provide an adequate speech structure, the student may be fitted with a device known as an obturator, or a **speech appliance**. An **obturator** is a plastic device worn in the mouth to cover any unclosed portions of the cleft and to aid the velopharyngeal mechanism in closing off the nasal passage. Speech problems associated with cleft palate are most often problems of resonance and articulation. The most common resonance problem exhibited by cleft palate speakers is hypernasality. **Hypernasality** is what many people refer to simply as a nasal quality, or some may say that hypernasal speakers sound as if they "talk through their nose." Hypernasality is the perceptual result of sound passing inappropriately into the nose. Recall from Chapter 2 that in English, the only sounds which are produced with the nasal cavity coupled with the oral cavity are <u>m</u>, <u>n</u>, and <u>ng</u>. Sound passing into the nose on any other phonemes cause the speaker to be perceived as excessively nasal. Hypernasality is most frequently heard on vowel sounds.

Articulation problems in cleft palate typically involve those consonants which require oral air pressure, i.e., stops (<u>p</u>, <u>b</u>, <u>t</u>, <u>d</u>, <u>k</u>, <u>g</u>), fricatives (<u>f</u>, <u>v</u>, <u>th</u>, s, z, sh), and affricates (ch, j [as in joy]). These articulation errors most often take one of two forms: nasal emission or compensatory articulations. **Nasal emission** refers to air escaping through the nose as a sound is produced. The result is often a "snorting" sound which distorts the target phoneme and reduces intelligibility. Compensatory articulations refer to changes in the way a sound is produced in order to adjust for structural inadequacy. **Compensatory articulations** exhibited by cleft palate speakers frequently involve moving the place of production farther back in the vocal tract to prevent the loss of air pressure through the nose. For example, rather than producing the s sound at the alveolar ridge, the cleft palate speaker may attempt to constrict the airflow by placing the tongue against the throat (pharynx), producing a compensation known as a pharyngeal fricative. Another common compensation used by cleft palate speakers is the glottal stop. In this production, which may be substituted for any or all stops, airflow is arrested, then suddenly released at the level of the vocal folds. The result is that words such as *battle* and *button* are produced as *baUHl* and *buUHn*. Once learned, these compensatory articulations may be difficult to eliminate. For that reason, early speech training places emphasis on correct placement to prevent the development and habituation of the compensatory productions. In addition to the articulation problems described here, students with clefts may also exhibit errors on nonpressure consonants such as l and r (Trost-Cardemone & Bernthal, 1993; Van Demark, 1964). Errors on nonpressure consonants may be part of a general delay in speech and language development.

Hearing Problems

Another factor that may contribute to communication problems and academic difficulties of students with cleft palate is an extremely high incidence of middle ear disease. This middle ear disease frequently results in a fluctuating bilateral (both ears) conductive hearing loss (Witzel, 1995). The incidence of middle ear disease in children with clefts has been reported to be as high as 100% (Paradise, Bluestone, & Felder, 1969). The middle ear disease and resulting hearing loss most likely result from an inability of the eustachian tube to properly ventilate the middle ear space, thus causing it to fill with fluid that may become infected. This condition, as you may remember from Chapter 10, is called *otitis media*. While surgical repair of the palate does seem to improve the situation in many children, in many others the hearing problems last through most of childhood and beyond (Gerson, 1990). Therefore, children with cleft palate are at risk for hearing loss not only during critical periods of speech and language development, but also during early school years when so much critical information is provided through the auditory channel. As was discussed in Chapter 10, mild-to-moderate conductive hearing losses, especially those which may come and go, do not always have obvious symptoms. The effects of a mild conductive hearing loss on language development have not been proven beyond a reasonable doubt. However, it is certainly a factor that must be kept in mind when discussing language development among children with cleft palate.

Language Problems

It is important to realize that children with clefts cannot be viewed as a homogeneous group when considering language abilities. Golding-Kushner (2001) indicates that there is a wide variety of language abilities among children with clefts and many exhibit normal language development. However, as a group, children with clefts are more likely than their noncleft peers to exhibit delayed language development (Broen, Devers, Doyle, Prouty, & Moller, 1998; Golding-Kushner, 2001; Scherer & D'Antonio, 1995). The reasons for this delay are not clear. There are several possible factors. As mentioned, the conductive hearing loss that is so common among these children may affect language development. Another possible factor is reduced language stimulation. Some children with cleft palates spend a great deal of time in hospitals and at home recovering from surgery. This is not an ideal situation for language stimulation. Some parents do not interact with their handicapped children in the same way as their nonhandicapped children, resulting in reduced language stimulation. Another factor that appears to play a role in language ability is the type of cleft. Children with isolated clefts of the palate with no involvement of the lip tend to exhibit more significant language problems than children with clefts that involve the lip (Golding-Kushner, 2001; Richman, 1980; Richman & Eliason, 1984). More than likely, the language delay seen in cleft palate children reflects an interaction of those and other factors yet to be defined. Regardless of the cause, it would appear that many children with clefts would benefit from early language intervention (Brookshire, Lynch, & Fox, 1984; Hahn, 1989). Such early intervention seems to be effective. In one particularly interesting study (Pecyna, Feeney-Giacoma, & Nieman, 1987), it was reported that cleft palate infants between the ages of 12 and 18 months received higher scores on a test of the concept of object permanence than a control group of noncleft peers. Pecyna and colleagues suggested that the superior performance by the cleft palate group may have been due to increased environmental stimulation by their parents.

Teachers should be aware that the potential for language problems exists among children with clefts. As discussed in Chapter 6, many children experience academic difficulty as a result of language problems, even when those problems are too subtle to be identified by standard language tests. Such may be the case with many students with clefts.

Academic Problems

Students with clefts of the lip and/or palate are at risk for learning disabilities, low school achievement, and grade retention (Broder, Richman, & Matheson, 1998; Richman & Eliason, 1986). In a study of school-age children with clefts and no other associated problems, Broder and colleagues (1998) reported that 46% of the children with clefts exhibited learning disabilities, 47% demonstrated deficient educational progress as measured by standardized tests, and 27% had repeated a grade. One area in which the academic problems of students with clefts can be seen is reading. Richman and Eliason (1986) reported that the rate of reading problems among cleft palate students is approximately 30%, as compared to about 5–15% in the general population. Richman, Eliason, and Lindgren (1988) reported that reading problems among cleft palate students decrease with age. The degree to which the reading problems decreased, however, was related to type of cleft. Students with clefts of the lip and palate exhibited essentially normal reading skills by age 13 years, while children with isolated clefts of the palate and no involvement of the lip maintained higher than average levels of reading problems. This, according to Richman and colleagues (1988), reflects a greater degree of language deficit in children with isolated clefts of the palate. In fact, more recent research (Millard & Richman, 2001) suggests that children with isolated clefts of the palate are not only more likely to exhibit learning problems, but are also more likely to experience anxiety and depression than children with clefts that involve the lip.

Richman and Ryan (2003) suggested that the reading problems exhibited by students with clefts are not the result of phonemic awareness deficits but may be related to deficits in short-term automatic memory. Therefore, Richman and Ryan suggest that sight word reading approaches should be avoided with this population in favor of phonics-based approaches within the context of meaningful stories.

Because of the language delays and academic problems noted among cleft palate students, parents, teachers, and speech-language pathologists often express concern over the cognitive development of these students. Several early studies reported that children with cleft palate, as a group, exhibited slightly lower IQ scores than their noncleft peers (Estes & Morris, 1970; Lewis, 1961; Means & Irwin, 1954). The results of these studies, however, may be misleading. Many of these early studies often included children with multiple disorders in addition to cleft palate, failed to separate findings for children with varying cleft types, and tended to use tests which relied heavily on verbal skills (Peterson-Falzone et al., 2001; Richman & Eliason, 1986; Strauss, 2004). More recent research has viewed children with clefts as a more heterogeneous group. Endriga and Kapp-Simon (1999) indicate that children with clefts and no other accompanying anomalies (syndromes) are at only a slightly higher risk for mental retardation (4–6% as opposed to 2% in the general population) but children with clefts as part of a syndrome are at higher risk. With regard to cleft type, it appears that children with isolated clefts of the palate score more poorly on IQ tests such as the Stanford-Binet and the Wechsler Intelligence Scale for Children (WISC) (Richman & Eliason, 1982; Peterson-Falzone et al., 2001). This variation by cleft type prompted Strauss (2004) to suggest that while it is important to periodically screen all children with clefts for cognitive delays, particular attention should be given to those children with isolated clefts of the palate.

Finally, the reduced IQ scores reported in earlier literature reflected the fact that children with clefts tend to do more poorly on tests of verbal IQ than on tests of performance IQ (Richman & Eliason, 1982; Strauss, 2004). This deficit on verbal tests may reflect language problems and specific learning disabilities rather than a generalized cognitive delay.

In addition to difficulties in language-based areas, the classroom performance of cleft palate students may be affected by social and emotional factors. There has never been evidence of a specific personality type associated with cleft palate students, nor has there been conclusive evidence that people with clefts exhibit psychopathology or severe emotional disturbance at a higher rate than the noncleft population (Strauss, 2004). There is, however, evidence of more subtle adjustment problems. Cleft palate students tend to be more withdrawn and inhibited, and tend to participate less in classroom activities than their noncleft peers (Endriga & Kapp-Simon, 1999; Kapp, 1979; Powers, 1986; Richman & Eliason, 1993; Richman & Harper, 1979). These characteristics reflect the necessity for children with clefts "to adjust and accommodate to a variety of speech-, education-, and appearance-related social and interpersonal challenges in their development" (Strauss, 2004, p. 167). Richman and Eliason (1986) suggest that these socioemotional variables may interact with cognitive variables to produce a greater vulnerability to academic problems.

SYNDROMES THAT INCLUDE CRANIOFACIAL ANOMALIES

Many craniofacial anomalies, including cleft lip and palate, occur as part of a syndrome. A **syndrome** is a collection of signs and symptoms that occur together and characterize a particular disease or condition. There are hundreds of syndromes that include craniofacial anomalies. Peterson-Falzone and colleagues (2001) indicate that there are approximately 350 syndromes which are associated with oral-facial clefting. There are many more syndromes that include craniofacial anomalies without clefts. Obviously, it is beyond the scope of this text to attempt to describe this plethora of conditions. In this chapter, we hope to provide a brief description of some of the more commonly occurring syndromes associated with craniofacial anomalies, to provide a brief glossary of medical terms used to describe some of the many malformations of the craniofacial structures, and to discuss the school adjustment of students with facial disfigurements. Table 11-1 lists syndromes which are frequently associated with craniofacial anomalies and provides a brief description of the primary signs related to each syndrome.

Table 11-2 describes some of the possible malformations of the craniofacial structure. The purpose of introducing these medical terms is to provide some idea of the variety of facial disfigurements that can occur and to familiarize teachers with terms that may find their way into students' files through reports from various professionals.

Table 11-1 Brief Descriptions of Syndromes That Include Craniofacial Anomalies

Apert syndrome: Premature closure of the skull resulting in disorders in the shape of skull and face, including excessive distance between the eyes, protrusion of the eyes, down-slanting of the eyes, midfacial deficiency or underdevelopment, webbing of the hands and feet, possible conductive hearing loss, and possible mental retardation.

Cornelia de Lange syndrome: Microcephaly, excessive body hair, low-set large ears, small nose, mental retardation, limb disorders.

Crouzon syndrome: Similar to Apert syndrome but less severe and no webbing of hands and feet.

Down syndrome: Flat face, upward-slanting eyes, some protrusion of tongue (may be due to small mouth and poor muscle tone of tongue), small ears, short fingers, mental retardation.

Goldenhar syndrome: Facial asymmetry due largely to underdevelopment of the vertical portion of the mandible on one side, lateral cleftlike extension of the mouth, underdeveloped facial muscles, deformed external ears, conductive hearing loss. Some forms of this condition may be referred to as hemifacial microsomia.

continues

Neurofibromatosis: Numerous tumors (progressive) occurring on internal and external structures. These tumors may result in severe deformity when they occur on the face. This is the condition depicted in the movie *Elephant Man*.

Oro-facial-digital syndrome (OFD) type II: Lobed tongue (the anterior portion of the tongue is divided into two or more rounded projections), more-than-normal number of digits, cleft lip, underdevelopment of the chin (mandible), malformation of the outer and possibly middle ear, conductive hearing loss.

Pierre Robin sequence: Extremely underdeveloped chin (mandible) which causes the tongue to be pushed back into the pharynx, possibly resulting in respiratory difficulty, cleft palate, or possible conductive hearing loss; may exist as an isolated condition or as part of several other syndromes.

Treacher Collins syndrome: Down slanting eyes, defects in the shape of the eye, underdeveloped cheek bones and mandible, defects in auditory canal and middle ear, conductive hearing loss, cleft palate.

Sources: Cohen, 1978; Jung, 1989; Peterson-Falzone et al., 2001; and Shprintzen, 1997.

Table 11-2 Selected Medical Terms Used to Describe Various Craniofacial Anomalies

Anecephaly	A condition in which the brain fails to develop
Anodontia	The absence of teeth
Atresia	An occlusion of an opening or passage. In communication disorders, it most commonly refers to an underdeveloped pinna that may result in occlusion of the external auditory canal.
Bifid	Divided into two parts. This most often refers to a divided uvula or tongue.
Brachycephaly	Reduction in the front to back dimension of the skull
Coloboma	Defect in the shape of the eye, which may involve the lower lid, iris, or retina
Craniosynostosis	A premature fusing together of the bones of the cranium
Heterochromia iridis	Different color eyes
Hirsutism	Excessive body hair
Hypertelorism	Excessive distance between the eyes
Macroglossia	An excessively large tongue
Microcephaly	Small head
Microglossia	A small tongue
Micrognathia	A severely underdeveloped mandible or chin

continues

Table 11-2 Continued

Microtia	Small outer ear
Oligodontia	Less than the normal number of teeth
Poliosis	Premature graying of the hair. If limited to a particular area, the term *poliosis circumscripta* may be used.
Proptosis	Bulging eyes
Synophrys	A growing together or confluence of the eyebrows

LEARNING PROBLEMS IN CHILDREN WITH CRANIOFACIAL ANOMALIES

The learning problems of students with craniofacial anomalies depend to a large extent on the degree of intellectual impairment. Some syndromes typically result in severe mental retardation, others result in milder degrees of retardation, and still others are not associated with any cognitive deficits. Because many of these students have more severe facial disfigurement than those with cleft palate only, social and emotional variables might play a more significant role in school adjustment.

Students with severe craniofacial anomalies do not appear to exhibit severe psychosocial disorders. Their social and emotional problems, like those of cleft palate children, tend to be more subtle and seem to be related to coping with social pressures. Pertschuk and Whitaker (1985) reported that children with craniofacial malformations demonstrated poorer self-concepts, increased levels of anxiety, and more introversion than a control group of children with normal facial structures. Teachers reported poorer classroom behavior among the craniofacial group, but parents did not observe such behavior problems at home.

One of the more troubling factors for children with craniofacial anomalies is the reaction of others to their appearance. In recent years, movies such as *Elephant Man* and *Mask* have dramatized this problem. The academic performance of children with craniofacial anomalies may be affected by the expectations of parents and teachers. Berscheid and Walster (1974) reported that teachers tend to view physically attractive students as having more acceptable behavior and higher mental abilities than less attractive students. This appears to hold true for students with craniofacial disorders. Richman (1979) compared teacher ratings of the intellectual ability of children with facial deformities to the IQ scores of those children. The results indicated that the intellectual abilities of children with noticeable facial disfigurements and above average IQs were underestimated by teachers. Parents also may have lower expectations of children with craniofacial anomalies, resulting in lower academic aspirations (Richman & Eliason, 1982). Children also tend to view students with craniofacial anomalies in a more negative fashion (Schneiderman & Harding, 1984; Tobiason, 1987). It is very difficult for a child to develop a good self-image and to achieve his or her potential when teachers, parents, and peers expect less of that student.

In addition to the syndromes listed in Table 11-1, there are three syndromes which, because of the unique speech and language problems as well as the presence of learning problems, merit special attention in this chapter. Those three conditions are velocardiofacial syndrome, fetal alcohol syndrome, and fragile X syndrome.

Velocardiofacial Syndrome (VCFS)

Also known as Shprintzen syndrome, DiGeorge syndrome, or 22q11.2 deletion syndrome (referring to the chromosome abnormality that is the source of the problem), this syndrome was first described in 1978 (Shprintzen et al., 1978). VCFS occurs in about one in every 1800 births, (Golding-Kushner, 2001) and is one of the most common syndromes associated with cleft palate (Shprintzen, 2000). The syndrome is characterized by several features including: cleft palate (often a submucous cleft), heart anomalies, a long nose with a bulbous tip, puffy eyelids, small ears, learning disabilities, ADHD, and delayed speech and language (Shprintzen, 1997). Also, many children with VCFS unfortunately develop mental illness including bipolar disorder, manic depression, and psychosis later in life (Golding-Kushner, 2001; Peterson-Falzone et al., 2001). As with most syndromes, not every child exhibits every symptom; however, language deficits are almost universal among VCFS children, and the language deficit is present from the onset of language (Scherer, D'Antonio, & Kalbfleisch, 1999). The delays in expressive language are greater than in receptive language, and the expressive speech and language delays are more severe than would be expected compared to their other developmental problems. Some VCFS children may be essentially nonverbal as late as age 3 years, and some may even be candidates for some form of augmentative (nonvocal) communication such as signing, picture boards, or computer-assisted devices (Scherer, et al., 1999; Scherer, 2003). D'Antonio, Scherer, Miller, Kalbfleisch, and Bartley (2001) concluded that young children with VCFS demonstrate speech production that is different from normal and may be specific to the syndrome. For example children with VCFS often exhibit a high number of glottal stops and have more hypernasality following repair of their cleft palate than children with clefts not associated with a syndrome (Scherer et al., 1999). Speech and language delays persist through elementary school; however, VCFS children appear to narrow the gap somewhat between their language skills and those of their peer age group as they grow (D'Antonio et al., 2001). Golding-

Kushner (2001) indicates that "The learning curve of children with VCFS may be more stepwise than smooth" (p. 147). This means that children may have some advances followed by plateaus with no discernable progress. This suggests that parents, speech-language pathologists, and teachers should not be discouraged by periodic lack of progress and should continue intervention and stimulation even when the VCFS child is moving ahead as rapidly as expected of other children. Golding-Kusner (2001) notes that because children with VCFS seem to learn best in frequent short sessions with much repetition, an SLP may want to see these children more frequently than other children on the caseload.

Regarding educational achievement, Golding-Kusner (2001) indicated that although most children with VCFS are of normal or borderline normal intelligence, learning disabilities are common. She states that the learning disabilities exhibited by VCFS children affect reading comprehension, math concepts, and tasks involving inferential reasoning and abstract thinking. Therefore, the learning problems of VCFS children may not be apparent until second or third grade when academic tasks become more complex. Because ADHD is also commonly reported among VCFS children, they are likely to demonstrate many of the problems associated with ADHD described in Chapter 12.

Fetal Alcohol Syndrome (FAS)

This syndrome is characterized by low birth weight, cleft lip or palate or both, microcephaly, and unusual facial features that may include a short nose and an underdeveloped midface area (Jung, 1989; Shprintzen, 1997). These children also frequently exhibit cognitive delays and ADHD. The problem results, as the name implies, from alcohol consumption by the mother during pregnancy. The severity of the symptoms associated with this syndrome vary widely and may be related to the amount of alcohol consumed and the regularity and timing of the alcohol consumption (Jung, 1989; Little & Streissguth, 1981). FAS is reported to occur at different rates in different parts of the world (Jung, 1989). In North America the incidence is reported to range from 0.5 to 3/1,000 births (Stratton, Howe, & Bataglia, 1996).

The communication abilities of children with FAS vary widely. However, some research has described the language of many FAS children as superficial (Abkarian, 1992; Streissguth, Bookstein, Sampson, & Barr, 1993). This means that a child may appear to have appropriate language in certain social situations, but when pressed to describe or explain more complicated concepts the language skills are inadequate. Such superficial language skills would tend to be exposed when increased academic demands are placed on children. This could be seen as early as early as second or third grade. This description of potential language problems is consistent with the fact that deficits in cognitive performance are beginning to be noted reliably (Stratton et al., 1996).

Fragile X Syndrome

Also known as Martin-Bell syndrome or X-linked mental retardation, this syndrome is among the most common inherited cause of cognitive delay and learning difficulties (Dew-Hughes, 2004; Paul, Cohen, Breg, Watson, & Herman, 1984). Because this condition is transmitted on the X (sex) chromosome, fragile X syndrome is transmitted by the mother and most typically affects males. However some females exhibit some of the symptoms associated with this syndrome. According to the Web site of the National Fragile X Foundation (2005) (http://www.fragilex.org/html/summary.htm), fragile X syndrome occurs in approximately 1 in 3,600 males and 1 in 4,000 to 6,000 females. About one-third of the carrier females also exhibit cognitive problems. Unlike VCFS and FAS, fragile X syndrome does not include a cleft lip or palate. However, it is characterized by atypical facial features including a long narrow face, large ears, and prominent jaw (Jung, 1989; Shprintzen, 1997). There is a high incidence of cognitive involvement in the condition although approximately 15% of males with fragile X syndrome are considered to have normal or above normal intelligence (Hagerman, 2004).

Children with fragile X syndrome typically show a speech and language delay and occasionally exhibit a rapid rate and stuttering or cluttering-like speech. Many children with fragile X tend to exhibit perseverative speech (continuing to repeat a word or phrase after it is no longer appropriate) and tangential speech (wandering from the topic) (Paul et al., 1984; Taylor, 2004). The perseverative speech may be related to an inability to organize tasks logically, impulsivity, vocabulary problems, or anxiety, all of which characterize this syndrome (Taylor, 2004). Taylor also suggests that tangential speech and inability to stay on topic may be related to these children's inability to organize tasks as well as attention problems also seen frequently in fragile X. In addition to the communication problems exhibited by children with fragile X syndrome, teachers often observe behavioral problems due to severe and persistent inattention, overactivity, and impulsiveness causing many fragile X children to be diagnosed as ADHD (Scerif & Cornish, 2004).

Some of the language and behavior of children with fragile X syndrome are suggestive of autism, and in fact approximately 15–25% of children with fragile

X meet the diagnostic criteria for autism. Cornish and Taylor (2004) indicate that research relating fragile X to autism is somewhat equivocal. Some authors view fragile X as part of the autism spectrum and others view the two as separate conditions. Regardless of the relationship between the two conditions, the presence of autism-like symptoms in children with fragile X syndrome complicates the language, behavioral, and educational profiles of these children.

Shyness along with attention deficits and perseverative and tangential speech typically make conversational skills a communicative weakness for children with fragile X. In spite of these communicative problems, children with fragile X are often described as friendly and helpful and demonstrate a desire to interact with peers (Sudhalter & Belser, 2004).

The habilitative process for students with craniofacial anomalies often is prolonged and typically involves surgeons, orthodontists, and speech-language pathologists. Teachers also make a significant contribution to the adjustment and development of these children, yet most teachers have very little training or experience with such students. Moran and Pentz (1991) interviewed members of a parent support group for children with craniofacial anomalies. The parent information was combined with a review of the literature, and resulted in the following suggestions.

SUGGESTIONS FOR TEACHERS

- Avoid self-fulfilling prophecies—Judge the child by his or her performance and objective measures of ability rather than by any preconceived notion based on physical appearance or speech quality.
- Consult with the SLP to know what level of speech proficiency can be expected—If the student's oral structure is inadequate, perfect speech can not be expected. On the other hand, teachers can be of great assistance by reminding the student to use newly acquired speech and language skills in the classroom setting.
- Refer any student with hypernasality or nasal emission to the SLP for evaluation—Some submucous clefts and other forms of velopharyngeal incompetence may have gone undetected during the preschool years.
- Be alert to the possibility of language-based learning disabilities—These problems may surface in reading and writing activities. Although the possibility of learning disabilities is particularly great in certain craniofacial syndromes such as VCFS, FAS, and fragile X, teachers should be alert to the possibility of such disorders even in children with nonsyndromic clefts of the palate.

- Watch for signs of middle ear problems and a mild hearing loss—See Chapter 10 for specific behaviors which indicate such a hearing loss.
- Encourage participation in classroom activities—Help to foster a feeling of "fitting in" with the rest of the class. Teachers should encourage, but not be overzealous in pressuring, the student with craniofacial anomalies to participate in classroom activities. Teachers must also be alert to any ridicule or teasing that the student with craniofacial anomalies might experience. While it is not possible to completely eliminate such behavior, measures must be taken to minimize it. Failure to do so, by default, condones ridicule and permits it to grow.
- Be prepared to help the student make up missed work—Children may miss several classes if secondary surgical procedures or extensive dental work are performed during the school year. An outline of assignments for the various subject areas and a supply of necessary texts and workbooks supplied to the parents, would be quite helpful. A brief follow-up by the teacher after the absences can help to identify any deficits that remain.

CONCLUSION

For the most part, children with craniofacial anomalies are just that: children. They may miss somewhat more school than others. They may look a little different. They tend to have a higher incidence of speech, language, and hearing problems than their classmates. They may struggle a bit with social and academic challenges. However, with a few adjustments and a little extra attention and respect, the overwhelming majority of students with craniofacial anomalies can do just fine in their school routine. The knowledgeable teacher can do a great deal to build and promote the environment in which a child can earn that attention and respect from both classmates and school personnel.

REFERENCES

Abkarian, G.G. (1992). Communication effects of prenatal alcohol exposure. *Journal of Communication Disorders, 25,* 221–240.

Berscheid, E., & Walster, E. (1974). Physical attractiveness. In S. Berkowitz (Ed.), *Advances in experimental psychology.* (Vol. 7). New York: Academic Press.

Broder, H.L., Richman, L.C., & Matheson, P. (1998). Learning disability, school achievement, and grade retention among children with cleft: A two-center study. *Cleft Palate Craniofacial Journal, 35,* 127–131.

Broen, P.A., Devers, M.C., Doyle, S.S., Prouty, J.M., & Moller, K.T. (1998). Acquisition of linguistic and cognitive skills by children with cleft palate. *Journal of Speech, Language, and Hearing Research, 41,* 676–700.

Brookshire, B.L., Lynch, J.I., & Fox, D.R. (1984). *A parent-child cleft palate curriculum: Developing speech and language.* Tigard, OR: C.C. Publications.

Bzoch, K.R. (2004). Introduction to the study of communicative disorders in cleft palate and related craniofacial anomalies. In K.R. Bzoch (Ed.), *Communicative disorders related to cleft lip and palate* (5th ed.). Austin, TX: PRO-ED.

Cohen, M.M. (1978). Syndromes with cleft lip and cleft palate. *Cleft Palate Journal, 15,* 306–328.

Cornish, K., & Taylor, J. (2004). Related conditions: Autism and attention deficit/hyperactivity disorder. In D. Dew-Hughes (Ed.), *Educating children with fragile X syndrome.* London: Routledge-Falmer.

D'Antonio, L.L., Scherer, N.J., Miller, L.L., Kalbfleisch, J.H., & Bartley, J.A. (2001). Analysis of speech characteristics in children with velocardiofacial syndrome (VCFS) and children with phenotypic overlap without VCFS. *Cleft Palate Craniofacial Journal, 35,* 455–467.

Dew-Hughes, D. (2004). *Educating children with fragile X syndrome.* London: Routledge-Falmer.

Endriga, M.C., & Kapp-Simon, K.A. (1999). Psychological issues in craniofacial care: State of the art. *Cleft Palate Craniofacial Journal, 36,* 3–11.

Estes, R.E., & Morris, H.L. (1970). Relationships among intelligence, speech proficiency, and hearing sensitivity in children with cleft palates. *Cleft Palate Journal, 7,* 763–773.

Gerson, C.R. (1990). Otologic disease in the cleft palate patient. In D. Kernahan, & S. Stark (Eds.). *Cleft lip and palate: A system of management.* Baltimore: Williams & Wilkins.

Golding-Kushner, K.J. (2001). *Therapy techniques for cleft palate speech and related disorders.* San Diego, CA: Singular.

Hagerman, R. (2004). Physical and behavioural characteristics of fragile X syndrome. In D. Dew-Hughes (Ed.). *Educating children with fragile X syndrome.* London: Routledge-Falmer.

Hahn, E. (1989). Directed home training perogram for infants with cleft lip and palate. In K. Bzocht (Ed.), *Communicative disorders related to cleft lip and palate* (3rd ed.). Boston: Little, Brown.

Jung, J.H. (1989). *Genetic syndromes in communication disorders.* Boston: Little, Brown.

Kapp, K. (1979). Self-concept of the cleft lip and/or palate child. *Cleft Palate Journal, 16,* 171–176.

LaRossa, D. (2000). The state of the art in cleft palate surgery. *Cleft Palate Craniofacial Journal, 37,* 225–227.

Lewis, R. (1961). A survey of the intelligence of cleft palate children in Ontario. *Cleft Palate Bulletin, 11,* 83–85.

Little, R.E., & Streissguth, A.P. (1981). Effects of alcohol on the fetus: Impact and prevention. *Canadian Medical Association Journal, 125,* 159–164.

Means, B., & Irwin, J. (1954). An analysis of certain measures of intelligence and hearing in a sample of the Wisconsin cleft palate population. *Cleft Palate Newsletter, 4,* 2–4.

Meyerson, M. (1990). Cultural considerations in the treatment of Latinos with craniofacial malformations. *Cleft Palate Journal, 27,* 279–288.

Millard, T., & Richman, L.C. (2001). Different cleft conditions, facial appearance, and speech: Relationship to psychological variables. *Cleft Palate Craniofacial Journal, 38,* 68–75.

Moran, M., & Pentz, A. (1991). Advising teachers of children with cleft lip/palate. Paper presented at the national convention of the American Speech-Language-Hearing Association, Atlanta, GA.

National Fragile X Foundation Web site. (2004). Retrieved from http://www.fragilex.org/html/summary.htm

Paradise, J., Bluestone, C., & Felder, H. (1969). The universality of otitis media in 50 infants with cleft palate. *Pediatrics, 44,* 35–42.

Paul, R., Cohen, D., Breg, R., Watson, M., & Herman, S. (1984). Fragile X syndrome: Its relation to speech and language disorders. *Journal of Speech and Hearing Disorders, 49,* 328–332.

Pecyna, P.M., Feeney-Giacoma, M.E., & Nieman, G.S. (1987). Development of the object permanence concept in cleft lip and palate and noncleft lip and palate infants. *Journal of Communication Disorders, 20,* 233–243.

Pertschuk, M.J., & Whitaker, L.A. (1985). Psychological adjustment and craniofacial malformations in childhood. *Plastic and Reconstructive Surgery, 75,* 177–182.

Peterson-Falzone, S.J., Hardin-Jones, M.A., & Karnell, M.P. (2001). *Cleft palate speech* (3rd ed.). St. Louis, MO: Mosby.

Powers, G.R. (1986). *Cleft palate.* Austin, TX: PRO-ED.

Richman, L.C. (1979). The effects of facial disfigurement on teachers' perception of ability in cleft palate children. *Cleft Palate Journal, 15,* 155–160.

Richman, L.C. (1980). Cognitive patterns and learning disabilities in cleft palate children with verbal deficits. *Journal of Speech and Hearing Research, 23,* 447–465.

Richman, L.C., & Eliason, M.J. (1982). Psychological characteristics of cleft lip and palate: Intellectual, achievement, behavioral, and personality variables. *Cleft Palate Journal, 19,* 249–257.

Richman, L.C., & Eliason, M.J. (1984). Types of reading disability related to cleft type and neuropsychological patterns. *Cleft Palate Journal, 21,* 1–6.

Richman, L.C., & Eliason, M.J. (1986). Development in children with cleft lip and/or palate: Intellectual, cognitive, personality, and parental factors. *Seminars in Speech and Language, 7,* 225–239.

Richman, L.C., & Eliason, M.J. (1993). Psychological characteristics associated with cleft palate. In K.T. Moller, & C.D. Starr (Eds.), *Cleft palate interdisciplinary issues and treatment: For clinicians by clinicians.* Austin, TX: PRO-ED.

Richman, L.C., Eliason, M.J., & Lindgren, S.D. (1988). Reading disability in children with clefts. *Cleft Palate Journal, 25,* 21–25.

Richman, L.C., & Harper, D. (1979). Self-identified personality patterns in children with facial or orthopedic disfigurement. *Cleft Palate Journal, 16,* 257–261.

Richman, L.C., & Ryan, S.M. (2003). Do the reading disabilities of children with cleft fit into current models of developmental dyslexia? *Cleft Palate Craniofacial Journal, 40,* 154–157.

Scerif, G., & Cornish, K. (2004). Development in the early years. In D. Dew-Hughes (Ed.), *Educating children with fragile X syndrome.* London: Routledge-Falmer.

Scheper-Hughes, N. (1990). Difference and danger: The cultural dynamics of childhood stigma, rejection and rescue. *Cleft Palate Journal, 27,* 301–307.

Scherer, N.J. (2003, October). Speech and language development in children with VCFS and children with clefts. Paper presented at the 16th Annual Cleft Lip and Palate Symposium, Children's Healthcare of Atlanta, Atlanta, GA.

Scherer, N.J., & D'Antonio, L. (1995, December). Longitudinal language development in 20–30 month children with cleft lip and/or palate. Paper presented at the annual convention of the American Speech-Language-Hearing Association, Orlando, FL.

Scherer, N.J., D'Antonio, L., & Kalbfleisch, J. (1999). Early speech and language development in children with velocardiofacial syndrome. *American Journal of Medical Genetics, 88,* 714–723.

Schneiderman, C.R., & Harding, J.B. (1984). Social ratings of children with cleft lips by school peers. *Cleft Palate Journal, 21,* 219–223.

Seagle, M.B. (2004). Primary surgical correction of cleft lip and palate. In K.R. Bzoch, *Communicative disorders related to cleft lip and palate* (5th ed.). Austin, TX: PRO-ED.

Shprintzen, R.J. (1997). *Genetics, syndromes, and communication disorders*. San Diego, CA: Singular.

Shprintzen, R.J. (2000). *Syndrome identification for speech-language pathologists: An illustrated pocket guide*. San Diego, CA: Singular.

Shprintzen, R.J., Goldberg, R.B., Lewin, M.L., Sidoti, E.J., Berkman, M.D., Argamaso, P.V., et al. (1978). A new syndrome involving cleft palate, cardiac anomalies, typical facies, and learning disabilities: Velo-cardio-facial syndrome. *Cleft Palate Journal, 15*, 56–62.

Strauss, R.P. (2004). Social and psychological perspectives on cleft lip and palate. In K.R. Bzoch (Ed.), *Communicative disorders related to cleft lip and palate* (5th ed.). Austin, TX: PRO-ED.

Slavkin, H.C. (1992). Incidence of cleft lips, palates rising. *Journal of the American Dental Association, 123*, 61–65.

Stratton, K., Howe, C., & Battaglia, F. (Eds.). (1996). *Fetal alcohol syndrome: diagnosis, epidemiology, prevention and treatment*. Washington, DC: National Academy Press.

Streissguth, A.P., Bookstein, F.L., Sampson, P.C., & Barr, H.M. (1993). The enduring effects of prenatal alcohol exposure on child development: Birth through seven years, a partial least squares solution. Ann Arbor, MI: University of Michigan Press.

Sudhalter, V., & Belser, R.C. (2004). Atypical language production of males with fragile X syndrome. In D. Dew-Hughes (Ed.), *Educating children with fragile X syndrome*. London: Routledge-Falmer.

Taylor, C. (2004). Speech and language therapy. In D. Dew-Hughes (Ed.), *Educating children with fragile X syndrome*. London: Routledge-Falmer.

Tobiason, J.B. (1987). Social judgments of facial deformity. *Cleft Palate Journal, 24*, 323–327.

Toliver-Weddington, G. (1990). Cultural considerations in the treatment of craniofacial malformations in African Americans. *Cleft Palate Journal, 27*, 289–293.

Trost-Cardemone, J.E., & Bernthal, J.E. (1993). Articulation assessment procedures and treatment decisions. In K.T. Moller, & C. Starr (Eds.), *Cleft palate interdisciplinary issues and treatment: For clinicians by clinicians*. Austin, TX: PRO-ED.

Van Demark, D.R. (1964). Misarticulations and listener judgments of the speech of individuals with cleft palates. *Cleft Palate Journal, 1*, 232–245.

Witzel, M.A. (1995). Communicative impairment associated with clefting. In R.J. Shprintzen, & J. Bardach (Eds.), *Cleft palate speech management: A multidisciplinary approach*. St. Louis, MO: Mosby.

TERMS TO KNOW

cleft lip

cleft palate

compensatory articulation

hypernasality

nasal emission

obturator

speech appliance

submucous cleft

syndrome

velopharyngeal insufficiency (VPI)

STUDY QUESTIONS

1. Describe the various speech, language, and hearing problems a student with cleft palate might exhibit.

2. Describe several things a teacher could do to facilitate the learning of a student with cleft palate.

3. Describe the possible negative reactions that students with craniofacial anomalies might encounter in a school setting and identify actions that teachers could take to deal with such reactions.

chapter twelve

Neurologic Impairments

INTRODUCTION

Speech and language deficits may be part of a more global condition in which the student has motor impairments, perceptual difficulties, cognitive deficits, behavioral problems, and the like. Problems of these types may be subtle or highly noticeable to peers and teachers. They most certainly will be educationally handicapping and necessitate teamwork among school personnel and health care professionals. Conditions discussed in this chapter, while not communication disorders per se, do have neurologic foundations that impact the students' speech-language skills and, ultimately, academic performance. We will provide an overview of neuromuscular problems such as cerebral palsy, dysarthria, and dysphagia; the neurologic and behavioral sequela to traumatic brain injury; and the multifaceted problems associated with the condition termed attention deficit disorder.

Students with these neurologic problems may need special education support services, yet most will be mainstreamed into regular classrooms. These students may present a challenge to the classroom teacher and require adaptation of physical facilities, knowledge of special equipment, use of technology, and modification of curricular activities. The conspicuousness of the student's condition also may strain social relations among peers. The teacher's understanding of a student's medical condition is paramount to structuring an optimal learning environment. This chapter will discuss some of the medical conditions affecting communication that a classroom teacher is likely to encounter.

THE NATURE OF NEUROLOGIC PROBLEMS

Damage to the nervous system may render muscular problems of weakness, incoordination, slowness, or even paralysis. The location and extent of nervous system damage is, of course, important, but the essence of the person's **neuromuscular problem** is movement based. If the damage to the brain occurred before, during, or after birth (during childhood), the person is diagnosed as having **cerebral palsy**. If the affected muscles include those involved in speech production or are limited to those involved in speech production (i.e., muscles of respiration, phonation, and articulation), the speech-language pathologist may refer to the condition as **dysarthria**. Actually, there are many types of dysarthria; the term simply means a **motor speech disorder**.

Dysarthria, particularly in adults and adolescents, may exist in the absence of cerebral palsy. In such cases, the dysarthria (motor speech condition) is usually due to some trauma (e.g., automobile wreck, stroke, near poisoning) or disease state (e.g., muscular dystrophy, myasthenia gravis, tumor invasion, multiple sclerosis, encephalitis, inherited degenerative disorders). The neuromuscular problems of cerebral palsy will be discussed followed by brief mention of a form of dysarthria (not associated with true cerebral palsy) that may be seen in school-aged students.

Cerebral Palsy

Cerebral palsy is a static encephalopathy, meaning there is nondegenerative damage to the brain. Cerebral palsy (CP) often is classified on the basis of at least two factors: the type of neuromuscular involvement, and the distribution of injury. Table 12-1 outlines the six major types of CP with respect to neuromuscular involvement: **spasticity, athetosis, ataxia, tremor, rigidity,** and **mixed**. Spasticity is by far the most common form of CP, whereas tremor and rigidity are infrequent in children. At the risk of oversimplification, physical therapists, occupational therapists, speech-language pathologists (SLPs), and special educators, often design intervention programs and han-

Table 12-1 The Major Types of Cerebral Palsy as Classified by Neuromuscular Involvement

Type	Neuromuscular Characteristics
Spasticity	Muscles of the limbs feel tight; increased muscle tone; hyperactive reflexes.
Athetosis	Limbs have involuntary purposeless movements; purposeful movements are contorted.
Ataxia	A lack of balance sensation; a lack of position sense in space; uncoordinated movements.
Tremor	Shakiness of the involved limbs; tremor might be noticed only in the attempt to use the limb (intention tremor). Continuous tremor at rest is not common in children but often accompanies brain disease in adults.
Rigidity	Perhaps a severe form of spasticity; in movement the rigid limb gives way as if it were a lead pipe or a cogwheel.
Mixed	A combination of neuromuscular symptoms; often spasticity and athetosis appear in children with quadriplegia.

dling techniques for these students based on the amount of muscle tone generally present (i.e., whether the student has high tone, low tone, or fluctuating tone). Classification based on the distribution of injury reflects the underlying extent of brain damage. Many classifying terms exist; three common forms of CP are hemiplegia, paraplegia, and quadriplegia. **Hemiplegia** is the most common type of CP and often occurs with spasticity. The arm and leg on the same side of the body are involved; the side of involvement is opposite to the side of brain damage. **Paraplegia** is the term used to describe involvement of both legs but with the arms usually unaffected. Brain damage is confined to a particular region within both hemispheres. When all four extremities are involved, the CP is called **quadriplegia**. The degree of motor involvement may or may not be equal in the extremities. Quadriplegia results from a wide area of brain damage.

The causes of cerebral palsy are many and varied. Suffice it to say that CP can result from brain damage occurring at any time during the developmental period (prenatal, natal, postnatal). Causes include faulty genetic factors, maternal infections, anoxia (lack of oxygen), trauma during delivery, childhood traumatic injuries, and infectious diseases.

The individual with CP often is multiply handicapped. The classroom teacher most certainly needs to know the student's strengths and weaknesses. Frequently occurring disabilities associated with cerebral palsy include the following list.

Epileptic Seizures

Massive convulsions with or without the loss of consciousness are known as grand mal seizures, whereas minor and fleeting seizures are petit mal or other partial types (Brumback, Mathews, & Shenoy, 2001). Persons with cerebral palsy have a propensity for epileptic seizures. It may be wise to check with the school nurse regarding what to do or not to do if a seizure occurs in the classroom. Also it is desirable to find out whether the student is on medication for seizure control and what the side effects of medication are likely to be, especially regarding activity level and attention span.

Orthopedic Problems

Abnormal muscle stresses may cause deformities and dislocations for which the student may need bracing, compensatory postures, or even surgery. Correct positioning of motorically involved students is critical for the educational environment. Teachers should consult with the appropriate school system personnel to learn optimal positioning and handling techniques for each individual student. The physical therapist, occupational therapist, special education teacher, school medical personnel, or even the SLP might be contacted in this regard. The IEP meeting provides an optimal time for the various disciplines to interact and discuss an appropriate course of action, including positioning and handling, for the student. Each team member should become familiar with the student's braces, wheelchair, restraint systems, and/or other specialized equipment to best work with the student.

Feeding and Nutritional Problems

Incoordination of muscles involved in chewing and swallowing may lead to feeding or nutritional problems. Often, with infants, specialized feeding programs must be developed, incorporating the use of special postures, techniques, utensils, and exercises. Throughout the child's growth and development, nutrition may continue to be a concern because of reduced food intake (due to problems in chewing and swallowing) and the fact that much caloric energy is consumed with involuntary movements. We will touch on dysphagia (swallowing disorders) again later in this chapter.

Communication Disorders

Cerebral palsy may encompass any or all of the speech production processes, leading to problems with air control (e.g., able to speak too few words per breath), voice production (e.g., phonatory spasms causing vocal strain or other quality changes), prosody (e.g., difficulty controlling pitch inflections and proportional stressing of syllables), and articulation (e.g., speech sounding slurred or imprecise). Solomon and Charron (1998) espouse that breathing problems are central to most forms of CP and warrant attention from the SLP. They advocate techniques for improved speech breathing and exhalatory control. In general, speech treatment seeks to normalize muscle movements, when possible, or to train compensatory movements to their best potential for improved intelligibility. Individuals with CP and very severe motoric involvement, however, may not be candidates for learning speech. In such cases, therapy is directed at training in the use of an augmentative or alternative communication mode, as will be discussed later in this chapter.

In addition to speech problems, the student may have delayed language abilities, perhaps due to the brain damage itself or due to the restricted environmental exposure afforded the child when young. Language intervention programs are likely parts of the total educational needs of the student with CP. Intervention strategies and collaborative learning, as discussed in the early chapters of this book, certainly apply to this type of student.

Cognitive Deficits

Deficits in cognition may parallel language delays. Presumably the brain damage that produces the motor movement problems also reduces the person's ability to assimilate stimuli and to organize it meaningfully (i.e., to think intelligently). However, it has been estimated that about 30–40% of individuals with CP are of average or above average intelligence (Mirenda & Mathy-Laikko, 1989) and so teachers should never underestimate the academic potential of a motorically involved student!

Perceptual Deficits

Perceptual deficits are many and varied. Visual defects stem from problems of eye movement; hearing loss also occurs frequently in cerebral palsied individuals. Often there is difficulty organizing sensory stimuli into some kind of meaning. Students may have figure-ground problems, visual-motor problems, and have inabilities shifting to abstract forms of behavior (staying instead at concrete, stereotyped, and predictive responses). Teachers should realize that perceptual problems may necessitate some adaptations in the classroom learning environment.

Dysarthria

As mentioned at the beginning of the chapter, motor speech disturbances often accompany certain disease states and/or may result from trauma to the peripheral nervous system, central nervous system, or both. In particular, dysarthria refers to an impairment in neuromuscular function of the respiratory, phonatory, and/or articulatory processes of speech. The degree of impairment can be so minimal that dysarthria would be difficult to detect during conversational speech, or the degree of impairment can be so severe that any speech produced is completely unintelligible. In such severe cases, alternative communication systems often are necessary. Muscular dystrophy is one disease encountered in school-aged youth that eventually results in severe dysarthria.

The Jerry Lewis Telethons, broadcast on television on Labor Day weekends for the past few decades, have made **muscular dystrophy** a household word. As a group of diseases, muscular dystrophy (MD) is anything but simple. There is progressive atrophy, or wasting away of the skeletal muscles throughout the body, without damage to the nerves. Onset is usually at an early age; often a waddling gait appears when a child begins to walk or first starts school. Muscle deterioration can progress rapidly, leaving the youngster on a bracing system for ambulation, or confined to a wheelchair by the teenage years. MD seems to be a familial disease, and it occurs more frequently in males than females. The widespread deterioration of muscles not only interferes with locomotion ability but also affects the muscles involved in respiration. Obviously, speech will become impaired as these muscles atrophy, but there is major concern for breathing adequacy. Treatment is multidisciplinary and directed toward relieving symptoms and slowing the progress of the disease. Unnecessary immobilization may accelerate the rate of deterioration (Jones, 1985). The student should be encouraged to lead as normal a life as possible.

Augmentative and Alternative Communication Modes

Speech-language pathologists have a responsibility to help motorically involved persons develop **augmentative or alternative communication (AAC)** strategies when the cerebral palsy or dysarthria is too severe to permit intelligible, conversational speech. The SLP may train the student to use an alternative communication method to speech or the SLP may train the student augmentatively, using a combination of spoken output and a communication device. According to the American Speech-Language-Hearing Association (2004) and others (McCormick & Wegner, 2003; Silverman, 1989), this responsibility includes the following aspects:

1. Identifying appropriate candidates for AAC
2. Selecting the communication mode or modes that will meet the student's communication needs
3. Securing necessary hardware and software (through school purchasing or leasing)
4. Teaching the student how to use the mode selected for encoding and transmitting messages
5. Developing intervention plans to promote the student's maximal functional communication
6. Working with the education team, especially the classroom teacher, to implement the intervention plan in all school settings (lunch, gym, art, etc.)
7. Periodically reassessing the student's cognitive, motor, sensory, and communication abilities to ensure that the mode selected and semantic choices provided initially continue to meet the student's communication needs.

In introducing an augmentative or alternative communication system, the SLP often encounters resistance from a variety of sources. It is important for families and school personnel to recognize that introduction of an augmentative and alternative communication system does not interfere with speech acquisition. To the contrary, there are many reports describing increased speech following implementation of such systems. This substantial literature, reviewed by Abrahamsen, Romski, and Sevcik (1989), documents that users of augmentative and alternative communication demonstrate positive gains in: (1) speech production and comprehension; (2) attention span; (3) task orientation; and (4) social skills.

Legislative provisions for assistive technology have been included in the Individuals with Disabilities Education Act (IDEA) and the Americans with Disabilities Act (ADA-PL101-336). As stated by McCormick and Wegner (2003), both laws require that individuals with disabilities obtain whatever assistive devices they need, including items such as battery-powered toys, hearing aids, wheelchairs, computers, eating systems, augmentative communication devices, special switches, and a wide range of other devices that have the potential to improve an individual's ability to learn, compete, work, and interact with others. School districts are required to foster education by providing assistive technology devices and services to eligible children.

Communication may be achieved through a variety of high-tech and low-tech augmentative or alternative systems, such as pointing to picture boards, using sign language, accessing a symbolic code (manually or electronically), typing a message on a computer screen, or using a machine that produces a synthetic or digital voice. The past few years have also seen an explosion of technologically advanced and miniaturized systems such as palmtop, hand-held, and tablet devices. Table 12-2 lists some Web resources for viewing what is commercially available; it also provides some basic sites for resources on the general subject of augmentative and alternative communication.

It may be helpful to think of all augmentative/alternative communication systems as having four primary components: symbols, aids, strategies, and techniques (American Speech-Language-Hearing Association, 2004). Depending on the student's cognitive and physical skills, the symbols used may range from actual objects, pictures of objects, universal icons (e.g., Minspeak's icons of thumbs up, thumbs down, stop sign, and so forth) (Van Der Merwe & Alant, 2004), and traditional orthography (printed word). Teachers and classroom peers need to become familiar with the symbols used by a particular student for communication to occur. Aids refer to devices used to

Table 12-2 A Sampling of Commercially Available Augmentative and Alternative Communication Devices and General Subject Information

Palmtop, handheld, tablet, or e-talk Dynavox systems are shown at www.enkidu.net or in the products section of www.dynavoxsystems.com

Assorted augmentative communication products, such as a picture–word boardmaker for the personal computer, a talking picture and word-processing program with over 8,000 pictures, or a tool for creating talking interactive activities for the class are shown at www.mayer-johnson.com

The American Speech-Language-Hearing Association provides basic information on augmentative and alternative communication at the following site; in particular, teachers and parents may be interested in the primer of terminology and articles on team approaches to evaluation and management. Visit www.asha.org/public/speech/disorders/augmentative-and-alternative.htm

The AAC Institute provides resources for people who rely on augmentative and alternative communication, their families, friends, educators, and professionals. The education/training information may be of particular interest through www.aacinstitute.org

Low-tech and high-tech products at www.communicationaids.com include the Crestwood line of communication boards, mounting kits, picture kits, talking aids, switches, amplifiers, and more.

Full-service hardware and software systems and support are provided by the Prentke Romich Company at www.prentrom.com

transmit or receive messages. These vary from the very simple and basic to complex technological systems. Strategies refer to ways in which symbols can be conveyed effectively. Techniques refer to the various ways messages can be transmitted—either through direct selection or scanning.

Classroom teachers must work with the SLP to understand the communication system and the ways to interact with the student. Teachers also need to be familiar with the device used by a particular student in case the teacher needs to make quick repairs to limit the student's downtime (Daniel, 2004). Although it is beyond the scope of this text to explain the intricacies of alternative devices (Glennen & DeCoste, 1997, is a thorough source), the SLP should be able to provide detailed assistance on the use of any student's particular system. Roles and responsibilities suggested for the classroom teacher on the AAC team are presented in Table 12-3.

Augmentative and alternative communication has become a vast subject and most all school systems have had or will have students needing such accommodations. It must be remembered that the primary role of ACC systems is to facilitate active participation and engagement in meaningful events in the daily lives of handicapped students. And, it is in this light that teachers and classroom peers must take the responsibility to become true conversational partners.

Table 12-3 Suggested Roles for the Classroom Teacher on the AAC Team

- Adapt the curriculum for the student using an AAC system.
- Write goals and objectives for the student user and maintain documentation.
- Informally assess and frequently reassess the cognitive abilities of the student (the school psychologist could assist with formal cognitive testing).
- Act as a liaison with the family and between all educational team members.
- Assess, and frequently reassess, the student's social capabilities.
- Provide for ongoing skill development.
- Identify content specific vocabulary to be programmed or added to the student's AAC system.
- Provide information about the student's motivation and attitude toward the AAC system.
- Determine the student's communication needs throughout the school day, working closely with the speech-language pathologist.
- Know the system well enough to use it within all settings across the curriculum.
- Provide training or instruction for classroom peers to use the device conversationally with the student.

Source: McCormick & Wegner, 2003.

According to Beukelman and Mirenda (1992), participation is a prerequisite to communication: without participation there is no one to talk to, nothing to talk about, and no reason to communicate. Maria, aged 3 years, is in a wheelchair and has limited use of her hands and semi-intelligible speech. The preschool teacher and SLP wish to enhance Maria's participation in small-group playtime. At present she just sits in her wheelchair and watches peers play in the toy kitchen or with blocks and other manipulable toys. Together the teacher and the SLP plan intervention strategies so that Maria's lap tray becomes a play surface: some toys have been adapted with Velcro so she can pick them up wearing a Velcro glove, and a smaller toy stove and sink have been purchased for use on the lap tray (instead of the large play kitchen furniture). Also the battery-operated blender has been adapted for switch activation. These adaptations to the play situation are generating two-way communication among Maria and her peers, allowing for much needed speech and language practice. The context-based communication is also aiding peers' understanding of Maria's speech as she simultaneously manipulates toys and real objects.

Tyrone's cerebral palsy has meant that he has long needed AAC systems for communicative interactions but now, in the second grade, his experiences with symbols and iconic encoding (such as Minspeak) are about to change. The AAC team, especially the speech-language pathologist and the classroom teacher, are transitioning Tyrone to learn orthography for reading and writing development. The vocabulary of the curriculum is becoming more diverse (in language arts, math, science, music, social studies) and Tyrone's thirst for knowledge and participation are growing too. The AAC team is supplying and training Tyrone with computer-based options involving an orthographic keyboard with speech synthesis, screen-reader software (for reading enlarged print texts entered into the system), and written literacy software (for Tyrone to compose and write). His typing skills, though slow and laborious, are sufficient for his total communication and educational advancement.

Swallowing Disorders of Dysphagia

The role and scope of practice in speech-language pathology includes the burgeoning area of evaluation and treatment of swallowing disorders, or **dysphagia** (ASHA, 2002). While pediatric swallowing and feeding disorders are not communication disorders per se, they do share some of the same anatomical structures and issues of neuromuscular control. Students with cerebral palsy or dysarthria are likely to present with dysphagia as well, and this presents another opportunity for the classroom teacher and speech-language pathologist to work collaboratively. Indeed, as in the example presented next, (Logemann & Sonies, 2004), the classroom teacher may be the person to suspect a problem and make a referral to the SLP.

A 5-year-old child was referred to the SLP in a public school because he refused to eat snacks with the other children and was noted to be uncoordinated and small for his age. On investigation with the family, it was discovered that the child had anoxia at birth, was diagnosed with mild cerebral palsy, and at one time had been diagnosed through imaging studies to have oropharyngeal dysphagia and gastroesophageal reflux. A feeding tube had once been used and later a private clinician had worked with the child on oral feeding. Later, it was said the child did not like to brush his teeth, would refuse certain foods, and generally was a picky eater. He often made nonnutritive chewing motions and sucked on clothing and soft toys. He was "floppy" and ill-coordinated during playtime at school, and so was not included in some tasks. At parties for children, he did not put anything into his mouth, preferring to smell or lick items rather than taste them. Upon evaluation of the child's strengths and weaknesses, the SLP determined that this student was a candidate for services, noting on the individualized education program (IEP) how the disabilities affected the child's participation in appropriate school activities. The parents obtained an updated swallowing study at the local medical facility and all parties involved determined that intervention was both safe and educationally necessary. The school SLP focused on oral (tactile) desensitization, behavior modification, and restructuring the environment at home (with the parents) and at school (with the classroom teacher).

Teacher Tips for Students with Neuromuscular Problems

Students with neuromuscular problems, such as cerebral palsy, dysarthria, and dysphagia present with multiple handicaps. In the past, the majority of these students were placed inappropriately into residential institutes or special day schools. With the advent of PL 94-142, IDEA, and the ADA, students with dysarthria and cerebral palsy are now educated in regular and special classes within public school systems. Many have sufficient intellectual capacity for education in the normal classroom setting. Classroom teachers, however, may need to provide these students with extra attention, understanding, and the willingness to modify or adapt academic assignments. The following suggestions are adapted from Eisenson and Ogilvie (1983), Phillips (1984), and from Sexson and Dingle (2001):

1. Help the student adjust to the group and instill a sense of belonging. Being socially accepted by classroom peers is difficult for the student who may look different, talk with slurred and labored speech, and walk with a staggered gait or not at all. Social adjustment problems may amplify during adolescence. School dances, first dates, sports, learning to drive a car, and acceptable speech are just some of the ways students with neuromuscular problems are "left out." Feeling depressed, discouraged, resentful, and rebellious are emotions common to youth with handicaps. As a teacher, recognize the need for referral to a counselor when a student's feelings become too negative.
2. Provide understanding, not sympathy or pity.
3. Encourage and provide opportunities for classmates to maintain contact and communication with the student.
4. Expect the student to perform tasks that are within his/her capabilities. Do not allow the handicapping condition to become an "excuse."
5. Speech is best when the student is relaxed. Set a casual, relaxed classroom atmosphere. Tasks that frustrate also tend to cause deterioration of speech intelligibility.
6. Support any specific educational accommodations needed, such as test conditions, note taking, large print, and so forth.
7. Modify the environment to suit the motorically involved student. For example, consider placing the student's desk (or other apparatus) in the most accessible location. With young children using augmentative communication devices, positioning of the device with other manipulables (crayons, clay, lunch, maps, globes) is critical and must be learned by teachers.
8. Frequently review the child's learning capabilities and formally evaluate (or refer for evaluation) as needed.
9. Help the child break assignments into discrete tasks to facilitate an organized and successful approach.
10. Be aware of any chewing or swallowing dysfunctions and, when appropriate, assist with safe intake approaches during classroom parties, snacks, and lunch.

11. Encourage participation in all regular classroom activities, yet allow for special considerations. For instance, a student who cannot hold a pencil well or write legibly may do much better typing class work on a typewriter or computer.

12. Be willing to assist the speech-language pathologist in providing speech and language stimulation, or to assist in communicating with alternative systems frequently throughout the school day. Students on an augmentative communication system often need much encouragement to use the device in the classroom and to interact with peers. A teacher's assistance is invaluable here.

STUDENTS WITH TRAUMATIC BRAIN INJURY

Youth and young adulthood represent age groups that are extremely vulnerable to **traumatic brain injuries** (**TBI**). Potentially dangerous pastimes these ages enjoy include: bicycling, skateboarding, trampolining, driving all-terrain vehicles, cruising in a car, gang activities, and so forth. The term **closed head injuries** (**CHI**) is used when the brain has been damaged in an accident, yet the skull has not been penetrated. In contrast, a bullet penetrates the skull and destroys a specific path through brain tissues. The resulting neurologic deficits from such an **open head wound** may be surprisingly minor if the bullet entered a not-so-critical area of the brain. Closed head injuries, on the other hand, often result in widespread damage and the neurologic disability often is quite extensive. Imagine the areas of widespread damage that might occur when a person's head impacts the dashboard or windshield of a car. The brain, suspended within the bony skull, continues its forward momentum despite impact, hitting the front of the bony skull (causing what is known as *coup* damage), and then rebounding with great force to hit the back of the bony skull (causing *contrecoup* injury). Damage also may occur as the brain moves and bends over rough bones at the base of the skull. All of this rotary movement of the brain tears or shears many blood vessels and nerve fibers. Unconsciousness, either brief or prolonged, may result from disruption of nerve fibers going to the brain stem. Loss of consciousness occurs in about 50% of children with brain injuries (Segalowitz & Lawson, 1995). Closed head injuries are the more common type of TBI and often are the result of motor vehicle accidents, falls, sports injuries, or abuse. Children and young adults tend to be involved in such injuries, with junior and senior high-school-aged students most vulnerable.

Following an accident, doctors initially work to control bleeding, maintain oxygen supply, and treat shock. There may be associated injuries in the abdomen, pelvis, and chest that need immediate attention. The brain damage sustained during the accident may be worsened by secondary complications such as brain swelling and bleeding into or around the brain. These complications, too, may result in death or may directly affect later neurologic function in a recovering patient. Predicting long-term outcomes and degree of disability is difficult. However, recovery tends to be good, though not necessarily complete, following most brain injuries (Brumback et al., 2001).

Once the patient is out of immediate danger, the rehabilitation team at the medical facility begins the rehabilitation program in earnest. Acute hospitalization often lasts a few weeks to a few months; some patients are discharged to specialized rehabilitation hospitals or centers for continued therapies. As soon as the student returns home, the public school system is responsible for ensuring that a homebound teacher is provided as well as speech-language services, physical therapy, and other support services as needed. Counseling is often a very important aspect of the initial adjustment for the student and family. The emotional state of the student and severity of injury are extremely important factors. Eventually, the decision regarding the appropriateness of a return to school is made, and the student may begin with only one or two classes per day. Reintegration of a a student with a head injury into the school is a challenge for the student, the family, and the entire educational system. The TBI student is likely to present with a myriad of problems. It has often been said that no matter how serious the physical disabilities are following an injury, the neuropsychological and behavioral abnormalities will be the most limiting factors in recovery and the major reason for stress within the family.

According to Brumback and colleagues (2001), studies of the long-term effects of brain injury on cognitive functioning in children following even mild brain injury have found that the most consistent impairments involve visuospatial skills and verbal abilities. Other reported effects include sleep disturbances, social difficulties, altered handedness pattern, attention disturbances, depression, and reading disorders.

The widespread nature of the brain damage may cause unusual kinds of behavior and learning patterns in the student. School systems typically have no specific programs for students with head injuries and, therefore, place them back into the same class schedule as before the accident. Such an inappropriate placement often results in emotional distress and academic failure. At other times, school systems will place students with head injuries into learning disability programs or classes for the mentally retarded. Again, placement often is inappropriate. Each student with TBI who returns to school will present with a unique combination of deficits. The educational team should be aware of the student's deficits and be prepared to plan for them with flexibility. Table 12-4 lists possible deficit areas of returning students, compiled from the writings of Blosser and DePompei (1994), DePompei and Blosser (1987), Griffith (1983), and from the definition of TBI provided by the federal Division of Special Education (*Federal Register*, 1992).

The list below of TBI characteristics may sound similar to other handicapped conditions, yet their interactions produce some unique needs and the necessity for specialized teaching strategies. The TBI student is not like the typical learning-disabled or multihandicapped student, and the educational plan should reflect an understanding of the differences. (For example, the reading teacher must not assume that teaching reading skills to a TBI student

Table 12-4 Neuropsychological and Behavioral Deficit Areas Often Present in TBI Students Returning to School

Physical	Impairments can exist in mobility, strength, coordination, vision, and/or hearing.
Communication	Problems may include deficits in processing and sequencing information, use of "confused" language, dysarthric articulation, prosody abnormalities, word-finding (anomia), reading, writing, computation, and abstraction difficulties.
Cognitive	Difficulties can be found with long- and short-term memory, thought processes, reasoning, conceptual skills, problem solving, decreased abstraction, decreased learning abilities, and mental fatigue.
Perceptual motor	Involvement can include visual neglect (of, say, half the printed page), visual field cuts, motor apraxia, motor speed, motor sequencing, distractibility, reduced hand–eye coordination, and spatial disorientation.
Behavioral-emotional	Problems can account for impulsivity, poor judgment, disinhibition, dependence, anger outburst, displacing aggressive behavior or bizarre/psychotic behavior, denial, depression, emotional lability, apathy, lethargy, poor motivation, poor initiative, inability to make decisions, and poor attention span.
Social	Impairments can result in the TBI student not learning from peers, not generalizing from social situations, behaving like a much younger child, withdrawing, becoming distracted in noisy surroundings, and becoming lost or disoriented even in familiar surroundings.

is like teaching to a student with developmental reading problems.) Blosser and DePompei (1994), Cohen, Joyce, Rhodes, and Welks (1985), and Rosen and Gerring (1986) cite some of the characteristic and frustrating differences between the TBI student and those with other handicaps:

1. Students with TBI have previous successful experiences in academic and social settings; they may retain the premorbid self-concept of being perfectly normal.
2. Discrepancies in ability levels may be more extreme. Learning problems may exist even though some skills remain relatively unaffected. For example, the level of reading comprehension may be 4 years lower than spelling ability.
3. There may be inconsistent patterns of performance. Uneven progress can occur because of continuing recovery. Programs must maintain flexibility to accommodate sharp and frequent improvements.
4. Students with TBI often learn more rapidly than learning disabled students. To "relearn" material, a reacquaintance with the process or concept may be all that is necessary.
5. Students with TBI may have more extreme problems with generalizing, integrating, or structuring information. More individualized instruction may be necessary. They may not be able to process even limited amounts of information; comprehension deteriorates markedly as the quantity and complexity of material increases.

The educational setting can be an ideal situation in which to continue the student's rehabilitation toward relearning and new learning. Structure is vitally important and must encompass social and academic activities. For such coordination to take place, all disciplines must work closely together. To assist in a student's smooth transition, the rehabilitation team members from the medical facility should be invited to participate with the educational team and the parents in the multidisciplinary evaluation and formulation of the individualized educational plan (IEP). A typical team for a student with TBI would include an SLP, physical therapist, occupational therapist, vocational rehabilitation counselor, parents, special education teacher, and classroom teacher(s). Much can be gained for the student when such open communication exists. Discussion about skills, needs, and problems related to reentry should be encouraged. For those students who are junior high or senior high-school age, vocational evaluation and training may become priority goals. If the student is no longer ambulatory, special transportation skills may become a need.

The SLP should be an active participant in planning for the reintegration of a student with a head injury into the school. This is true because the SLP possesses an understanding of language and learning problems as well as other specific skills that will benefit the reentry process. These skills, as cited by DePompei and Blosser (1987), include the following:

1. In-depth understanding of anatomy and physiology as it relates to language processing
2. Ability to observe and diagnose subtle communication deficits and hidden inadequacies of the communication system
3. Proficiency in objective evaluation procedures
4. Ability to establish remediation goals based upon hierarchical approach, working from a simple to complex continuum
5. Understanding of the process for teaching judgment, organization, planning, and problem solving
6. Understanding of the communication requirements necessary for task performance at various academic levels
7. Awareness of the impact communication deficits can have on school success
8. Awareness of the pragmatic skills necessary for social interaction and communication
9. Understanding of physical environmental factors that can interfere with learning and communication

Blosser and DePompei (1994) provide excellent examples of cognitive-communicative interventions using functional outcome-based plans. These plans are useful by both SLPs and classroom teachers. Concrete examples are provided for goals such as developing cognitive skills for math, adapting amount of auditory information for enhanced receptive language, increasing ability to respond to questioning and engage in concise conversations (expressive language), taking turns and self-monitoring aspects of pragmatic language, and so forth.

Teacher Tips for Students with TBI

As discussed by Cohen (1991) and by Cohen and his colleagues (1985), strategies are procedures that help a student clarify, organize, remember, and express information. Strategies help structure and emphasize parts of the learning process that a student with a head injury previously performed automatically. This treatment approach is also endorsed by Snow and Hooper (1994). It is suggested that the teacher spend time teaching the student *how* to use these strategies and *why* they should be used. At first, the teacher uses strategies to structure the environment or the student's behavior (e.g., blocking out everything but the sentence the student is to read). The teacher then cues the student to apply the compensatory strategies in specific situations. The ultimate goal is for the student to use the strategies independently (e.g., to take out a marker and use it to keep the place when reading). Thus programming should progress from the point at which the teacher implements strategies to the point at which the student is expected to use them independently. Table 12-5 presents some of the cognitive-communicative problems that a student with a head injury demonstrates and strategies that can be used to compensate for them. The SLP and teacher should work collaboratively on identifying problems and useful strategies for each particular TBI student.

The following list of techniques and classroom adaptations also can be implemented to help the student (Blosser & DePompei, 1994; DePompei & Blosser, 1987). Educators working with a TBI student should use as many of these techniques as possible during classroom activities.

1. Plan many small group activities to facilitate learning of appropriate interaction skills.
2. Clarify verbal and written instructions in the following ways:
   a. Alert the student to the important topic or concept being taught ("I'm going to tell a story, and then we'll discuss where it takes place.").
   b. Accompany verbal instructions with written instructions.
   c. Repeat instructions and redefine words and terms.
   d. Verbally explain written instructions or assign a "classroom buddy" to do so.
3. Privately ask the student to repeat information and/or answer a few key questions to be sure that important information presented has been understood. Care should be taken, however, not to cause stress in students who have difficulty responding to direct questions.
4. Use pauses when giving classroom instructions to allow time for processing information.
5. Because response time is often delayed, provide the student with ample time to respond verbally and to complete in-class and home assignments.

Table 12-5 Compensatory Strategies for Cognitive Problems in a Classroom Setting

Attending problems: Student may be unable to attend to auditory and visual information. He or she may do such things as talk out of turn or change the topic, be distracted by noise in the hall, fidget, or poke others. It is important to note that the student may maintain eye contact and appear to be listening and actually not be attending.

Strategies:
- Remove unnecessary distractions such as pencils and books. Limit background noise at first and gradually increase it to more normal levels.
- Provide visual cues to attend (e.g., have a sign on student's desk with the word or pictured symbol for behaviors, such as *look* or *listen*). Point to the sign when the student is off task.
- Limit the amount of information on a page.
- Adjust assignments to the length of the student's attention span so that he or she can complete tasks successfully.
- Focus the student's attention on specific information: "I'm going to read a story and ask *who* is in the story."
- Both partners in a communication dyad should reduce utterance length, reduce sentence complexity, reduce rate of speech (or increase pause time), and vary intonation patterns to emphasize key words.

Difficulties with language comprehension or following directions: Student may have difficulty understanding language that is spoken rapidly, is complex, or is lengthy.

Strategies:
- Limit amount of information presented, perhaps to 1–2 sentences.
- Reduce rate of delivery.
- Use more concrete language.
- Teach student to ask for clarification or repetitions or for information to be given at a slower rate.
- Give prompts and assistance such as using pictures or written words to cue students or pairing manual signs, gestures, or pictures with verbal information.
- Act out directions: If the student is to collect papers and put them in a designated spot, demonstrate how this should be done.
- Use cognitive mapping: Diagram ideas in order of importance or sequence to clarify content graphically. This also helps students to see part–whole relationships.
- See also strategies listed under memory and attending that can be used to improve language comprehension.

Memory problems: Student may be unable to retain information he or she has heard or read and may not remember where to go or what materials to use.

Strategies:
- Include pictures or visual cues with oral information, since this multisensory input strengthens the information and provides various ways to recall it.

continues

Table 12-5 *continued*

- Use visual imagery. Have student form a mental picture of information that is presented orally. Retrieval of the visual images may trigger the recall of oral information.
- Use verbal rehearsal. After the visual or auditory information is presented, have the student "practice" it (repeat it) and *listen to himself or herself* before acting on it.
- Limit the amount of information presented so that the student can retain and retrieve it.
- Provide a matrix for the student to refer to if he or she has difficulty recalling information (such as a number fact chart).
- Have the student take notes or record information on tape.
- Underline key words in a passage for emphasis.
- Provide a log book to record assignments or daily events.
- Provide a printed or pictured schedule of daily activities, locations, and materials needed.
- Role-play or pantomime stories or procedures to strengthen the information to be remembered.
- Write down key information to be remembered, such as who, what, and when. Help the student develop note-taking skills.

Retrieving information that has been stored in memory and word-finding difficulties:

Strategies:

- Have student gesture or role-play. He or she may be able to act out a situation that has occurred but not have adequate verbal language to describe it.
- Provide visual or auditory cues: "Is it _ or _?" or give the beginning sound of a word.
- Include written multiple choice cues or pictures in worksheets.
- Teach student to compensate for word-finding problems by describing the function, size, or other attributes of items to be recalled.

Difficulties organizing and sequencing information: Student may have difficulty understanding, recognizing, displaying, or describing a sequence of events presented orally or visually.

Strategies:

- Limit the number of steps in a task.
- Present part of a sequence and have student finish it.
- Show or discuss one step of the sequence (lesson) at a time.
- Give general cues with each step: "What should you do first? Second?"
- Have student repeat multistep directions and listen to self before attempting a task.
- Present information in chunks or help student group it.
- Provide pictures or a written sequence of steps to remember: Tape a cue card to the desk with words or pictures of materials needed for a lesson, then expand original written directions. For example, if the direction was "Underline the words in each sentence in which *ou* or *ow* stands for the vowel sound. Then write the two words that have the same vowel sound," change it to "(1) Read the sentence; (2) underline *ou* and *ow* words; (3) read the underlined words; (4) find the two words that have the same vowel sounds; (5) write these two words on the lines below the sentence."

- Introduce information with attention-getting words.
- Tell student how many steps are in a task: "I'm going to tell you three things to do." (Hold up three fingers.)
- Act out a sequence of events to clarify information.
- Provide sample items describing how to proceed through parts of a worksheet.
- Number the steps in a written direction and have the student cross off each step as it is completed.
- Teach student to refer to directions if he or she is unsure of the task.

Thought disorganization: Student has difficulty organizing thoughts in oral or written language. Students may not have adequate labels or vocabulary to convey a clear message; he or she may tend to ramble without getting to the point.

Strategies:
- Attempt to limit impulsive responses by encouraging the student to take "thinking time" before answering.
- Have student organize information by using categories, such as who, what, when, and where. (Emphasize each of these separately if necessary.) This strategy can be used in an expanded form to write a story.
- Teach student a sequence of steps to aid in verbal organization: have the student use cue cards with written pictured steps when formulating an answer.
- Focus on one type of information at a time (e.g., the main idea).
- Decrease rambling by having student express a thought "in one sequence."

Problems with generalization: Student learns a skill or concept but has difficulty applying it to other situations (e.g., may count a group of coins in a structured mathematics lesson but not be able to count money for lunch).

Strategies:
- Teach the structure or format of a task (e.g., how to complete a worksheet or mathematics problem).
- Maintain a known format and change the content of a task to help student see a relationship: Two pictures are presented and student must say if they are in the same category, or have the same initial sound; a worksheet format requires filling in blanks with words or numbers.
- Change the format of the task: Have student solve mathematics facts on a worksheet as well as on flash cards.
- Have completed sample worksheets in a notebook serve as models indicating how to proceed.
- Demonstrate how skills can be used throughout the day. For example, discuss how the student relies on the clock or a schedule to get up in the morning, begin school, or catch a bus.
- Role-play situations that simulate those that the student may encounter, emphasizing the generalization of specific skills taught; for example, completing school assignments and going to the store may involve the same strategies of making a list or asking for help.

Sources: Blosser & DePompei, 1994; Cohen, 1991; Cohen, Joyce, Rhoades, & Welks, 1985.

6. Avoid figurative, idiomatic, ambiguous, and sarcastic language when presenting lessons (example: "You're a ham.").

7. Select a classroom buddy to keep the student aware of instructions, transitions, and assignments.

8. Permit the student to use assistive devices such as a calculator, tape recorder, and/or computer.

9. Help the student formulate and use a system for maintaining organization. Require the student to carry a written log of activities, schedule of classes, list of assignments and due dates, and room locations. Frequently monitor the student's use of the organization system.

10. Schedule a specific time for rest and/or emotional release. Encourage the student to share any problems being experienced.

11. Plan extracurricular activities based on the student's physical and emotional capabilities as well as interests.

12. Structure the physical environment of the classroom to decrease distractions and permit ease of movement by carefully planning seating and furniture arrangements.

13. Modify and individualize the student's assignments and tests to accommodate special needs. Examples of modifications include reducing the number of questions to be answered or amount of material to be read, permitting the student to tape record the teacher's lectures or responses to test questions, and changing the format of a task.

14. Develop resources to accompany textbook assignments. For example, use pictures and written cues to illustrate important information and concepts. Assign review questions at the end of chapters. Write new vocabulary. Present a summary of a chapter on tape or paper. Go over errors made on tests to let the student know where and why errors occurred.

15. Establish a system of verbal or nonverbal signals to cue the student to attend, respond, or alter behavior (examples include calling the student's name, touching, written signs, or hand signals).

Above all, access the team of specialists who are serving the student (SLP, occupational therapist, physical therapist, vocational rehabilitation counselor, and course or special education teachers). As a teacher, ask for these consultants to come and help work through problems, especially in the early phases as the student is adjusting. Also, it is important to remember to keep in close contact with the parents regarding the student's attitude, stamina, emotional ability, self-concept, perceptions of peer relations, use of medication (many students are seizure-prone), and other important but frequently changing characteristics of the student.

ATTENTION DEFICIT/HYPERACTIVITY DISORDER

An increasing number of students who exhibit learning and behavior problems are being diagnosed as having **Attention Deficit/Hyperactivity Disorder (ADHD)**. Although not a communication disorder as such, ADHD results in a complex pattern of interrelated problems in attention, behavior, organization, peer interactions, and social competence that affect the student's ability to communicate effectively and to perform many of the tasks expected in the classroom. It is not our purpose here to provide a detailed discussion of the neurologic research on this disorder; however, it is important that teachers realize that the condition of ADHD stems from a neurologic basis. The American Psychiatric Association (1994) recognizes three types of ADHD. One type is characterized by a combination of inattention and hyperactivity–impulsivity. A second type has inattention as a predominant symptom and children with the third type primarily exhibit hyperactivity and impulsivity. ADHD is not well understood by many classroom teachers, and the children exhibiting this disorder are even less well understood. In fact, Jordan (1992) stated the following:

> It would be accurate to say that most persons who have ADHD or ADD are among the most seriously misunderstood individuals within our culture. They live most of their developmental years being misunderstood and failing to understand the world around them (p. 42).

Children with ADHD have, over the years, been assigned to a number of different diagnostic categories including learning disabilities, minimal brain dysfunction, and hyperactivity. These children also have been, and in many instances still are, frequently accused of being lazy, inattentive, disobedient, or just plain dumb. Even when a diagnosis of ADHD has been made, many teachers fail to understand that this is a neurologic disorder that cannot be changed in a short period of time with a system of behavior-contingent rewards and punishments. Scolding, detention, or other punishments are no more likely to make ADHD students improve their attention and memory than they are to make wheelchair-bound students walk.

Students with ADHD usually have average or above average intelligence. But these students are likely to experience difficulty in the classroom as a result of problems in the following areas:

- Organization and memory
- On task behavior
- Time management
- Rigidity
- Inappropriate and out-of-proportion reactions
- Problems with peer relationships
- Frustration resulting from failed socialization and academic difficulties
- General immaturity

Children with ADHD tend to operate on their own schedules, which are different from those of their age peers and certainly different from those that adults try to impose upon them. This is true in terms of maturation and readiness to deal with various concepts as well as in the time required to complete tasks.

When no accommodations are made for their disorder, students with ADHD experience a myriad of difficulties in the classroom, as discussed in the following section.

Problems Frequently Encountered by ADHD Students

Inability to Follow Verbal Directions

Because of an inability to process connected speech quickly, to focus attention on the spoken message, to separate important information from less important information, and to remember a sequence of instructions, students with ADHD frequently have difficulty doing what they are asked to do. Jordan (1992) reported that students with ADHD comprehend only about 30% of the information presented to them through the auditory channel. As a result, these children are frequently confused about what they are to do. Some may ask for instructions to be repeated. Many ADHD students, however, will not admit to the teacher and their classmates that they did not understand the instructions because of the emotional sensitivity that accompanies this disorder and because of past negative experiences with an exasperated teacher or the snickering of classmates. These students simply go ahead and do the wrong thing.

Inability to Finish Assignments

Because of an inability to stay on task, students with ADHD simply cannot complete most tasks as quickly as their peers. This is true of tests as well as written assignments and class projects. Unfortunately, instead of providing more time for the ADHD student, teachers frequently respond to unfinished tasks with punishment such as detention or missed rewards, which does nothing more than increase the student's frustration.

An interesting pattern noted in the work of many students with ADHD is a deterioration in performance as the task progresses. It is not unusual to see a student with ADHD make the majority of errors on the second part of a spelling or math test. It seems that they can focus their attention for a while, but not for the duration of the test (Jordan,1992).

Other reasons for problems with timed tasks include the inability to hold one piece of information in memory while processing another part of the problem, having to rely on finger counting or other manipulatives to perform basic addition and subtraction, and agonizing over choices in multiple choice or true–false test formats.

Poorly Organized and Messy Assignments

Assignments prepared by students with ADHD frequently reflect the lack of organization and scattered attention that characterize the disorder. Any assignment that requires a certain orderly progression will be extraordinarily challenging for these students. Whether it is placing in logical sequence the events which led to the Revolutionary War, conducting and/or describing a science project, or solving a multistep mathematics problem, the student with ADHD will have difficulty with the organization and execution. Written work is typically characterized by numerous erasures with resulting ripped and crinkled papers, misspelling, and punctuation errors (see Figure 12-1). Artwork often resembles that of a much younger child. These students often have notebooks and desks that are in such disarray that they cannot find the materials needed to complete assignments. Sometimes they cannot find the assignments they have completed to turn in to the teacher.

Difficulties with Homework

Homework is a particularly challenging part of school for students with ADHD. First, there is the formidable task of remembering exactly what it is

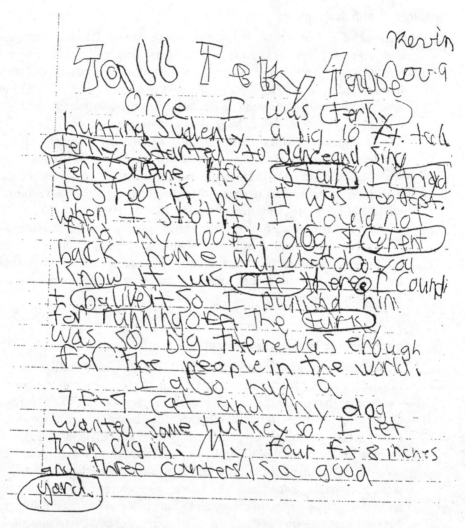

Figure 12-1 A Story Written by a Fifth-Grade Student with ADHD. Notice the Writing, Phonetic Spelling, and Incomplete Erasures. The Story is Supposed to be as Follows.

Tall Turkey

Once I was turkey hunting. Suddenly a big 10 ft. turkey started to dance and sing, "Turkey in the Straw." I tried to shoot it, but it was too fast. When I shot it, I could not find my 100 ft. dog. I went back home, and what do you know, it was right there. I couldn't believe it, so I punished him for running off. The turkey was so big there was enough for the people in the world. I also had a 7 ft. 7 cat and my dog wanted some turkey so I let them dig in. My four ft 8 inches and three quarters is a good guard.

they are to do. Even when they can remember what the task is they frequently forget to bring home the texts or other materials required to complete the task. A typical dialogue between parent and a child with ADHD might go something like this:

Parent: How was school today?

Child: OK.

Parent: Do you have any homework?

Child: We have a test tomorrow.

Parent: In which class are you having a test?

Child: I forget.

Parent: Well, which teacher told you that you were having a test?

Child: I think it was Mrs. Smith.

Parent: Well, Mrs. Smith teaches social studies. Is your test in social studies?

Child: I guess.

Parent: Where is your social studies book?

Child: I left it at school. Oh, Mrs. Jones says I have to miss storytime tomorrow because I didn't do my chapter summary.

Parent: We did your chapter summary last night. Why didn't you hand it in?

Child: I couldn't find it.

Parent: AAAGGHH!

Another problem with homework is that it takes students with ADHD far longer than other students to complete the homework assignments. What might be a half-hour homework assignment for most students may take two hours or more for the student with ADHD.

Many ADHD students take medication such as Ritalin to help them focus attention. The effects of the medication typically wear off by homework time. The parents are faced with the choice of giving the child more medication so he or she can do the homework, or trying to get an unmedicated child to focus attention on the assignment that may be only partially understood to begin with.

Interpersonal Skills

Many students with ADHD have difficulty relating to peers and, sometimes, interacting appropriately with adults. These students tend to be less mature than students of similar chronological age and are often more comfortable and more successful when interacting with younger children. As a result, ADHD students are frequently social outcasts among their age peers. Many ADHD students are very sensitive and react to this social ostracism in a negative and often inappropriate or immature fashion. Their reaction then tends to reinforce their status as an outsider. Because they have difficulty with impulse control, students with ADHD are also prone to lash out in both a verbally and physically aggressive manner against those whom they feel are treating them unjustly. To make matters worse, students with ADHD, once committed to a course of action, are often unable to alter that course regardless of the circumstances. For example, most students know better than to retaliate against another student when a teacher is looking. Students with ADHD, however, seem unable to suppress their behavior and are more likely to be "caught in the act." This social frustration combines with academic difficulty experienced by many students with ADHD to make school a very unpleasant place.

Accommodations to Help the Student with ADHD

Students with ADHD are entitled to accommodations under a variety of federal laws, including the Rehabilitation Act of 1973, the Individuals With Disabilities Education Act of 2004 (IDEA), and the Americans With Disabilities Act of 1992 (ADA). The effects of ADHD on academic performance vary among individuals. As a result, many children with ADHD may not qualify for services under IDEA. Those students, as indicated in Chapter 1 of this text, may still be eligible for services under section 504 of the Rehabilitation Act of 1973. Section 504 is a civil rights statute that requires that schools not discriminate against students with disabilities and that they provide students with reasonable accommodations. If a student is eligible for accommodations under section 504, the school must develop a 504 plan. One significant difference between a 504 plan and an IEP is that regulations governing 504 plans do not specify the frequency with which a plan should be reviewed and do not specify the rights of parents to be involved in the development of the plan (Children and Adults with Attention-Deficit/Hyperactivity Disorder, 2001).

Some of the possible accommodations which may prove helpful to ADHD students whether they are covered by federal legislation or not are included in the following lists:

Homework

1. Provide an assignment notebook which is *checked daily by the teacher.*
2. Check to ensure that appropriate books and materials are taken home.
3. Textbooks and other materials can be supplied to the parents.

4. Establish a "buddy system" where a reliable student is assigned to help remind the student with ADHD what the assignments are and which materials need to be taken home.
5. Notify parents of upcoming tests and assignments.
6. Establish a voice mail system at the school, where parents call to check on assignments.
7. Reduce the amount of homework for students with ADHD, perhaps assigning every other math problem or half of the questions at the end of the chapter.

Classroom Activities

1. Check to see if the student with ADHD is on task and gently remind him or her when attention wanders.
2. Physical proximity to the teacher often serves as a reminder for the child to stay on task.
3. Provide additional time to complete tasks.
4. Check to be sure that the student understands directions. Do not simply ask, "Is that clear?" but say something like, "Show/tell me how you are going to do this."
5. Help older students to develop note-taking skills.
6. Help the student to maintain an organized notebook. Notebooks with dividers and pockets may help students with ADHD to organize assignments and notes.
7. Allow students to tape record lectures.
8. In schools where students change classrooms, an attempt should be made to keep these changes to a minimum for students with ADHD.
9. Consider alternative test methods:
   a. Consider allowing the ADHD student to take tests alone rather than with the rest of the class.
   b. Avoid computer scan sheets.
   c. Avoid writing test items on the blackboard.
   d. Avoid using faded or poor quality copies of tests.
   e. Print or type test questions; avoid using cursive.
10. Be aware of potential difficulty with multistep tasks.
11. Do not assume that students with ADHD will draw appropriate conclusions.
12. Identify the best learning avenue. Some children may be better visual learners than auditory, some better auditory than visual.

In addition to the general suggestions above, Kline, Silver, and Russell (2001) provide the following suggestions that are specific to children who exhibit predominantly inattentive type ADHD and those who exhibit predominantly hyperactivity–impulsivity type. For children who have problems with inattention and distractibility Kline, Silver, and Russell suggest:

1. Shorten the task, or break one task into several smaller parts.
2. For rote tasks use shorter more frequent sessions rather than fewer longer sessions.
3. Use hand signals to remind the student to refocus.

For children who exhibit the predominantly hyperactive–impulsive type ADHD, Kline, Silver, and Russell (2001) suggest:

1. When possible, allow nondisruptive, directed movement in the classroom or standing during seat work.
2. Use activity as a reward.
3. Teach substitute verbal or motor responses that the child may use while waiting his or her turn.
4. Allow the student with ADHD to doodle with paper clips or other items while waiting or listening to instructions.

Socialization and Behavior

1. Be aware of the behavior problems that may result from ADHD.
   a. Inability to inhibit responses
   b. Overreaction
   c. Immaturity
2. Avoid situations that tend to exacerbate behavior problems.
   a. Boisterous group activities
   b. Use preferential seating on the schoolbus, in the cafeteria, at assemblies, etc.
3. Help students manage peer relations.
   a. Students with ADHD are often "easy marks" for teasing and bullying.
   b. Students with ADHD tend to retaliate without regard for consequences.

Medications

As mentioned earlier, many students with ADHD may take one of several available medications to help control the symptoms of ADHD. In spite of what many people think, these medications are not designed to sedate these children. Instead they are intended to increase the production or decrease the absorption of certain chemicals in the brain known as neurotransmitters (Kline, Silver, & Russell, 2001). In general, stimulants such a Ritalin or Dexedrine stimulate the production of neurotransmitters, and nonstimulants such as Strattera block the absorption of the neurotransmitter making it last longer in the child's system (Eli Lily Corporation, 2004). All medications have potential side effects and all must be given in the appropriate dosage. Teachers should be aware of any children in their class who are taking medication on a regular basis and should be aware of the possible side effects of those medications. Some things that teachers may be able to notice as well as or better than others in the child's environment are: signs that the medication is wearing off too soon, irritability (sometimes a rebound effect associated with the wearing off of the medication), appetite suppression, sluggishness, drowsiness, stomach pain, and behavior change when child forgets medication. Teachers should report the presence of any possible side effects to the parents or the school nurse (in schools where a nurse is on staff). Such reports by teachers can be quite helpful to the physician in determining the best medication and the most appropriate dosage.

REFERENCES

Abrahamsen, A.A., Romski, M.A., & Sevcik, R.A. (1989). Concomitants of success in acquiring an augmentative communication system: Changes in attention, communication, and sociability. *American Journal on Mental Retardation, 93*(5), 475–496.

American Psychiatric Association (1994). *Diagnostic and statistical manual of mental disorders* (4th ed.). Washington, DC: Author.

American Speech-Language-Hearing Association. (2002). Roles and responsibilities of speech-language pathologists with respect to evaluation and treatment for dysphagia. ASHA *Supplement, 22*, 73–87.

American Speech-Language-Hearing Association. (2004). Roles and responsibilities of speech-language pathologists with respect to augmentative and alternative communication: Technical report. *ASHA Supplement, 24*, 93–95.

Beukelman, D., & Mirenda, P. (1992). *Augmentative and alternative communication: Management of severe communication disorders in children and adults*. Baltimore: Paul H. Brooks.

Blosser J., & DePompei, R. (1994). *Pediatric brain injury: Proactive intervention*. San Diego, CA: Singular.

Brumback, R., Mathews, S., & Shenoy, S. (2001). Neurological disorders. In F. Kline, L. Silver, & S. Russell (Eds.), *The educator's guide to medical issues in the classroom* (pp. 49–64). Baltimore: Paul H. Brookes.

CHADD. (2001). Educational rights for children with ADHD-CHADD, Fact sheet #4. Retrieved March, 2005, from www.chadd.org/fs/fs4.pdf

Cohen, S.B. (1991). Adapting educational programs for students with head injuries. *Journal of Head Trauma Rehabilitation, 6*, 56–63.

Cohen, S.B., Joyce, C.M., Rhoades, K.W., & Welks, D.M. (1985). Educational programming for head-injured students. In M. Ylvisaker (Ed.), *Head injury rehabilitation: Children and adolescents,* San Diego, CA: College-Hill Press.

Daniel, D. (2004). AAC in the schools: Moving students along a communication continuum. *The ASHA Leader, 9*(10), 16–17.

DePompei, R., & Blosser, J. (1987). Strategies for helping head-injured children successfully return to school. *Language, Speech, and Hearing Services in Schools, 18,* 292–300.

Denckla, M. (1991). *Brain behavior insights through imaging.* Paper presented at the Learning Disabilities Association National Conference, Chicago, IL.

Eisenson, J., & Ogilvie, M. (1983). *Communicative disorders in children* (5th ed.). New York: Macmillan.

Eli Lily Corporation. (2004). Web site. Retrieved from www.strattera.com/pdf/teachers_guide.pdf

Federal Register. (1992). Traumatic brain injury (Vol. 57, No. 189).

Glennen, S.L., & DeCoste, D.C. (1997). *Handbook of augmentative and alternative communication.* San Diego, CA: Singular.

Griffith, E.R. (1983). Types of disability. In M. Rosenthal, E.R. Griffith, M.R. Bond, and J.D. Miller (Eds.), *Rehabilitation of the head-injured adult.* Philadelphia: F.A. Davis.

Jones, H.R. (1985). Diseases of the peripheral motor-sensory unit. *Clinical Symposia, 37*(2), 22–25.

Jordan, D.R. (1992) *Attention deficit disorder.* Austin, TX: PRO-ED.

Kline, F.M., Silver, L.B., & Russell, S.C. (2001). *The educator's guide to medical issues in the classroom.* Baltimore: Paul H. Brookes.

Logemann, J., & Sonies, B. (2004). Grand rounds dysphagia. *The ASHA Leader, 9*(13), 4–5, 18–19.

McCormick, L., & Wegner, J. (2003). Supporting augmentative and alternative communication. In L. McCormick, D.F. Loeb, & R.L. Schiefelbusch (Eds.), *Supporting children with communication difficulties in inclusive settings* (2nd ed.). Boston: Pearson Education.

Mirenda, P., & Mathy-Laikko, R. (1989). Augmentative and alternative communication application for persons with severe congenital communication disorders: An introduction. *Augmentative and Alternative Communication, 5,* 3–13.

Phillips, P. P. (1984). *Speech and hearing problems in the classroom.* Lincoln, NE: Cliffs Notes.

Rosen, C.D., & Gerring, J.P. (1986). *Head trauma: Educational re-integration.* San Diego, CA: College-Hill Press.

Segalowitz, S.J., & Lawson, S. (1995). Subtle symptoms associated with self-reported mild head injury. *Journal of Learning Disabilities, 28,* 309–319.

Sexson, S.B., & Dingle, A.D. (2001). Medical disorders. In F. Kline, L. Silver, & S. Russell (Eds.), *The educator's guide to medical issues in the classroom* (pp. 28–48). Baltimore: Paul H. Brookes.

Silverman, F.H. (1989). *Communication for the speechless* (2nd ed.). Englewood Cliffs, NJ: Prentice-Hall.

Snow, J., & Hooper, S. (1994). *Pediatric traumatic brain injury.* Thousand Oaks, CA: Sage.

Solomon, N.P., & Charron, S. (1998). Speech breathing in able-bodied children and children with cerebral palsy: A review of the literature and implication for clinical intervention. *American Journal of Speech-Language Pathology, 7*(2), 61–78.

Van Der Merwe, E., & Alant, E. (2004). Associations with Minspeak icons. *Journal of Communication Disorders, 37*(3), 255–274.

TERMS TO KNOW

ataxia
athetosis
attention deficit disorder (ADD)
augmentative or alternative communication (AAC)
cerebral palsy
closed head injury (CHI)
dysarthria
dysphagia
hemiplegia
mixed (cerebral palsy)

motor speech disorders
muscular dystrophy
neuromuscular problems
open head wound
paraplegia
quadriplegia
rigidity
spasticity
traumatic brain injury (TBI)
tremor

STUDY QUESTIONS

1. Why are many persons with cerebral palsy multiply handicapped? Discuss some of the most frequent types of handicapping conditions, especially as may affect the educational process.

2. Speech may or may not be affected in neuromuscular disorders. Discuss the speech characteristics and problem areas typically noted in these individuals when speech is moderately to severely affected.

3. Speech may be so severely affected in neuromuscular disorders that intelligible speech is not a reasonable expectation. Discuss as many alternative methods of communication as you can.

4. Discuss why placing a closed head injured student back into the class schedule held before the accident often is not appropriate. Why is placement in special classes for the learning disabled or mentally retarded also inappropriate?

5. Discuss some specific strategies and techniques that classroom teachers can employ in working with closed head injured students.

6. Describe accommodations that would appropriate for a student with attention deficit disorder, and discuss how such accommodations might be implemented in a regular classroom setting.

chapter thirteen

Communication Disorders and Academic Success

If education were a monetary system, the currency would no doubt be language. There are certain groups of students that you will encounter in this textbook that have a weakness in the area of language. The obvious ones, of course, are those students who had language disorders during their preschool years, and these linguistic difficulties have simply persisted into the early grades. Other groups that may not be as obvious are those children with phonological disorders, learning disabilities, attention deficit disorder, and students who have experienced traumatic brain injury. We have specific chapters that deal with all of these groups, but we wanted to devote a single portion of this text to how these language-based disorders affect a student's academic performance. Also, we wanted to illustrate some recent research that suggests working on language goals and metalinguistic abilities may play a significant role in a student's academic achievement, especially in terms of reading.

STUDENTS WITH LANGUAGE PROBLEMS: THE HIGH-RISK GROUPS

It is important to emphasize that certain groups of school-age students have a tendency to exhibit problems with language. If the teacher and speech-language pathologist carefully examine these high-risk groups, the bulk of older students with language disorders will be detected and appropriately served. Certainly, however, this does not mean that a student who is not included in these groups is immune to a language disorder, and anyone who manifests symptoms of language disturbance should be referred for evaluation. We include this section because the underlying language problems of students are sometimes overlooked, and teachers may tend to focus their efforts on symptoms rather than the underlying problems. For instance, a student who has difficulty learning to read and write may also have subtle problems with producing spoken language and comprehension of complex sentences uttered by others. If the teacher knows that there are certain groups of students who have been shown in research to exhibit more pervasive language problems than simply those seen in one modality (e.g., reading, writing, and such), then appropriate referrals can be made. This will allow the speech-language pathologist (SLP) to address any underlying language problem that exists. These major groups are discussed next.

Students with a History of Preschool Language Delay

If a student had a language delay as a preschooler, sometime after school entrance he or she is at high risk to experience difficulties on language-based tasks. This does not occur because the SLP has done a poor job of treatment during the preschool period. In fact, many of these students may have been dismissed from treatment because they have remediated all of the symptoms that they were enrolled to correct. In many cases, they were enrolled for problems with semantics, syntax, phonology, and morphology, and when the problems no longer exist, they are dismissed. In other cases, the student is not dismissed from treatment, but simply continues therapy upon school entrance because goals have not been reached. We must remember that these students, for want of a better word, exhibited a "weakness" in the area of language. They had trouble learning to talk and using language rules appropriately.

When the SLP completes treatment on such a child, one would think that the problem has been solved. Perhaps, the problem would have been solved if the young child were in an environment where his or her linguistic system was not taxed any further by forcing the use of more and more complex language operations. But we know that when a child enters school, there is an emphasis on learning to read, write, and speak in far more complex ways than children have dealt with prior to school entrance. Much of the teaching and learning is done through the use of language, with the teacher explaining things, and the student having to listen and try to understand them. We will address some of the stresses and strains of typical school curricula in a later section, but for now it is enough to mention that, upon school entrance, students are subjected to significant increases in the complexity, speed, and expectations with which they use language. For a student with a history of language problems, these increased expectations and complexities may be inordinately difficult. The very things (language rules) in which the student has experienced a weakness as a preschooler are the areas that are emphasized and prized in early elementary grades.

A number of longitudinal investigations have been done in an effort to follow up students with a history of preschool language disorders. In essence, these studies examined clinical records to determine the students who had received treatment for language impairment as preschoolers, and then they located these same students once they had reached school age. For example, Strominger and Bashir (1977, p. 3) studied 40 such students and found that "no child was found without residual deficits" (p. 3). Most of the students had difficulties with spoken and written language and reading. They state, "The child who evidences early disruption of language acquisition is at the highest risk for future educational failure or difficulty in reading and written language" (p. 4). They emphasize that the language problems do not disappear, but simply become more subtle and are manifested differently when a student becomes older. This, of course, is due in part to the concomitant increases in the complexity of the educational curriculum coupled with the weakness in the language area. Aram and Nation (1980) examined 63 students who had a history of preschool language problems. Four to 5 years after their initial evaluation, problems persisted in 80% of the group. About half of the students had persisting speech-language problems, while the other half demonstrated normal language, but had difficulties in reading and math. King, Jones, & Lasky (1982) did a 15-year study of 50 preschool language-disordered students who ranged in age from 13 to 20 years at follow-up. The majority had histories of academic problems (failed grades, special placements, and so on), and almost half of them had persisting communication problems. Hall and Tomblin (1978) found that 50% of the preschool language-impaired children they studied longitudinally showed persistent language problems into adulthood. We could cite many other studies which show that children with language problems often experience academic difficulties throughout their time in school (Bashir, Kuban, Kleinman, & Scavuzzo, 1983). Parents of children with a history of language disorders should be routinely counseled regarding the increased possibility of language-based academic difficulties as the child progresses through the educational system.

Students with Learning and/or Reading Disabilities

Maxwell and Wallach (1984, p. 25) state: "Research and clinical data from a variety of sources and orientations continue to suggest that the largest percentage of learning and reading-disabled children have language problems." Wiig and Semel (1976) have said, after reviewing the literature in this area, that 75–85% of students with learning disabilities have experienced language delays and that some of these perpetuate into adulthood. As these references indicate, the research is quite clear on the occurrence of language problems in learning- and reading-disabled populations. Some publications refer to such students as "language-learning disabled," a nomenclature that reflects the far-reaching effect of language on the disorder (Wallach & Butler, 1994). In school systems, the speech-language pathologist is most interested in screening the students who are receiving special services for learning or reading disabilities. This is because there is a reasonable chance that their problems in the areas of reading and writing may stem from an underlying difficulty with language in general.

Students Who Are Academically At Risk

If a student has not been found to have a language problem, learning disability, or reading disturbance through formal testing, no special services are typically provided by the school system. In early elementary grades, of course, there are different levels of reading instruction and some special services (the "Chapter One" reading programs, for example), but as children become older, there is less emphasis on teaching basic skills such as reading. Simon (1985) refers to students who have significant academic difficulties but do not qualify for special services in learning disabilities, reading, or speech-language as students who have "fallen between the cracks" in the educational system. Simon further indicates that if these students are given in-depth testing for language abilities, a significant percentage (about 50%) exhibit gaps in their ability to perform age-appropriate linguistic tasks.

Hill and Haynes (1992) studied fourth-grade children who were rated by their teachers as "academically at risk." These children repeatedly earned grades below C in their academic coursework and were in the low reading group. The children had no history of speech or language problems and were currently receiving no remedial services of any kind. Hill and Haynes administered three language tests to the academically at-risk children and their normally achieving peers. The tests focused on pragmatics, metalinguistics, and the language typically used by teachers in giving classroom directions. It was found that over 50% of the academically at-risk children scored low enough on the three language tests to warrant enrollment in treatment.

Thus, the third major population in the school system that is at risk for language problems is the group that is often earning poor grades, experiencing grade retention, and may be receiving no special services. It could be that their language problems are subtle enough that they are either not referred or not identified by routine screenings and evaluation techniques.

CURRICULUM AND TEACHING IMPACT ON STUDENTS WITH LANGUAGE PROBLEMS

Using language in the home environment is quite different from communication in a school setting. Even children who have gone to daycare facilities prior to school entrance have not been subjected to the pressure of using the level of language demanded in most kindergartens. This section attempts to bring to a conscious level the types of communication seen in classroom settings. It is through an understanding of the typical communicative milieu in the classroom that teachers can appreciate the profound disadvantage this setting presents to a student with borderline or deficient language skills.

The School Culture

Prior to school entrance, children have a limited number of daily routines with which they are familiar. These routines allow the child to understand events in the environment and even help the child to determine how to act in certain situations (Tattershall & Creaghead, 1985). Many of these routines, however, are not an integral part of the school experience, and the child entering school must make the appropriate adjustments to existing routines and learn new ones. While the preschooler knows routines such as going to the store, visiting grandma, dinnertime, bedtime, discipline, and party behaviors, there are new school routines such as following directions, question asking, taking turns, and such that may be foreign to the child. Also, the child may be accustomed to routines that include no other children or only one or two peers. The preschool child lives in a supportive environment where family members and friends are familiar with his or her abilities, accomplishments, preferences, and behavioral tendencies. Many times, the familiarity with the child's tendencies can compensate for any language deficiencies in the child. In the classroom, however, there are many other potential interactants and different rules for interaction. In addition, the child, his or her history, his or her preferences, and his or her abilities are virtually unknown to the teacher and other students. The student must learn the classroom routine and the teacher must learn about the new children in his or her classroom. Creaghead and Tattershall (1985) state, "A sixth-grade teacher was asked the following question in early September, 'What is the hardest thing about starting school?' Her answer was, 'teaching the children my routine.'" This would be even more difficult with younger students. Another complication is that teachers' expectations change from year to year, which makes the adjustment to school even more difficult for students. Tattershall and Creaghead (1985) quote a study by Baron, Baron, and MacDonald (1983) in which teachers of various grades were asked about the skills children should possess for kindergarten and first grade. Prerequisite skills for kindergarten were:

1. Say his full name, his parents' full names, his address, and his phone number.
2. Talk loud enough.
3. Recognize his name in print.
4. Listen and sit quietly while others are talking.
5. Share, take turns, and play by the rules.

Contrast this with the expectations for "desirable abilities" the very next year in first grade:

1. The ability to attend to a task for at least 10 minutes.
2. The ability to express themselves orally with teachers and peers.
3. The ability to retell the plot and describe the main character after listening to a story.
4. The ability to follow basic procedures for reading—left to right, top to bottom.
5. The ability to count objects and count aloud to 10.
6. The ability to say the alphabet in order.
7. The ability to see letter-to-sound relationships.
8. The ability to identify beginning sounds.
9. The ability to print their own names legibly. (Tattershall & Creaghead, 1985, p. 32).

As the grades progress toward secondary school, language-based abilities such as the following become increasingly important:

- The ability to work independently
- Organizational skills
- Taking responsibility for work assignments
- Using the library
- Developing appropriate study habits
- Thinking and problem solving using language and mathematics
- Performing group problem solving
- The ability to discuss opinions
- Discriminating fact from opinion
- The ability to develop arguments for a number of issues

There are many more changes in expectations, and students are expected to learn more sophisticated skills each year, sometimes with no direct explanation, but just by inference based on teacher and peer behavior.

In the school environment, there are even different communication rules that must be learned in addition to the rules of proper behavior (sit in your seat, don't talk to your neighbor, raise your hand). Question sequences are different from the typical routine experienced at home. For instance, many researchers (Mehan, 1978; Sinclair & Coulthard, 1975) have reported that school questions typically form a 3-level sequence which is composed of the following:

1. The question (What letter is at the beginning of the word *cat*?)
2. The answer (C)
3. The teacher's evaluation of the response (That's right, David).

There are at least three differences between question routines existing at home and at school. First, home questioning usually has a 2-part sequence (typically the evaluation portion is not included, although it can be). Second, questions at home are most often asked to obtain "real" information from the child. Questions in the classroom are more to demonstrate knowledge that is already known to the teacher and most of the class. Finally, teachers spend significantly more time in questioning behavior than do parents.

Another difference in the classroom is the routine for turn allocation. Especially in the lower grades, the teacher usually chooses the speaker (child) and the child talks to the teacher (typically in an answering mode).

The child rarely gets to address communications to other students unless he or she "sneaks" these communications during activities like arts and crafts that are not designed for such interactions. Then, the teacher does not always reinforce the interactions. Thus, the speaker selection and interactions are not natural in the classroom.

Topic selection and maintenance also are different in the classroom setting. The teacher almost always chooses the topic of conversation, selects who will take turns, maintains the topic, and changes the topic, when he or she sees fit. This is different from topic management in the natural environment, which is more arbitrary.

The purpose of this section has been to show that the student entering school must learn a host of new routines, both verbal and nonverbal, and is faced with significantly different and more complex expectations than previously experienced at home. This requires a significant adjustment for the young child, and if a language disorder exists, the adjustment may be even more difficult or impossible. If the student with a language disorder has difficulty abstracting the rules for classroom participation, he or she may be faced with negative feedback. One can imagine how the routines can become even more complicated in the higher grades where the student is confronted with several different teachers in the same day, all with different expectations and modifications of the basic school routine. For a student with a language disorder, this may be insurmountable.

Teacher Talk

Many studies have focused on the types of language teachers use in the classroom. Nelson (1984) summarizes data that were gathered on teacher language in first, third, and sixth grades. The major variables that Nelson examined were grammatical complexity of sentences, rate of speaking (speed), and fluency (pauses, hesitations). She found that the syntactic complexity increased with grade level, which made the language used in sixth grade more complex than in first grade. There was also more pausing and dysfluency as the grade level increased. Finally, the rate of speech in syllables per second (sps) increased from first (4.5 sps), to third (5.4 sps), and sixth (5.3 sps) grades. Interestingly, in an earlier study, Nelson (1976) found that a rate of 5 syllables per second increased comprehension problems among normal children up to the age of 9 years. We know that students with language disorders have difficulty with a number of aspects of linguistic material. For instance, more complex sentences are more difficult to understand for normal as well as language-impaired students. Many studies have shown that students with language learning-disabilities have trouble with rapid auditory processing of information. The incorporation of teacher dysfluencies, hesitations, and false starts serves only to add to the confusion as the grade level increases. Wallach and Miller (1988, p. 43) address another aspect of teacher talking:

> Teachers make great use of rhetorical questioning in their teaching. Teachers, after approximately fourth grade, make frequent use of nonliteral language such as idioms, analogies, similes, sarcasm, and indirect polite forms (Nelson, 1984; Stephens & Montgomery, 1985). Many children are able to handle some aspects of nonliteral language by age 8, but many nonliteral forms are acquired as late as 13 years old. Adolescents with language learning disabilities are especially vulnerable as language becomes more abstract.

Cuda and Nelson (1976) found that first-grade teachers use a high number of statements to direct attention and gain behavioral control of their classrooms. At the first-grade level there is an emphasis on "how to do" reading, writing, and mathematics, using concrete materials with much assistance from the physical context in the classroom. By third grade, the teachers focus more on content subjects such as social studies, science, and geography than on the how-to aspects. Verbal instruction increases in importance as grade level rises, and by sixth grade, students are almost exclusively concentrating on content areas, using reading and writing as tools for learning. Therefore, after the first few grades in elementary school the basic skills of reading, writing, and spoken language are assumed by the teacher to be acquired, and no review of these important requisites is provided. Sturm and Nelson (1997, p. 271) state: "One of the many challenges in inclusive classrooms is monitoring and assisting the comprehension of lower-functioning students without reducing the level of interaction for others."

Curriculum and Materials

A very important concept that many teachers are unaware of is called metalinguistics. This concept is critical to classroom teaching and the performance of students with normal language and language disorders. Many of you have not even heard of the concept, yet, if we could think of only one concept in this chapter that you should remember, it probably would be the concept of metalinguistics. Often, people have difficulty grasping the notion of metalinguistics, so we provide several examples here. VanKleek (1984) describes metalinguistics as:

> Specifically, we will be concerned here with the developmental unfolding in the child of this ability to focus upon and think about the language (i.e., what its parts are and how those parts relate to each other) (VanKleek, 1984, p. 128).

Walter and Miller (1988) further define metalinguistics as:

> Explicit language knowledge, sometimes defined under the general term metalinguistics, involves the ability to make conscious judgments about one's language. Adult language users are capable of making many metalinguistic judgments. They can decide whether sentences are grammatical, they can correct written language, and they can decide whether words have equivalent meanings. Children demonstrate metalinguistic ability when they tell us the first sound in *dog*, when they circle all the pictures that begin with the k sound, and when they tell us whether a sentence looks all right. The 3-year-old boy who says, "The zebra looks like a horse, but he has funny stripes" would be unable to tell us how many words are in the sentence or how many sounds are in the word *zebra*, because the word and sound judgments require metalinguistic ability, which is a later acquisition. This shows how one can be quite capable of talking (as reflected in the zebra sentence) without being able to talk about talking (Wallach & Miller, 1988, p. 9).

So, what does all this have to do with classroom teaching and students with language disorders? The first point that teachers need to realize is that much of their time in the early grades is spent teaching metalinguistic skills. For instance, Wallach and Miller (1988, p. 9) state:

> School activities . . . also require a great deal of metalinguistic ability. Even in the early grades, children are asked to compare sentences, to count the number of words in a sentence, to listen for the first sound in a word, to identify a rhyming word, and to decide which sentence is the "proper" way to say something. The discovery that the alphabet corresponds with particular sounds requires rudimentary metalinguistic ability. In addition standardized tests and intervention materials have a metalinguistic focus."

VanKleek (1984, p. 187) writes:

> It appears that verbal intelligence measures require that the child focus on and consciously manipulate language. Such tests often contain subtests in which children are asked to give definitions, rhyme, solve anagrams, check secret codes, complete verbal analogies, etc. Such an assessment tells us far more about a child's metalinguistic skills than how he or she functions using language in social interactions.

Thus, we can easily see that elementary schoolteachers are dealing with metalinguistics on a daily basis. There are several important things that teachers need to be aware of, however, concerning metalinguistics. The first is that metalinguistic ability develops, as all language skills do, on a maturational timetable. That is, a child must have reached a particular level of linguistic maturity to perform and understand metalinguistic tasks. It should be noted that many normal students do not acquire the ability to segment syllables into phonemes until they are about 6 years of age. Yet, many students are involved in phonics programs either before or at the same time as these skills are developing. Also, the appreciation of figurative language and abstract language use may not be understood until well after age 8 years, yet authorities have reported that abstract and figurative language (analogies, dual word meanings) occurs in teacher utterances even at the first-grade level (Cuda & Nelson, 1976). If these skills are later developing ones for normal language students, then they are clearly going to cause extreme difficulty for language-impaired youngsters. In fact, many studies indicate students with language learning disabilities have particular trouble with metalinguistic tasks (Baker, 1982; Hook & Johnson, 1978; Nippold & Fey, 1983; Simon, 1985). Nelson (1984) provides an example of the complexity of an actual teacher directive that relies heavily on metalinguistic ability:

> What kind of animal do you see at the very top? And where is the rabbit? He's sitting on a radio. Did you ever see a real rabbit sit on a radio? What does *rabbit* begin with? *R*, all right. And what about the thing he's sitting on? Say the word. *Radio*. Radio and rabbit both begin with the letter *r*. OK, can you see how that letter is made? The capital *R* is how many spaces? Two spaces tall. And the small *r*? After your name is made at the space at the top, will you make a capital *R* and a small *r* on the lines that are shown right beside the rabbit?

Note that in the above example the student must mentally shift from one metalinguistic task to another (location of sounds in words, capital versus small letters, the correspondence between sounds and letters, the physical configurations that differentiate capital from small letters). The student also is asked to describe the picture, reflect on metalinguistic issues, and then to actually perform a writing task. You also should note that the instructions for the writing task (the last sentence in the example) form a very complex sentence that reverses the order of events in time (After your name is made in the space at the top, will you make . . ."). Finally, the instructions for the writing task are stated in the form of a question (polite form) rather than a directive. This type of indirect request is often very difficult for a student with a language impairment student to understand.

Often, even the textbooks used by classroom teachers are infested with complex and sometimes incomprehensible instructions written by "experts" in the educational process (Creaghead & Donnelly, 1982; Lasky & Chapandy, 1976; Nelson, 1984). The classroom teacher often is encouraged by the textbook to read such directives verbatim to the students.

Reading: A Language-Based Skill

While we are discussing curriculum issues, it is pertinent to mention the teaching of reading, which is an important language skill. There are a variety of approaches to teaching reading and we are certainly not experts in this area. However, we have observed that reading, as a language skill, is particularly difficult to learn for children with language disorders. Catts & Kamhi (2005, p. 115) state:

> The research reviewed in these studies clearly demonstrates that language deficits are closely associated with reading disabilities. In many cases, these language deficits precede and are causally linked to reading problems. Reading is a linguistic behavior, and, as such, it depends on adequate language development. Many children with reading disabilities have developmental language disorders that become manifested as reading problems upon entering school.

As in many academic realms and areas of professional practice the popularity of certain teaching methods ebbs and flows according to the tenor of the times. Fifty years ago the rule was phonics programs for reading instruction. Then, in the 1980s the "whole language" movement affected reading instruction and phonics training fell out of favor in many school systems. Now the pendulum is swinging back toward an emphasis on phonological awareness. Some approaches use a highly metalinguistic approach (phonics) coupled with reading material that emphasizes decoding of written words. One can imagine that this type of approach may be extremely difficult for a student with metalinguistic deficits, yet, these skills may be the key to learning to read for such a child. Other approaches (e.g., whole language) emphasize meaning and comprehension of the written material and have less emphasis on phonemic awareness. They emphasize that language in any form (speaking, writing, reading, and listening) has real communicative value. This awareness provides an incentive for the various uses of language, since all of the content areas in school will depend upon what language communicates, not on how effectively one can "play with" sounds, letters, words, and sentences. It is easy to see that children with language disorders may benefit greatly from a whole language approach to reading instruction because it makes reading meaningful and relevant to their daily life instead of focusing on phonetic aspects. We are learning, however, that even if the whole language approach is used, children with language disorders still can benefit greatly from phonological awareness training to improve their reading ability (Kaderavek & Justice, 2004). The lesson here is that the teacher and SLP should work together to determine the most effective strategy for each student on the caseload, especially when that student is having difficulty with reading as well as oral communication. The teacher who is willing to consider a variety of approaches or a combination of methods in instruction is far more likely to succeed with students having communication impairments.

Much literature has suggested that reading difficulties may have a linguistic basis (Casby, 1988; Catts & Kamhi, 1986; Catts & Kamhi, 2005). These same sources advocate that the SLP take on an increased role in working with students having reading problems (see Chapter 6 for specific examples and references). It is important to identify students as early as possible who are at risk for reading and other literacy difficulties. Justice, Invernizzi, and Meier (2002) describe the design and implementation of an early literacy screening protocol for use in public school systems. The goal of the screening protocol is to examine early literacy skills and offer help to students before they fail at learning how to read. Justice and colleagues (2002) recommend that teachers and SLPs both participate in the literacy screening program as members of an educational team. The specific targets of literacy screening include written language awareness, phonological awareness, letter-name knowledge, letter-sound correspondence, literacy motivation, and home literacy. Once a student has been identified as having difficulty with these important emergent literacy skills, a remediation program can be initiated. Recently, emergent literacy intervention programs have been developed for use in school environments that involve cooperation of teachers and SLPs (Justice & Kaderavek, 2004; Kaderavek & Justice, 2004). Kaderavek and Justice (2004) recommend an "embedded-explicit" approach to teaching emergent literacy. The "embedded" part of the approach is conducted by the classroom teacher in the normal classroom routines that involve a print-rich environment, adult-child book sharing, and an emphasis on literacy in play. The "explicit" part of the approach is conducted by the SLP and may involve direct service delivery or work with the entire class or small groups in which specific training on phonological awareness, print concepts, alphabet knowledge, and letter-sound correspondence are directly targeted. In another example of intervention, work in the areas of metacognition, metalinguistics, phonology, and language use patterns was targeted in a collaborative (teacher and SLP) effort by Fleming and Forester (1997). They found that "integrating reading and language instruction proved to be mutually beneficial for both skill areas" (p. 180). Payoffs for collaboration between the teacher and SLP can even be found in treatment of articulation and phonological disorders. Stewart, Gonzalez, and Page (1997) found that children with articulation disorders "learned to read sight words incidentally during articulation training, and this learning generalized beyond printed words on cards to printed words on a list" (p. 115). Thus, we need to begin to think in terms of multiple payoffs from our interactions with students. How can the SLP work with the student on communication and positively affect his or her academic performance and reading and writing abilities? How can the teacher enhance academic performance and at the same time facilitate better communication strategies? Answers to these questions will come from increased collaborative efforts and communication between teachers and speech-language pathologists.

IMPACT OF PHONOLOGICAL DISORDERS

Phonology is the aspect of language that deals with the organization and use of sounds within that language. Three academic skills: reading, writing, and spelling, each require that students have some degree of mastery of the sound system of their language. Therefore, one might expect that students who exhibit phonological problems would be likely also to exhibit problems with reading, writing, and spelling. Most of the research investigating the relationship between speech sound errors and academic performance has focused on reading. The results of this research, especially earlier research, have been somewhat equivocal. For example, some studies (FitzSimons, 1958; Ham, 1958; Winitz, 1969) reported a significant relationship between reading problems and articulation disorders. On the other hand Everhart (1953), Flynn and Byrne (1970), and Hall (1938) reported no significant differences in the articulation abilities of good and poor readers. One possible reason for the lack of consensus among these early studies might be that the investigators failed to take into account the difference between "articulation" problems and "phonological" problems. Remember, that speech sound production has two aspects: the motor-based aspect of speech sound production known as articulation, and the linguistic rule-based aspect generally referred to as phonology. The inability of a student to make correct motor movements to produce speech sounds may not have a significant affect on reading, writing, or spelling. However, if a student's phonological disorder reflects an underlying problem in the organization of the sound system, it would be reasonable to expect this underlying problem to surface in one or more of those academic skills related to the sound system. The distinction between the possible effects of structurally based articulation disorders and phonological disorders on reading was investigated by Stackhouse (1982). She compared the reading and spelling abilities of children exhibiting articulation problems related to cleft lip and palate with those of children with expressive phonological problems not related to structural anomalies. Stackhouse reported that the children with cleft lip and palate did not differ significantly in reading and spelling ability from a group of normally developing children. However, the children with expressive phonological impairments performed significantly more poorly in reading and spelling than the normally developing control group. In a later work, Stackhouse (1997) stated that it appears that children who exhibit an isolated articulatory difficulty relating to a physical abnormality may be no more likely to have reading impairments than those with normally developing speech. Catts and Kamhi (2005) discuss the relationship between reading problems and the broader area of phonological processing, which includes phonological awareness, memory, production, and retrieval. They state that there is much evidence to suggest that a phonological processing deficit is at the core of the reading problems in dyslexia.

Another confounding factor in the research exploring the relationship between reading, writing, and spelling and expressive phonology is the presence of coexisting language disorders. Catts (1991) reported that children with phonological and language impairments were much more likely to exhibit reading problems than were children with phonological problems only. The relationship between phonology and the other components of language is complex. Our current understanding of this relationship may be summarized as follows:

1. Many, but not all, children with phonological disorders also exhibit language disorders (Stoel-Gammon & Dunn, 1985).
2. Children with severe phonological disorders are more likely to exhibit a co-occurring language disorder than children with milder disorders (Bernthal & Bankson, 2004).
3. Phonology disorders co-occur with disorders of syntax more frequently than with other language disorders (Stoel-Gammon & Dunn, 1985).
4. Comprehension of language structures is usually not affected by phonology disorders (Shriberg, 1982).

It would seem then that research designed to investigate the relationship between reading and phonology must take into account the presence of coexisting language disorders. Here is a word of caution, however. Because language disorders are frequently more subtle and less obvious than phonological disorders, teachers must be aware of the potential for a language disorder in any child who exhibits a moderate to severe disorder of phonology. Therefore, a child with a phonological disorder should be considered at risk for problems in reading and spelling.

There is a growing body of research suggesting that **phonological awareness** may be yet another link between phonological disorders and reading ability. Another term, **phonemic awareness**, is also used in the literature. Although some authors make a distinction between phonological and phonemic awareness, these terms will be considered synonyms for purposes of this chapter. As described in Chapter 3, phonological awareness refers to the explicit understanding of the sound structure of language, including the awareness that words are composed of syllables and phonemes (Catts, 1991). The link between phonological awareness and reading has been well established (Adams, 1990; Blachman, 1991; Catts, 1991; Catts & Kamhi, 2005; Ehri, Nunes, Willows, Schuster, Yaghoub-Zadeh, & Shanahan, 2001). Several studies have indicated that many children with phonological problems perform more poorly on phonological awareness tasks than do children of similar age with normal phonological skills (Cowan & Moran, 1997; Magnusson & Naucler, 1990; Webster & Plante, 1992). Bird, Bishop, and

Freeman (1995) reported that children with persisting speech sound production problems often have literacy and phonological awareness problems.

Several different types of tasks have been used to measure phonological awareness. These tasks include rhyming activities, segmenting words into phonemes or syllables, producing words after the first or last sounds have been changed or deleted (e.g., "What does *fat* become if we take away the f sound?") and comparing the length of spoken words (e.g., when asked, "Which word is longer: *whale* or *mosquito*?" children with poor phonological awareness may respond that *whale* is longer because the object it represents is longer). All of these measures, to one extent or another, appear to be predictors of reading ability (Blachman, 1991; Catts, 1991; Magnusson, 1991). That is to say children who have difficulty on the phonological awareness tasks also frequently prove to be poor readers. Catts and Kamhi (2005) state that children with more severe phonological disorders, who have broad-based language impairments, and who perform poorly on tests of phonological awareness are most at risk for reading disabilities.

Certainly the research on the possible relationships among phonology, phonological awareness, and reading should hold some interest for teachers. However, of even more importance to teachers are the reports of several investigators who have demonstrated that training in tasks designed to develop phonological awareness appears to facilitate learning to read (Blachman, 1991; Ehri et al., 2001). The relationship of phonological awareness to reading has resulted in many school systems reevaluating the way reading is taught. Several years ago, many school systems incorporated so-called whole language approaches to teaching reading. Whole language approaches tend to deemphasize or eliminate specific training in awareness of sounds (Hall & Moats, 2002). Mounting evidence that training in phonological awareness may greatly facilitate learning to read has resulted in reading programs that place greater emphasis on the awareness of sounds. Adams (1990), after reviewing the literature on this subject, concluded that, "The evidence is compelling: Toward the goal of efficient and effective reading instruction, explicit training of phoneme awareness is invaluable" (p. 331). Ehri and colleagues (2001) after conducting a meta-analysis of existing literature concluded that phonemic awareness instruction improved word reading as well as comprehension. Ehri and colleagues also reported that both normally developing children as well as children with reading disabilities benefited from phonemic awareness instruction. This is certainly one area in which speech-language pathologists, classroom teachers, and reading teachers can engage in a mutually beneficial collaborative effort to improve both the phonological and reading skills of students.

Several approaches to teaching phonological awareness to kindergarten and first-grade students are provided by Blachman (1991), Blachman, Ball, Black, and Tangel (2000), Goldsworthy (1998), and Lindamood and Lindamood (1998). These interventions include techniques based on categorizing words according to the sounds they contain, segmenting words into their phonemic components, and rhyming activities. Such techniques have been demonstrated to result in improved reading and/or spelling skills (Blachman, 1991; Ehri et al., 2001). There have been no studies to date, however, which demonstrate whether children with phonological disorders perform better in one type of reading instruction than another.

The relationship between phonological disorders and spelling is even less clear than reading. Intuition tells us that a child who has problems processing sounds for speech production may have problems processing sounds for written production. Research, however, has not conclusively proved or disproved the prevailing clinical intuition.

One reason that the literature may be somewhat less clear than we would like regarding the relationship between phonological ability and spelling may once again be the concept of phonological awareness. There is extensive recent literature that demonstrates a relationship between phonological awareness and spelling (Apel, Masterson, & Hart, 2004; Ball & Blachman, 1991; Ehri et al., 2001; Lombardino, Bedford, Fortier, Carter, & Brandi, 1997; Tangel & Blachman, 1992). Clarke-Klein (1994) suggested that children who have phonetic errors (e.g., spell *candle* as *candol*, or *square* as *skwar*) likely do not have phonological awareness problems and are no more likely than other children to have phonological problems. However, children who show nonphonetic or bizarre spelling patterns (e.g., spell *smoke* as *scoteser*, or *crayons* as *carinsteds*) are more likely to have phonological awareness problems. Clarke-Klein (1994) suggested that children who have histories of severe expressive phonological deviations are at risk for these unusual or bizarre spelling errors. Lombardino and colleagues (1997) suggested that children who do not exhibit expected spelling patterns should be provided with phoneme awareness training.

In summary, there appears to be a significant relationship between expressive phonological ability and reading, writing, and spelling. However, the exact nature of that relationship is not entirely clear. It would appear that children with a phonological disorder as opposed to a simple motor-based articulation disorder are at risk for reading, writing, and spelling problems. This is particularly true in situations in which the phonological problem is accompanied by a language problem. A critical link between phonology and reading and spelling might be phonological awareness. Poorly developed phonological awareness is characteristic of many students with phonological problems as well as of students with reading problems. The assessment and development of phonological awareness skills in young children provides many marvelous opportunities for collaborative efforts among speech-language pathologists, classroom teachers, and reading specialists.

IMPACT OF HEARING IMPAIRMENT

Many of the effects of hearing loss on classroom performance should be obvious. If a student cannot hear instructions, examples or assignments, his or her performance will likely be incorrect or inappropriate. You know from the information presented in Chapter 10 that students with a sensorineural loss may hear some sounds but not others, resulting in those students hearing the teacher's speech in a garbled or distorted fashion. These obvious problems can be addressed through the technology and suggestions provided in Chapter 10. There are, however, more subtle academic problems for students with hearing impairments. These more subtle problems are determined largely by the extent to which the hearing loss disrupts the student's ability to process language. Sometimes this critical link between language skill and academic achievement by hearing-impaired students is not apparent to teachers who are unaccustomed to working with this population.

It is not possible to provide a specific list of language problems which constitute a "language of the hearing-impaired." As Lahey (1988, p. 67) stated:

> To know that a child is hearing-impaired does not tell the clinician what the child needs to know about language. Considerable variability is found among these children . . . variability that is not easily predicted given levels of hearing loss, mean length of utterance, grade in school, nonverbal IQ, or age at onset.

It is, however, reasonable to assume that most hearing-impaired students will have some language problems that affect their academic performance. Tye-Murray (1998) identified some of the more common types of problems exhibited by hearing-impaired students in language form, content, and use. These are presented in Table 13-1.

Because it is a language problem that underlies most of the hearing-impaired student's academic difficulty, it is not surprising that most of these

Table 13-1 Common Language Problems Exhibited by Hearing-Impaired Speakers

Problems of language form

Overuse of nouns and verbs with rare use of adverbs, prepositions, and pronouns

Omission of function words

Limited number of words per sentence

Sentences mostly in a simple subject-verb-object structure

Omission of plural and past tense markers

Incorrect ordering of words in a sentence

Problems of language content

Limited vocabulary

Difficulty with words that have multiple meanings or that can be used as more than one part of speech

Difficulty understanding idioms

Difficulty with synonyms and antonyms

Problems of language use (pragmatics)

Asking inappropriate questions

Problems with conversational turn-taking

Failure to acknowledge hearing a message

Inappropriate shifts in topic

Source: Adapted from Tye-Murray, 1998.

students have their greatest problem with language-based skills, especially reading and writing (Allen, 1986; Berg, 1986; Jensema, 1975; Marschark, Lang, & Albertini, 2002). Allen (1986) reported that the average reading and writing level of deaf high-school students is at the third- or fourth-grade level. Quigley and Thomure (1968) reported that hearing-impaired elementary and secondary students demonstrated scores of from 1 to 3 years below those of normal hearing peers on the word meaning, paragraph meaning, and language subtests of the Stanford Achievement Test. Marschark and colleagues (2002) indicate that although the literacy skills of students with severe and profound hearing impairments has improved in more recent years, a large discrepancy between hearing and deaf peers remains. They indicate that many deaf students graduating from high school are reading at levels comparable to hearing students who are 5 to 9 years younger.

Davis (1974) reported a "discouragingly low performance" by hard-of-hearing children on the Boehm Test of Basic Concepts. Several studies have reported that hearing-impaired children demonstrate delays in syntactic ability (Davis & Blasdell, 1975; Pressnell, 1973; Quigley, Wilbur, Power, Montanelli, & Steinkamp, 1976; Wilcox & Tobin, 1974). There is evidence that even mild hearing loss can affect language development and, therefore, academic skills. Holm and Kunze (1969) administered a battery of language development tests to children age 5 to 9 years. One group had fluctuating mild hearing losses due to persistent otitis media. The other group was a matched peer group of children with no history of middle ear problems. The authors reported that the otitis media group received lower scores than the control group on all tasks involving the reception or processing of auditory information or the production of a verbal response.

Dobie and Berlin (1979), through the use of simulated hearing loss, demonstrated that even mild losses of 20 dB could result in the student failing to hear plural and past tense word endings and inflections indicating a question. The lag between hearing-impaired and normal-hearing students tends to increase with the degree of hearing loss (Jensema, 1975; Quigley & Thomure, 1968) and with age (Berg, 1986; Brackett & Maxon, 1986; Kodman, 1963). The latter finding reflects the fact that, as students progress through the grade levels, they face more complex language-based tasks.

In recent years, early identification and early intervention (in the form of language stimulation and amplification) have resulted in dramatic improvement in the educational achievement of hearing-impaired students. Paul and Quigley (1987) state that recent studies suggest that the academic lag reported for hearing-impaired children is not as great as that indicated earlier. Such improvement, as a result of early language training, underscores the fact that the academic deficit seen among these students reflects their language difficulties rather than any generalized intellectual deficit.

Although early identification and intervention makes the picture considerably brighter for the hearing-impaired student in the classroom, the teacher must continue the momentum by doing such things as ensuring that the student's hearing aid is in working order, making maximum use of assistive listening devices, incorporating slight modifications in teaching style to accommodate the hearing-impaired student, and making the best use of the support personnel available in any particular school system.

REFERENCES

Adams, M. (1990). *Beginning to read: Thinking and learning about print.* Cambridge: MIT Press.

Allen, T.E. (1986). Patterns of academic achievement among hearing-impaired students: 1974 and 1983. In A.N. Schildroth, & M.A. Karchmer (Eds.), *Deaf children in America.* Boston: Little, Brown.

Apel, K., Masterson, J.J., & Hart, P. (2004). Integration of language components in spelling: Instruction that maximizes students' learning. In E.R. Silliman & L.C. Wilkinson (Eds.), *Language and literacy learning in schools* (pp. 292–315). New York: Guilford Press.

Aram, D., & Nation, J. (1980). Preschool language disorders and subsequent language and academic difficulties. *Journal of Communication Disorders, 13,* 159–170.

Baker, L. (1982). An evaluation of the role of metacognitive deficits in learning disabilities. *Topics in Learning and Learning Disabilities, 2,* 27–35.

Ball, E., & Blachman, B. (1991). Does phoneme awareness training in kindergarten make a difference in early word recognition and developmental spelling? *Reading Research Quarterly, 26,* 49–66.

Baron, B., Baron, C., & MacDonald, B. (1983). *What did you learn in school today?* New York: Warner Books.

Bashir, A., Kuban, K., Kleinman, S., & Scavuzzo, A. (1983). Issues in language disorders: Considerations of cause, maintenance, and change. In J. Miller, D. Yoder, & R. Shiefelbusch (Eds.), *Contemporary Issues in Language Intervention*, ASHA Reports 12, The American Speech-Language-Hearing Association; Rockville, MD.

Berg, F.S. (1986). Characteristics of the target population. In F.S. Berg, J.L. Blait, S.H. Viehweg, & A. Wilson-Vlotman (Eds.), *Educational audiology for the hard of hearing child.* Orlando, FL: Grune & Stratton.

Bernthal, J.E., & Bankson, N.W. (2004). *Articulation and phonological disorders* (5th ed.). Boston: Allyn & Bacon.

Bird, J., Bishop, D., & Freeman, N. (1995). Perception and awareness of phonemes in phonologically impaired children. *European Journal of Disorders of Communication, 27,* 289–311.

Blachman, B. (1991). Early intervention for children's reading problems: Clinical applications of the research in phonological awareness. *Topics in Language Disorders, 12,* 51–65.

Blachman, B., Ball, E., Black, R., & Tangel, D. (2000). *Road to the code: A phonological awareness program for young children.* Baltimore: Paul H. Brookes.

Brackett, D., & Maxon, A.B. (1986). Service delivery alternatives for the mainstreamed hearing-impaired child. *Language, Speech, and Hearing Services in Schools, 17,* 115–125.

Casby, M. (1988). Speech-language pathologists' attitudes and involvement regarding language and reading. *Language, Speech, and Hearing Services in Schools, 19,* 352–361.

Catts, H. (1991). Early identification of reading disabilities. *Topics in Language Disorders, 12,* 1–16.

Catts, H., & Kamhi, A. (1986). The linguistic basis of reading disorders: Implications for the speech-language pathologist. *Language, Speech, and Hearing Services in Schools, 17,* 318–328.

Catts, H.W., & Kamhi, A.G. (2005). *Language and Reading Disabilities* (2nd ed.). Boston: Allyn & Bacon.

Clarke-Klein, S. (1994). Expressive phonological deficiencies: Impact on spelling and development. *Topics in Language Disorders, 14,* 40–45.

Cowan, W., & Moran, M. (1997). Phonological awareness skills in children with articulation disorders in kindergarten to third grade. *Journal of Children's Communication Development, 8,* 31–38.

Creaghead, N., & Donnelly, K. (1982). Comprehension of superordinate and subordinate information by good and poor readers. *Language, Speech, and Hearing Services in Schools, 13,* 177–186.

Creaghead, N., & Tattershall, S. (1985). Observation and assessment of classroom pragmatic skills. In C. Simon (Ed.), *Communication skills and classroom success: Assessment of language-learning disabled students.* San Diego, CA: College-Hill.

Cuda, R., & Nelson, N. (1976). Analysis of teacher speaking rate, syntactic complexity, and hesitation phenomena as a function of grade level. Presented at the annual meeting of the American Speech-Language-Hearing Association, Houston, TX.

Davis, J. (1974). Performance of young hearing-impaired children on a test of basic concepts. *Journal of Speech and Hearing Research, 17,* 342–351.

Davis, J., & Blasdell, R. (1975). Perceptual strategies employed by normal-hearing and hearing-impaired children in the comprehension of sentences containing relative clauses. *Journal of Speech and Hearing Research, 18,* 281–295.

Dobie, R.A., & Berlin, C.I. (1979). Influence of otitis media on hearing and development. *Annals of Otology, Rhinology, and Laryngology, 88* (Suppl. 60), 48–53.

Ehri, L., Nunes, S., Willows, D., Schuster, B., Yaghoub-Zadeh, Z., & Shanahan, T. (2001). Phonemic awareness instruction helps children learn to read: Evidence from the National Panel's meta-analysis. *Reading Research Quarterly, 36,* 250–287.

Everhart, R. (1953). The relationship between articulation and other developmental factors in children. *Journal of Speech and Hearing Disorders, 18,* 332–338.

FitzSimons, R. (1958). Developmental, psychosocial, and educational factors in children with nonorganic articulation problems. *Child Development, 29,* 481–489.

Fleming, J., & Forester, B. (1997). Infusing language enhancement into the reading curriculum for disadvantaged adolescents. *Language, Speech, and Hearing Services in Schools, 28*(2), 177–180.

Flynn, P., & Byrne, M. (1970). Relationship between reading and selected auditory abilities of third-grade children. *Journal of Speech and Hearing Research, 13,* 731–740.

Goldsworthy, C.L. (1998). *Sourcebook of phonological awareness activities.* San Diego, CA: Singular.

Hall, M. (1938). Auditory factors in functional articulatory speech defects. *Journal of Experimental Education, 7,* 110–132.

Hall, P., & Tomblin, J. (1978). A follow-up study of children with articulation and language disorders. *Journal of Speech and Hearing Disorders, 43,* 227–241.

Hall, S.L., & Moats, L.C. (2002). *Parenting a struggling reader: A guide to diagnosing and finding help for your child's reading difficulties.* New York: Broadway Books.

Ham, R. (1958). Relationship between misspelling and misarticulation. *Journal of Speech and Hearing Disorders, 23,* 294–297.

Hill, S., & Haynes, W. (1992). Language performance in low achieving elementary school students. *Language, Speech, and Hearing Services in Schools, 23,* 169–175.

Holm, V.A., & Kunze, L.H. (1969). Effect of chronic otitis media on language and speech development. *Pediatrics, 43,* 833–839.

Hook, P., & Johnson, D. (1978). Metalinguistic awareness and reading strategies. *Bulletin of the Orton Society, 28,* 62–78.

Jensema, C.J. (1975). *The relationship between academic achievement and demographic characteristics of hearing-impaired children and youth.* Series R, No. 2. Washington, DC: Gallaudet College, Office of Demographic Studies.

Justice, L., Invernizzi, M., & Meier, J. (2002). Designing and implementing an early literacy screening protocol: Suggestions for the speech-language pathologist. *Language, Speech, and Hearing Services in Schools, 33,* 84–101.

Justice, L., & Kaderavek, J. (2004). Embedded-explicit emergent literacy intervention I: Background and description of approach. *Language, Speech, and Hearing Services in Schools, 35,* 201–211.

Kaderavek, J., & Justice, L. (2004). Embedded-explicit emergent literacy intervention II: Goal selection and implementation in the early childhood classroom. *Language, Speech, and Hearing Services in Schools, 35,* 212–228.

King, R., Jones, C., & Lasky, E. (1982). In retrospect: A fifteen year follow-up report of speech-language disorders in children. *Language, Speech, and Hearing Services in Schools, 13,* 24–32.

Kodman, F. (1963). Education status of the hard-of-hearing child in the classroom. *Journal of Speech and Hearing Research, 28,* 297–299.

Lahey, M. (1988). *Language disorders and language development.* New York: MacMillan.

Lasky, E., & Chapandy, A. (1976). Factors affecting language comprehension. *Language, Speech, and Hearing Services in Schools, 7,* 159–168.

Lindamood, C., & Lindamood, P. (1998). *The Lindamood Phoneme Sequencing Program for reading, spelling and speech* (3rd ed.). Austin, TX: PRO-ED.

Lombardino, L., Bedford, T., Fortier, C., Carter, J., & Brandi, J. (1997). Invented spelling: Developmental patterns in kindergarten children and guidelines for early literacy intervention. *Language, Speech, and Hearing Services in Schools, 28,* 333–343.

Magnusson, E. (1991). Metalinguistic awareness in phonologically disordered children. In Y. Mehmet (Ed.), *Phonological disorders in children* (pp. 87–120). New York: Routledge.

Magnusson, E., & Naucler, K. (1990). Reading and spelling in language-disordered children— Linguistic and metalinguistic prerequisites: Report on a longitudinal study. *Clinical Linguistics and Phonetics, 4,* 49–61.

Marschark, M., Lang, H., & Albertini, J. (2002). *Educating deaf students: From research to practice.* New York: Oxford University Press.

Maxwell, S., & Wallach, G. (1984). The language-learning disabilities connection: Symptoms of early language disability change over time. In G. Wallach, & K. Butler (Eds.), *Language learning disabilities in school-age children.* Baltimore: Williams & Wilkins.

Mehan, H. (1978). Structuring school structure. *Harvard Educational Review, 48,* 32–64.

Nelson, N. (1976). Comprehension of spoken language by normal children as a function of speaking rate, sentence difficulty and listener age and sex. *Child Development, 47,* 299–303.

Nelson, N. (1984). Beyond information processing: The language of teachers and textbooks. In G. Wallach, & K. Butler (Eds.), *Language learning disabilities in school-age children.* Baltimore: Williams & Wilkins.

Nippold, M., & Fey, M. (1983). Metaphoric understanding in pre-adolescents having a history of language acquisition difficulties. *Language, Speech, and Hearing Services in Schools, 14,* 171–180.

Paul, P.V., & Quigley, S.P. (1987). Some effects of early hearing impairment on English language development. In F.N. Martin (Ed.), *Hearing disorders in children.* Austin, TX: PRO-ED.

Pressnell, L. (1973). Hearing-impaired children's comprehension and production of syntax in oral language. *Journal of Speech and Hearing Research, 16,* 12–21.

Quigley, S., & Thomure, R. (1968). *Some effects of hearing impairment on school performance.* Urbana, IL: University of Illinois, Institute for Research on Exceptional Children.

Quigley, S., Wilbur, R., Power, D., Montanelli, D., & Steinkamp, M. (1976). *Syntactic structures in the language of deaf children.* (Final Report Project No. 232175). US Dept. of Health, Education and Welfare, National Institute of Education.

Shriberg, L. (1982). Programming for the language component in developmental phonological disorders. *Seminars in Speech, Language, and Hearing, 3,* 115–126.

Simon, C. (1985). The language-learning disabled student: Description and assessment implications. In C. Simon (Ed.), *Communication skills and classroom success: Assessment of language-learning disabled students.* San Diego, CA: College-Hill.

Sinclair, J., & Coulthard, R. (1975). *Towards an analysis of discourse: The English used by teachers and pupils.* Oxford, UK: Oxford University Press.

Stackhouse, J. (1982). An investigation of reading and spelling performance in speech disordered children. *British Journal of Disorders of Communication, 17,* 53–60.

Stackhouse, J. (1997). Phonological awareness. In B.W. Hodson, & M.L. Edwards (Eds.), *Perspectives in applied phonology.* Gaithersburg, MD: Aspen.

Stephens, M., & Montgomery, A. (1985). A critique of recent relevant standardized tests. *Topics in Language Disorders, 5,* 21–45.

Stewart, S., Gonzalez, L., & Page, J. (1997). Incidental learning of sight words during articulation training. *Language, Speech, and Hearing Services in Schools, 28*(2), 115–126.

Stoel-Gammon, C., & Dunn, C. (1985). *Normal and disordered phonology on children.* Austin, TX: Pro-Ed.

Strominger, A., & Bashir, A. (1977). A nine-year follow-up of language delayed children. Presented at the annual convention of the American Speech-Language-Hearing Association, Chicago, IL.

Sturm, J., & Nelson, N. (1997). Formal classroom lessons: New perspectives on a familiar discourse event. *Language, Speech, and Hearing Services in Schools, 28*(3), 255–273.

Tangel, D., & Blachman, B. (1992). Effect of phoneme awareness instruction on kindergarten children's invented spelling. *Journal of Reading Behavior, 24,* 223–258.

Tattershall, S., & Creaghead, N. (1985). A comparison of communication at home and school. In D. Ripich, & F. Spinelli (Eds.), *School discourse problems.* San Diego, CA: College-Hill.

Tye-Murray, N. (1998). *Foundations of aural rehabilitation: Children, adults, and their family members.* San Diego, CA: Singular.

VanKleek, A. (1984). Metalinguistic skills: Cutting across spoken and written language and problem-solving abilities. In G. Wallach, & K. Butler (Eds.), *Language learning disabilities in school-age children.* Baltimore: Williams & Wilkins.

Wallach, G., & Butler, K. (Eds.). (1994). *Language learning disabilities in school-age children and adolescents.* New York: Merrill.

Wallach, G., & Miller, L. (1988). *Language intervention and academic success.* San Diego, CA: College-Hill.

Webster, P., & Plante, A. (1992). Effects of phonological impairment on word, syllable, and phoneme segmentation and reading. *Language, Speech, and Hearing Services in Schools, 23,* 176–182.

Wiig, E., & Semel, E. (1976). *Language disabilities in children and adolescents.* Columbus, OH: Merrill.

Wilcox, J., & Tobin, H. (1974). Linguistic performance of hard-of-hearing and normal hearing children. *Journal of Speech and Hearing Research, 17,* 286–293.

Winitz, H. (1969). *Articulatory acquisition and behavior.* New York: Appleton-Century-Crofts.

TERMS TO KNOW

phonemic awareness   phonological awareness

Index